2013
YEAR BOOK OF
NEUROLOGY AND NEUROSURGERY®

The 2013 Year Book Series

Year Book of Critical Care Medicine®: Drs Dries, Zanotti-Cavazzoni, Latenser, Martinez, Rincon, and Zwank

Year Book of Emergency Medicine®: Drs Hamilton, Bruno, Handly, Minczak, Quintana, and Ramoska

Year Book of Endocrinology®: Drs Schott, Apovian, Clarke, Eugster, Meikle, Oetgen, Ovalle, Schteingart, and Toth

Year Book of Hand and Upper Limb Surgery®: Drs Yao, Adams, Isaacs, and Rizzo

Year Book of Medicine®: Drs Barker, Garrick, Gersh, Khardori, LeRoith, Panush, Talley, and Thigpen

Year Book of Neonatal and Perinatal Medicine®: Drs Fanaroff, Benitz, Donn, Neu, Papile, and Van Marter

Year Book of Neurology and Neurosurgery®: Drs Klimo, Minagar, Gandhi, Liu, Panagariya, Rezania, Riel-Romero, Riesenburger, Robottom, Schwendimann, Shafazand, and Yang

Year Book of Obstetrics, Gynecology, and Women's Health®: Drs Dungan and Shulman

Year Book of Oncology®: Drs Arceci, Bauer, Chiorean, Gordon, Lawton, Murphy, Thigpen, and Tsao

Year Book of Ophthalmology®: Drs Rapuano, Cohen, Flanders, Hammersmith, Milman, Myers, Nagra, Nelson, Penne, Pyfer, Sergott, Shields, Talekar, and Vander

Year Book of Orthopedics®: Drs Morrey, Huddleston, Rose, Swiontkowski, and Trigg

Year Book of Otolaryngology-Head and Neck Surgery®: Drs Sindwani, Balough, Franco, Gapany, and Mitchell

Year Book of Pathology and Laboratory Medicine®: Drs Raab and Bissell

Year Book of Pediatrics®: Dr Stockman

Year Book of Plastic and Aesthetic Surgery™: Drs Miller, Boehmler, Gosman, Gutowski, Ruberg, Salisbury, and Smith

Year Book of Psychiatry and Applied Mental Health®: Drs Talbott, Ballenger, Buckley, Frances, Krupnick, and Mack

Year Book of Pulmonary Disease®: Drs Barker, Jones, Maurer, Spradley, Tanoue, and Willsie

Year Book of Sports Medicine®: Drs Shephard, Cantu, Feldman, Galea, Jankowski, Janssen, Lebrun, and Nieman

Year Book of Surgery®: Drs Behrns, Daly, Fahey, Hines, Howe, Huber, Klodell, Mozingo, and Pruett

Year Book of Urology®: Drs Andriole and Coplen

Year Book of Vascular Surgery®: Drs Gillespie, Bush, Passman, Starnes, and Watkins

2013 The Year Book of NEUROLOGY AND NEUROSURGERY®

"Published without interruption since 1902"

Neurology

Editor

Alireza Minagar, MD, FAAN, FANA

Professor of Neurology, Louisiana State University Health Sciences Center, Shreveport, Louisiana

Neurosurgery

Editor

Paul Klimo, Jr, MD, MPH

Neurosurgeon, Semmes-Murphey Neurologic and Spine Institute, Memphis, Tennessee

ELSEVIER
MOSBY

2013 The Year Book of NEUROLOGY AND NEUROSURGERY®

"Published without interruption since 1902"

Neurology

Editor
Alireza Minagar, MD, FAAN, FANA
Professor of Neurology, Louisiana State University Health Sciences Center, Shreveport, Louisiana

Neurosurgery

Editor
Paul Klimo, Jr, MD, MPH
Neurosurgeon, Semmes-Murphey Neurologic and Spine Institute, Memphis, Tennessee

ELSEVIER
MOSBY

ELSEVIER
MOSBY

Senior Vice President, Content: Linda Belfus
Editor: Jessica McCool
Production Supervisor, Electronic Year Books: Donna M. Skelton
Electronic Article Manager: Mike Rainey
Illustrations and Permissions Coordinator: Dawn Vohsen

2013 EDITION

Composition by TNQ Books and Journals Pvt Ltd, India
Printing/binding by Sheridan Books, Inc.

Editorial Office:
Elsevier
1600 John F. Kennedy Blvd.
Suite 1800
Philadelphia, PA 19103-2899

International Standard Serial Number: 0513-5117
International Standard Book Number: 978-1-4557-7279-7

Printed and bound by CPI Group (UK) Ltd, Croydon, CR0 4YY
Transferred to digital print 2013

Associate Editors

Chirag D. Gandhi, MD, FAANS
Associate Professor of Neurological Surgery and Radiology; Director, Endovascular Neurosurgery Fellowship Program, New Jersey Medical School, Newark, New Jersey

James K. Liu, MD
Director, Center for Skull Base and Pituitary Surgery; Assistant Professor, Neurological Surgery and Otolaryngology-Head and Neck Surgery, Department of Neurological Surgery, Neurological Institute of New Jersey, University of Medicine and Dentistry of New Jersey, New Jersey Medical School, Newark, New Jersey

Ashok Panagariya, MD, DM, FRCP
Professor Emeritus Neurology, University Hospital and SMS Medical College, Jaipur, India

Kourosh Rezania, MD
Assistant Professor of Neurology, Department of Neurology, University of Chicago Medical Center, Chicago, Illinois

Rosario Maria S. Riel-Romero, MD, FAAP, FAAN
Professor of Neurology and Pediatrics, Louisiana State University Health Sciences Center, School of Medicine in Shreveport, Shreveport, Louisiana

Ron Riesenburger, MD
Assistant Professor of Neurosurgery, Tufts Medical Center, Boston, Massachusetts

Bradley J. Robottom, MD
Co-Director of Clinical Research, Raleigh Neurology Associates, Raleigh, North Carolina

Robert Schwendimann, MD
Department of Neurology, Louisiana State University Health Sciences Center, Shreveport, Louisiana

Shirin Shafazand, MD, MS, FCCP, D.ABSM
Associate Professor of Medicine, University of Miami, Miller School of Medicine, Division of Pulmonary Critical Care and Sleep Medicine, Miami, Florida

Isaac Yang, MD
Attending Neurosurgeon and Assistant Professor, UCLA Department of Neurosurgery, University of California Los Angeles; Principal Investigator, UCLA Jonsson Comprehensive Cancer Center, UCLA Brain Tumor Program, David Geffen UCLA School of Medicine, Los Angeles, California

Table of Contents

Journals Represented

Journals represented in this YEAR BOOK are listed below.

Acta Paediatrica
AJNR American Journal of Neuroradiology
American Journal of Hypertension
American Journal of Kidney Diseases
American Journal of Otolaryngology
American Journal of Respiratory and Critical Care Medicine
Anaesthesia and Intensive Care
Anesthesia & Analgesia
Annals of Otology Rhinology & Laryngology
Archives of Disease in Childhood
Archives of General Psychiatry
Archives of Neurology
Archives of Physical Medicine and Rehabilitation
Brain
British Medical Journal
Chest
Childs Nervous System
Circulation
Clinical Journal of Sport Medicine
Clinical Neurology and Neurosurgery
Clinical Nuclear Medicine
Cornea
Drugs
Epilepsia
European Journal of Obstetrics & Gynecology and Reproductive Biology
European Journal of Paediatric Neurology
European Journal of Radiology
Headache
International Journal of Radiation Oncology *Biology* Physics
JAMA Pediatrics
Journal of Clinical Endocrinology & Metabolism
Journal of Clinical Investigation
Journal of Clinical Neuroscience
Journal of Clinical Psychopharmacology
Journal of Clinical Rheumatology
Journal of Computer Assisted Tomography
Journal of Emergency Medicine
Journal of General Internal Medicine
Journal of Neuro-Oncology
Journal of Neurological Sciences
Journal of Neurology, Neurosurgery, and Psychiatry
Journal of Neurosurgery
Journal of Neurosurgery Pediatrics
Journal of Neurosurgery Spine
Journal of the American Medical Association
Lancet
Laryngoscope

Mayo Clinic Proceedings
Neurology
Neuroradiology
Neurosurgery
New England Journal of Medicine
Otolaryngology-Head and Neck Surgery
Otology & Neurotology
Pediatric Emergency Care
Pediatric Infectious Disease Journal
Pediatric Neurology
Pharmacotherapy
Seizures
Sleep
Spine
Stroke
Thorax
World Neurosurgery

Standard Abbreviations

The following terms are abbreviated in this edition: acquired immunodeficiency syndrome (AIDS), cardiopulmonary resuscitation (CPR), central nervous system (CNS), cerebrospinal fluid (CSF), computed tomography (CT), deoxyribonucleic acid (DNA), electrocardiography (ECG), health maintenance organization (HMO), human immunodeficiency virus (HIV), intensive care unit (ICU), intramuscular (IM), intravenous (IV), magnetic resonance (MR) imaging (MRI), ultrasound (US), and ribonucleic acid (RNA).

Note

The Year Book of Neurology and Neurosurgery is a literature survey service providing abstracts of articles published in the professional literature. Every effort is made to ensure the accuracy of the information presented in these pages. Neither the editors nor the publisher of the Year Book of Neurology and Neurosurgery can be responsible for errors in the original materials. The editors' comments are their own opinions. Mention of specific products within this publication does not constitute endorsement.

To facilitate the use of the Year Book of Neurology and Neurosurgery as a reference tool, all illustrations and tables included in this publication are now identified as they appear in the original article. This change is meant to help the reader recognize that any illustration or table appearing in the Year Book of Neurology and Neurosurgery may be only one of many in the original article. For this reason, figure and table numbers will often appear to be out of sequence within the Year Book of Neurology and Neurosurgery.

Introduction

The face of neurological science has been altered significantly over the past decade and with the recent project to allocate more funding to research on the human central nervous system, we will witness more fundamental improvement of our understanding of the scientific mechanisms behind neurological diseases. With a bright future for neurology and neuroscience, there is an increasing need to connect clinicians and basic scientists around the globe to share their knowledge and exchange novel ideas. Each year, a new volume of the Year Book of Neurology and Neurosurgery is presented to our avid readers worldwide to fulfill our academic commitment to spread the science and stimulate other bright minds to look beyond what we have already discovered. Each volume of this fabulous book contains the abstracts of the best research papers from the highest-ranking academic neurological journals, selected by our dedicated team of contributors. The latest findings, the most informative papers, and the best practical articles are selected for review to provide our readers with the opportunity to keep themselves informed of the latest scientific advances in different fields of neuroscience and clinical neurology.

While preparing this annual publication, I had the great opportunity to work with and learn from some of the brightest academic physicians, who generously provided us with their timely and insightful reviews. We always remain grateful to these dedicated physicians who use this platform to share their valuable views with our readers and promote the spirit of thinking and research. This book is the result and product of these great collaborators. I also would like to take advantage of this opportunity and express my appreciation to Mrs. Jessica McCool and other hardworking employees of the Elsevier medical publishing team for their continuous work on this annual review to keep it running and improve its quality. It is our wish that our readers find this book useful for their scientific purpose and continue their academic mission to teach others and find cures for previously incurable neurological diseases.

Alireza Minagar, MD, FAAN, FANA

NEUROLOGY

ALIREZA MINAGAR, MD, FAAN, FANA

1 Epilepsy and Other Seizure Disorders

A rapid course through the five electrographic stages of status epilepticus
Pender RA, Losey TE (Loma Linda Univ, CA)
Epilepsia 53:e193-e195, 2012

A 54-year-old woman was transferred to a university hospital for severe sepsis and multiorgan failure. A complex partial seizure was noted and she was placed on continuous electroencephalography (EEG). During EEG monitoring she developed generalized convulsive status epilepticus. After consultation with family it was decided not to escalate treatment due to her overall medical condition. She proceeded sequentially through the five stages of status epilepticus, described by Treiman et al. (1990) over 22 h and 30 min and then developed electrocerebral silence. This case is significant in that it is the first report of a single individual experiencing all five stages of status epilepticus displayed on a continuous EEG. The case further demonstrates the rapid progression of status epilepticus and exemplifies the need for prompt treatment.

► Convulsive status epilepticus is generally defined as continuous, convulsive seizures lasting greater than 5 minutes or 2 or more seizures between which a patient does not return to baseline. Pender and Losey describe the case of a severely ill 54-year-old woman who underwent continuous electroencephalography (EEG) and the evolution of 5 different EEG stages of status epilepticus documented in the nearly 23 hours of EEG monitoring. The first stage was characterized by discrete seizures with ictal slowing. Subsequently, the second stage was characterized by merging of the seizures and, thereafter, by continuous ictal activity. The third stage shows ictal periods interrupted by short periods of diffuse suppression. The fourth period follows with the presence of periodic epileptiform activity on a flat background. The fifth and final stage shows electrocerebral silence that preceded death. The report suggests the rapid evolution of status epilepticus and the need for prompt recognition and intervention.

R. Riel-Romero, MD

Alcohol and drugs in epilepsy: Pathophysiology, presentation, possibilities, and prevention

Leach JP, Mohanraj R, Borland W (Southern General Hosp, Glasgow, UK; Salford Royal Hosp, Manchester, UK; Gartnavel General Hosp, Glasgow, UK)
Epilepsia 53:48-57, 2012

The potentially serious outcomes from ingestion of and dependence on toxins make this an important topic for epileptologists. We must be aware of the potential for harm from compounds that may be freely available, yet patients may try to conceal their use. Problematic compounds may cause seizures either acutely or on withdrawal: Their use may reduce effectiveness of antiepileptic drugs, or may simply promote and enhance chaotic lifestyles. Any or all of these factors may worsen seizure control or even directly cause seizures. This article highlights the pathophysiology behind provoked seizures, provides clues to diagnosis, and then outlines the steps that clinicians should take to reduce the deleterious effects of toxic compounds.

▶ The use of alcohol, drugs, and other toxic compounds by patients with seizures hampers the ability of physicians to care for them. The authors of this article reviewed the effects of alcohol, amphetamines, benzodiazepines, cannabis, cocaine, heroin or opiates, γ-hydroxybutyrate, and ketamine on epilepsy. They discussed the acute and chronic management of patients with epilepsy whose seizures are exacerbated by the use of these toxic compounds. This is a useful overview of a medical issue that clinicians who care for patients with epilepsy often face. In particular, the authors included a table listing the approximate detection period in the urine for the different drugs, which is helpful in assessing timing and severity of illicit drug use among these patients.

R. Riel-Romero, MD

Advanced Treatments for Childhood Epilepsy: Beyond Antiseizure Medications

Joshi SM, Singh RK, Shellhaas RA (Univ of Michigan, Ann Arbor)
JAMA Pediatr 167:76-83, 2013

A substantial minority of children with epilepsy have continued seizures despite adequate trials of standard antiseizure medications. To maximize seizure control and thereby optimize their neurodevelopmental outcomes, alternate nonmedication therapies should be considered for these patients. Dietary therapies, including the ketogenic diet and its variations, have been available for years. With a recent resurgence in popularity and expansion of indications, these treatments can lead to freedom from seizures or a significantly reduced seizure burden for a large number of patients. For carefully selected individuals, resective epilepsy surgery may offer the best hope for a cure. For others, palliation may be achieved through additional surgical approaches, such as corpus callosotomy and multiple subpial transections, or through neurostimulation techniques, such as the vagus nerve stimulator. In this review, we present these nonmedication approaches to treatment-resistant childhood epilepsy, with attention to patient selection and the potential risks and benefits.

▶ Medically refractory epilepsy can be addressed by a variety of alternative treatments. This article reviews the current alternative therapies, including dietary therapies, surgical treatment, and neurostimulation. Among the dietary therapies discussed were the ketogenic diet, modified Atkins diet, and the low-glycemic diet. The authors discussed the presurgical evaluation for drug-resistant epilepsy, resective procedures including hemispherectomy, and the various palliative surgeries including corpus callosotomy and multiple subpial resection. Among the neurostimulation procedures, vagus nerve stimulation and anterior thalamic nuclei stimulation were discussed. This article is a good, basic review of the current alternative treatments for drug-resistant epilepsy.

R. Riel-Romero, MD

Dilemmas in the interpretation of diagnostic accuracy studies on presurgical workup for epilepsy surgery

Burch J, Marson A, Beyer F, et al (Univ of York, UK; Univ of Liverpool, UK; et al)

Epilepsia 53:1294-1302, 2012

We conducted a systematic review to determine which noninvasive technologies should be used in the workup for epilepsy surgery to identify structural or functional abnormalities to help locate the site of seizure onset. The review focused on patients where there was insufficient confidence, in either the decision to go to surgery or the site at which surgery should be conducted, after the initial clinical examination. The majority of the studies identified were single-gate diagnostic accuracy studies; none were randomized controlled trials, and only one reported the effect of the test results on the deision making process. It became apparent that the data derived from diagnostic accuracy studies could not be used to answer the review question. This article focuses on the methods used to extract data from the diagnostic accuracy studies, the difficulties interpreting the resulting data, why such studies are not an appropriate study design in this setting, and how the evidence-base can be improved.

▶ Epilepsy surgery is an underutilized method of treatment for medically refractory seizures. Kwan and Brodie, in their seminal article in the *New England Journal of Medicine*, stated that only 47% of patients will become seizure free after the first antiepileptic and if a second antiepileptic drug (AED) is used, only an additional 14% of patients will become seizure free, and only 3% will become seizure free if more than 1 AED is used.[1] Hence, epilepsy surgery should be considered sooner in many patients who fail on AEDs. The decision on when and how to proceed with surgery, however, requires analysis of several datasets.

Epilepsy specialists can certainly be aided in this process if the diagnostic accuracy of the tests used in epilepsy surgery evaluation is known. This article reviews the utility of noninvasive techniques, such as high-definition electroencephalogram, volumetric magnetic resonance imaging (MRI), functional MRI, magnetic resonance spectroscopy, single photon emission tomography (SPECT) scan, subtraction ictal SPECT coregistered MRI, positron emission tomography, magnetoencephalography (MEG), and MRI and MEG coregistered, in assessing the decision for doing or not doing surgery. The authors conclude that data from diagnostic accuracy studies are seriously limited and cannot be used to address this important clinical issue.

R. Riel-Romero, MD

Reference

1. Kwan P, Brodie M. Early identification of refractory epilepsy. *N Engl J Med.* 2000; 342:314-319.

Diagnosis and management of the epilepsies in children: a summary of the partial update of the 2012 NICE epilepsy guideline

Appleton RE, Freeman A, Cross JH (Alder Hey Children's NHS Foundation Trust, Liverpool, UK; Queen Alexandra Hosp, Portsmouth, UK; UCL-Inst of Child Health, London, UK)

Arch Dis Child 97:1073-1076, 2012

The epilepsies of childhood are a heterogeneous group of disorders with different causes, treatments and outcomes. The choice of anti-epileptic drug is largely determined by its effectiveness in a specific epilepsy syndrome, or seizure type(s) if a syndrome cannot be readily identified, and the drug's safety profile. There are minimal randomised controlled trial data to help inform this decision. In January 2012, the National Institute for Health and Clinical Excellence (NICE) published its partially revised and updated clinical guideline on the pharmacological treatment of the epilepsies in children and adults. This partial update provides additional data and also specific recommendations that improve the evidence base for the use of specific anti-epileptic drugs in treating the epilepsies of childhood.

▶ This interesting article from the United Kingdom is a 2012 update on the clinical guidelines published by the National Institutes of Health and Clinical Excellence (NICE) regarding the pharmacologic treatment of epilepsy in children and adults. It is fascinating to see how these guidelines were developed compared with similar guidelines published by other health organizations in the United States such as the American Academy of Neurology. Of note, the article states that previous NICE guidelines established in 2004 did not find a difference in efficiency between the newer and the older antiepileptic drugs (AEDs). This update also provides helpful evidence on the best first-line and adjunctive treatments for all seizure types, including refractory focal, generalized tonic-clonic, partial seizures, and absence seizures based on cost-effectiveness and efficacy. The newer AEDs evaluated included pregabalin, rufinamide, zonisamide, stiripentol, eslicarbazepine, corticosteroids, and the ketogenic diet. Rather than using the traditional levels of evidence, the NICE used the Grade of Recommendations, Development, and Evaluation system to evaluate outcomes. In the final analysis, recommendations were similar to guidelines generated by most US-based groups. Lamotrigine was the most effective, and carbamazepine was second in line.

R. Riel-Romero, MD

Epileptic encephalopathies (including severe epilepsy syndromes)

Covanis A (Childrens Hosp "Agia Sophia," Athens, Greece)

Epilepsia 53:114-126, 2012

Epileptic encephalopathies represent a group of devastating epileptic disorders that appear early in life and are characterized by pharmacoresistant generalized or focal seizures, persistent severe electroencephalography (EEG) abnormalities, and cognitive dysfunction or decline. The ictal and interictal epileptic discharges are age-specific and are the main etiologic factors causing cognitive deterioration. This is most obvious in the idiopathic group. In the symptomatic group, the most common causes are structural, congenital, or acquired and rarely some metabolic disorders. In certain cases, clinical and EEG abnormalities persist and may evolve from one type to another as the child grows older. Various factors trigger and sustain the underlying pathophysiologic process and the ongoing epileptic and epileptiform activity during the most critical periods of brain maturation, perpetuating their deleterious effect on the brain. Immune-mediated mechanisms may have a role, suggested by certain encephalopathies responding to immune-modulating treatments and by the finding of various autoimmune antibodies. The chance of a better cognitive outcome improves with early diagnosis and treatment that is appropriate and effective. Current antiepileptic drugs are, in general, not effective: we urgently need new trials in this very special epileptic category. This article briefly reviews the most common epileptic encephalopathies and analyzes the most important clinical issues.

▶ This article is an excellent review of the different epileptic encephalopathies, the clinical presentations, and typical encephalographic (EEG) findings. These were classified based on the age of occurrence, such as neonatal, infancy, and early childhood epileptic encephalopathies. Among those presenting during the newborn period as a typical burst-suppression pattern on EEG are Ohtahara syndrome and early myoclonic encephalopathy. In infancy, West syndrome, Dravet syndrome, epilepsy in infancy with migrating focal seizures, and myoclonic encephalopathy in nonprogressive disorders are discussed. During childhood, the authors describe the clinical features and typical EEG findings in epileptic encephalopathy with continuous spike-and-wave during sleep (CSWS) including Landau-Kleffner syndrome (LKS). The authors' discussion of the differential diagnoses of events similar to infantile spasms, such as

Fejerman syndrome and colic, is helpful, as is their discussion on the relationships between LKS and CSWS and benign rolandic epilepsy. Three syndromes in which sleep physiology is disturbed were illustrated. Lennox-Gastaut syndrome and the antiepileptic drugs commonly used to treat it were also discussed. The entity of fever-induced refractory epileptic encephalopathy was described by the authors, who suggest an underlying autoimmune cause.

R. Riel-Romero, MD

Antiepileptic Drugs 2012: Recent Advances and Trends

Sirven JI, Noe K, Hoerth M, et al (Mayo Clinic, Phoenix, AZ)

Mayo Clin Proc 87:879-889, 2012

There are now 24 antiepileptic drugs (AEDs) approved for use in epilepsy in the United States by the Food and Drug Administration. A literature search was conducted using PubMed, MEDLINE, and Google for all English-language articles that discuss newly approved AEDs and the use of AEDs in epilepsy in the United States from January 1, 2008, through December 31, 2011. Five new agents were identified that have come onto the market within the past 2 years. Moreover, 3 trends involving AEDs have become clinically important and must be considered by all who treat patients with epilepsy. These trends include issues of generic substitution of AEDs, pharmacogenomics predicting serious adverse events in certain ethnic populations, and the issue of the suicide risk involving the entire class of AEDs. This article discusses the most recent AEDs approved for use in the United States and the 3 important trends shaping the modern medical management of epilepsy.

▶ This article is an excellent review of the antiepileptic drugs (AEDs) that were approved by the US Food and Drug Administration (FDA) for the treatment of epilepsy in 2012. These drugs included vigabatrin, rufinamide, lacosamide, clobazam, and ezogabine. For the pediatric neurologist, vigabatrin is particularly useful as an alternative treatment for infantile spasms in cases of corticotropin failure.

The authors present the seminal clinical trials on which FDA approval was based for each drug discussed. The readers can then judge for themselves the practical implications of the trials (ie, whether these were clinically meaningful), in particular for rufinamide, which is approved for Lennox-Gastaut syndrome, wherein the endpoint was a 32.7% reduction in total seizure frequency in 138 patients with at least 90 seizures a month. The article also enumerates the more important adverse effects of each of the drugs, including irreversible peripheral vision constriction in 30% of patients taking vigabatrin, QT interval shortening with rufinamide, dizziness and PR prolongation with lacosamide, and urinary retention, neuropsychiatric symptoms, and QT interval shortening with ezogabine. The authors also discuss the issue of Stevens-Johnson syndrome occurring in Asians with the HLA-B*1502 marker and in Europeans with the HLA-B*3101 marker. The discussion on the small relative risk of 1.8% for suicide or suicidal ideation in patients taking AEDs was useful, as was the concern regarding generic drug substitution of AEDs.

R. Riel-Romero, MD

Benign childhood focal epilepsies

Guerrini R, Pellacani S (Children's Hosp A. Meyer-Univ of Florence, Italy)
Epilepsia 53:9-18, 2012

The idiopathic focal epilepsies comprise a group of syndromes characterized by focal-onset seizures for which there is no detectable structural brain abnormality and for which there is a proposed functional mechanism for the epilepsy and electroencephalography (EEG) abnormalities. This group includes benign rolandic epilepsy (BRE), benign epilepsy with occipital paroxysms (both early onset and late-onset types), idiopathic photosensitive occipital lobe epilepsy, and some less well-defined syndromes. The limits of the early onset idiopathic occipital epilepsy syndrome are not clear, and perhaps this entity represents part of a larger syndrome group of "autonomic" age-related epilepsies. The term "idiopathic" implies absence of a structural brain lesion and a genetic propensity to seizures. The term "benign" implies that the epileptic seizures are easily treated or require no treatment, show remission without sequelae with ultimate and definitive remission before adulthood, do not have severe or exceedingly disturbing seizures, and have no associated serious intellectual or behavioral disturbances. It may be that a syndrome is benign only when it can be recognized early with reasonable certainty, thereby avoiding unnecessary investigations, overtreatment, and lifestyle restrictions. Although BRE has such characteristic clinical and EEG features to make early recognition possible, this is less constantly so in the other focal idiopathic epilepsy syndromes, where the term "benign" may be inappropriate. Mild and selective neuropsychological impairment may occur even in those with typical syndromes but it is unclear whether such selective deficits outlast the active phase of epilepsy. Sometimes the clinical course may be complicated by obvious cognitive and language impairments. In such cases, the term benign is obviously inappropriate, even when seizures are rare. In most patients with the typical focal idiopathic epilepsy syndromes, medication is not necessary.

▶ This article from Florence, Italy, is an excellent review of the most common idiopathic focal epilepsies, including benign rolandic epilepsy (BRE), benign epilepsy with occipital paroxysms (both early and late types), and idiopathic photosensitive occipital lobe epilepsy. The authors reinforce the observation that some of the reportedly benign focal epilepsies may actually be less benign insofar as cognition may not be fully spared. For instance, children with BRE may have subtle impairments in attention and visuomotor skills. The same is true for benign epilepsy with occipital paroxysms, wherein 20% may have specific learning difficulties and abnormal visual perception. Another interesting point raised in this article is the association between atypical forms of rolandic epilepsy, such as the pseudo-Lennox syndrome, and the disturbances in sleep physiology, such as patterns similar to continuous spike and wave in sleep. The authors point out that in BRE clinical remission may precede normalization of electroencephalogram. One other interesting point raised in this article is that exacerbation of seizures by focusing on television and video games occurs not only in primary generalized epilepsies but also in idiopathic photosensitive epilepsy, which is a focal epilepsy syndrome.

R. Riel-Romero, MD

Antiglutamic Acid Decarboxylase Antibodies in Children With Encephalitis and Status Epilepticus

Lin J-J, the CHEESE Study Group (Chang Gung Univ, Taoyuan, Taiwan)
Pediatr Neurol 47:252-258, 2012

Encephalitis may present with seizures or status epilepticus, and the etiology is usually presumed. Specific antibodies to ion channels, receptors, and other synaptic proteins were identified during the past decade. However, only a few studies investigated antiglutamic acid decarboxylase antibodies and antibodies to cell membrane ion channels or surface antigens in pediatric encephalitis and status epilepticus. We examined antibodies to glutamic acid decarboxylase and cell membrane ion channels or surface antigens in acute-phase serum from 17 children with encephalitis and status epilepticus. Antiglutamic acid decarboxylase antibody titers were compared with those of control children manifesting therapy-resistant epilepsy. Antiglutamic acid decarboxylase antibody titers were significantly higher in those with encephalitis and status epilepticus than in those with therapy-resistant epilepsy. No patient demonstrated antibodies to cell membrane ion channels or surface antigens. Six children exhibited positive antiglutamic acid decarboxylase antibodies. One child died, three manifested postencephalitic epilepsy with neurologic deficits, and two recovered well. Higher antiglutamic acid decarboxylase antibody titers were evident in the children with encephalitis and status epilepticus. Clinicians should be aware of the potential role of antiglutamic acid decarboxylase antibodies in children with encephalitis and status epilepticus.

▶ Most physicians are initially less likely to think of autoimmune encephalitis as a cause of status epilepticus. However, it is increasingly apparent that many patients, especially children, may have an autoimmune etiology underlying status epilepticus. It is quite common to encounter patients whose standard workup includes cerebrospinal, serological, and neuroimaging studies yielding no clues. This article reinforces the idea put forth by others that antineuronal antibodies, specifically anticarboxylase antibodies, should be sought in cases where no clear cause could be found. The presence of such antibodies raises the option of immunomodulatory therapy for these patients. It behooves clinicians to have a high index of suspicion for autoimmune encephalitis, especially in cases of acute onset of illness presenting with status epilepticus with an unrevealing evaluation. Moreover, in such adult patients, the search for antineoplastic antibodies and a primary neoplasm should be undertaken as well.

R. Riel-Romero, MD

Cardiac autonomic dysfunction in drug naïve hot water epilepsy

Meghana A, Sathyaprabha TN, Sinha S, et al (Natl Inst of Mental Health and Neuroscience (NIMHANS), Bangalore, India)

Seizure 21:706-710, 2012

Purpose.—This study aimed to characterize the role of autonomic nervous system dysfunction in hot water epilepsy (HWE). Heart rate variability (HRV) has been established as a good index of cardio-autonomic regulation.

Methodology.—Forty-five patients with HWE (age: 24.6 ± 10.1 years; M:F = 37:8) and 45 age and gender matched controls (age: 24.17 ± 10.37 years; M:F = 37:8) were studied. Five minutes resting lead II electrocardiogram (ECG) was obtained (AD instruments) under standard conditions and analyzed for time and frequency domain HRV parameters using LabChart software.

Result.—Patients with hot water epilepsy showed significant increase in LF nu (Low frequency normalized unit) and LF/HF denoting an interictal increase in sympathetic activity. In addition, reductions were noted in parasympathetic function [RMSSD (root mean square successive difference of RR intervals), HF (High frequency) nu and LF/HF].

Conclusion.—This study has demonstrated an impaired sympatho-vagal balance characterized by increased sympathetic activity and reduced parasympathetic activity in patients with HWE. The present study supports the notion that the hypothalamus is involved in both, the pathogenesis of HWE and autonomic regulation.

▶ Sudden, unexpected death in epilepsy has been in the forefront of many discussions regarding the care of patients with seizures, more so those with medically refractory epilepsy. One of the theories behind the possible cause of this phenomenon is that of impaired autonomic functioning in patients with epilepsy that can be exacerbated by the type of antiepileptic medications they take. Heart rate variability (HRV) is a parameter that assesses the integrity of the autonomic nervous system. These authors examined 45 patients with hot water epilepsy (HWE) using routine electrocardiograms to assess high-frequency domains' HRV, such as root mean square successive difference of the RR intervals and number of successive NN intervals that vary by more than 50 microseconds using LabChart software. In their study, the authors demonstrated impaired sympathovagal balance with increased sympathetic activity and decreased vagal tone, suggesting that an autonomic hypothalamic dysfunction is present in patients with HWE.

R. Riel-Romero, MD

Dramatic weight loss with rufinamide

Mourand I, Crespel A, Gelisse P (Gui de Chauliac Hosp, Montpellier, France)
Epilepsia 54:e5-e8, 2013

Rufinamide (RUF) is a novel antiepileptic drug considered as second-line therapy in the treatment of Lennox-Gastaut syndrome. Treatment-emergent adverse events (AEs) have consisted mainly of drowsiness, irritability, vomiting, and loss of appetite. RUF is considered as a "weight-neutral" drug. We found clinically significant weight loss in 7 of 15 consecutive adult patients (47%; 3 male, 4 female, aged 18–31 years) treated with RUF as add-on therapy (800–2,400 mg/day: 23.5–57.1 mg/kg/day). The body mass index (BMI) decreased by 7.3–18.7%. Two patients were obese class I before RUF. Five patients (71%) were underweight before RUF (mild in one case, moderate in two cases, and severe in two cases). Four of these patients stopped RUF because of this adverse effect. RUF was recommenced in two patients using a lower and slower dosing strategy; one patient showed improvement in seizure control and no weight loss but RUF was re-stopped in the second patient because of continued weight loss. Despite of weight loss, RUF was continued in two other patients because it reduced seizure activity. We primarily related weight loss to reduced food intake, that is, loss of appetite and nausea, although in two patients no obvious loss of appetite was reported. RUF can cause clinically significant weight loss in adult patients, even at low dose. This AE can affect patients who are already underweight. There is a possibility that lower starting doses and slower escalation might minimize weight loss, but further information is required to determine whether this is the case.

▶ Rufinamide (RUF) is new antiepileptic that had been approved by the US Food and Drug Administration for the adjunctive treatment of Lennox-Gastaut syndrome. Side effects have included vomiting, headache, and somnolence, and changes in weight have been reported to be insignificant. This article reports that 7 of 15 consecutive adult patients treated with RUF at doses of 800 to 2400 mg per day had clinically significant weight loss with a decrease in body mass index of 7.3% to 18.7%. In 2 patients, RUF was restarted at a lower dose and at a slower pace with one patient showing improvement and no weight loss, but in the other RUF had to be discontinued a second time because of weight loss. The authors suggest that weight loss can occur as an adverse effect of RUF therapy. This is important information that can be relayed to patients with seizures, especially those with pre-existing weight issues and those already on topiramate and/or zonisamide who are considering adding RUF to their medication regimen.

R. Riel-Romero, MD

A randomized controlled trial of flunarizine as add-on therapy and effect on cognitive outcome in children with infantile spasms

Bitton JY, Sauerwein HC, Weiss SK, et al (Sainte-Justine Hosp (CHU Sainte-Justine), Montreal, Quebec, Canada; Univ of Toronto, Ontario, Canada; et al)

Epilepsia 53:1570-1576, 2012

Purpose.—Cognitive impairment is observed commonly in children with a history of infantile spasms (IS). The goal of this study was to prospectively examine the effect on cognitive outcome of a neuroprotective agent used as adjunctive therapy during treatment of the spasms.

Methods.—In a randomized controlled trial, patients received a standardized therapy plus flunarizine or placebo. The standardized treatment consisted of vigabatrin as first-line therapy. Nonresponders were switched to intramuscular synthetic adrenocorticotropic hormone (sACTH depot) after 2 weeks and, if necessary, to topiramate after two additional weeks. The Vineland Adaptive Behavior Scale (VABS) and Bayley Scales of Infant Development (BSID) were used as outcome measures 24 months after the intervention.

Key Findings.—Sixty-eight of 101 children diagnosed over 3 years in seven centers in Canada received either adjunctive flunarizine or placebo. Sixty-five of the 68 children (96%) became spasm-free within 8 weeks and no late relapse occurred. Bayley and Vineland results were available at baseline and at 24 months in 45 children. There was no significant difference in the BSID developmental quotient between the flunarizine- and placebo-treated children at baseline (44.3 ± 35.5 vs. 30.9 ± 29.8; $p = 0.18$) or 24 months later (56.9 ± 33.3 vs. 46 ± 34.2; $p = 0.29$). However, the 10 flunarizine-treated children with no identified etiology had a better outcome than the eight controls at 24 months on both the Vineland Scale (84.1 ± 11.3 vs. 72.3 ± 9.8; $p = 0.03$) and the Bayley Scale (87.6 ± 14.7 vs. 69.9 ± 25.3; $p = 0.07$).

Significance.—Our study failed to demonstrate a protective effect of flunarizine on cognitive outcome in a cohort of children with IS. An analysis of subgroups suggested that flunarizine may further improve cognitive outcome in children with no identified etiology.

▶ Infantile spasms (IS) are one of the most devastating seizure types in childhood, as these are usually associated with development arrest or regression. Any therapeutic option in controlling spasms or salvaging development should be strongly considered. Using a randomized, placebo-controlled trial design, the authors of the study evaluated the effect of flunarizine on the cognitive outcome of children using the Vineland Adaptive Behavior Scale and Bayley Scales of Infant Development (BSID) 24 months after intervention. Although flunarizine was tolerated, it did not significantly improve cognitive outcome in children with infantile spasms. This was interesting to note, as in this study, 96% (65 of 68) of the patients had control of spasms within 2 months of treatment with either vigabatrin, adrenocorticotropic hormone, or other antiepileptics, suggesting that cognitive outcome may not be entirely dependent on spasm control. However, 10 of the flunarizine-treated patients who had cryptogenic IS scored 17 points higher on BSID, suggesting that cryptogenic IS may be a subset more amenable to therapy with neuroprotective agents.

R. Riel-Romero, MD

Acute EEG findings in children with febrile status epilepticus: Results of the FEBSTAT study

Nordli DR Jr, For the FEBSTAT Study Team (Children's Memorial Hosp, Chicago, IL; et al)

Neurology 79:2180-2186, 2012

Objective.—The FEBSTAT (Consequences of Prolonged Febrile Seizures) study is prospectively addressing the relationships among serial EEG, MRI, and clinical follow-up in a cohort of children followed from the time of presentation with febrile status epilepticus (FSE).

Methods.—We recruited 199 children with FSE within 72 hours of presentation. Children underwent a detailed history, physical examination, MRI, and EEG within 72 hours. All EEGs were read by 2 teams and then conferenced. Associations with abnormal EEG were determined using logistic regression. Interrater reliability was assessed using the κ statistic.

Results.—Of the 199 EEGs, 90 (45.2%) were abnormal with the most common abnormality being focal slowing (n = 47) or attenuation (n = 25); these were maximal over the temporal areas in almost all cases. Epileptiform abnormalities were present in 13 EEGs (6.5%). In adjusted analysis, the odds of focal slowing were significantly increased by focal FSE (odds ratio [OR] = 5.08) and hippocampal T2 signal abnormality (OR = 3.50) and significantly decreased with high peak temperature (OR = 0.18). Focal EEG attenuation was also associated with hippocampal T2 signal abnormality (OR = 3.3).

Conclusions.—Focal EEG slowing or attenuation are present in EEGs obtained within 72 hours of FSE in a substantial proportion of children and are highly associated with MRI evidence of acute hippocampal injury. These findings may be a sensitive and readily obtainable marker of acute injury associated with FSE.

▶ The FEBSTAT (Consequences of Prolonged Febrile Seizures) study is a prospective, long-term, multicenter study designed to evaluate the outcome of febrile status epilepticus (FSE) and the predictors of outcome using serial magnetic resonance images, electroencephalograms (EEGs), and clinical follow-up. Results obtained during the study included the EEG findings in children during the acute phase of FSE, which is within 72 hours of the FSE. According to the authors, of the 119 EEGs obtained, 90 (45.2%) showed focal slowing or attenuation seen more commonly over the temporal areas. Only a small proportion 13 (6.5%) showed epileptiform discharges. Of note, whenever focal slowing or attenuation was seen, it was usually ipsilateral to the side of seizure lateralization and the side of hippocampal T_2 signal abnormality and more often seen on the right side than the left side. The authors suggest that this may be a marker for possible acute neuronal injury subsequent to the FSE, again lending credence to the hypothesis that FSE may be a risk factor for subsequent temporal lobe epilepsy.

R. Riel-Romero, MD

Lamotrigine Serum Concentration in Children With Epilepsy

Heyman E, Lavie R, Lahat E, et al (Assaf Harofeh Med Ctr, Zerifin, Israel; et al)
Pediatr Neurol 47:427-430, 2012

The correlation between lamotrigine serum concentration, efficacy, and toxicity in children is controversial. The database of the Clinical Pharmacology Laboratory at Assaf Harofeh Medical Center was retrospectively searched to identify lamotrigine serum concentrations in children aged 2-19 years with refractory epilepsy who received lamotrigine as monotherapy or polytherapy from 2007-2010. Data collected included age at epilepsy onset, additional antiepileptic drugs, lamotrigine dose, monthly seizure frequency before and after lamotrigine treatment, and side effects. Sixty blood samples were collected from 42 children aged 10.1 ± 4.9 years (range, 2-20 years). Seizure types included complex partial ($n = 28$), simple partial ($n = 7$), absence ($n = 2$), and generalized tonic-clonic ($n = 23$). Decreased seizure frequency was observed in 38 (63.3%) patients. No correlation with lamotrigine serum concentration was evident, but seizure frequency was significantly influenced by age and lamotrigine dose. Side effects were reported in 21 (35%) patients. Only diplopia was significantly correlated with lamotrigine serum concentration. Lamotrigine was more effective at lower doses and in older children. Lamotrigine serum concentration correlated significantly with diplopia, but not with other side effects or with clinical efficacy. Overall, lamotrigine is effective and safe in children with refractory epilepsy.

▶ Lamotrigine is a broad-spectrum antiepileptic drug approved for both adjunctive and monotherapy treatment for partial-onset seizures in adult patients and generalized seizures of the Lennox-Gastaut type of both pediatric and adult patients. It is one of the drugs commonly used by neurologists worldwide with excellent efficacy based on postmarketing reports. The aim of this retrospective study was to determine the correlation between lamotrigine serum concentration, efficacy, and adverse effects in pediatric patients. Sixty blood samples from 42 children were collected. The lamotrigine dose used ranged from 40 to 400 mg/d and serum levels were from 0.3 to 19.1 μg/mL. Lamotrigine levels and the dose-to-weight ratio were lower in those who were seizure free compared with other patients. Moreover, the decrease in seizure frequency was found to be significantly influenced by age. A drawback to the study was that the authors did not speculate on possible reasons behind these findings. Interestingly, only diplopia was significantly correlated with lamotrigine serum concentrations.

R. Riel-Romero, MD

Feasibility of antiepileptic drug withdrawal following extratemporal resective epilepsy surgery

Menon R, Rathore C, Sarma SP, et al (R. Madhavan Nayar Ctr for Comprehensive Epilepsy Care, Trivandrum, Kerala, India)

Neurology 79:770-776, 2012

Objective.—To identify the rate of successful antiepileptic drug (AED) withdrawal after resective surgery and the predictors of postwithdrawal seizure recurrence in patients with extratemporal epilepsy.

Methods.—We retrospectively analyzed the postoperative AED profile of 106 consecutive patients who had completed 2 or more years after resections involving frontal, parietal, and occipital lobes for AED-resistant epilepsy. To identify the potential predictors of seizure recurrence, we compared the attributes of recurred and nonrecurred groups by univariate and multivariate analyses.

Results.—We attempted AED withdrawal in 94 (88.7%) patients. Forty-four (41.5%) patients had seizure recurrence while reducing AED, of which 14 (31.8%) did not become seizure-free subsequently. On multivariate analysis, an abnormal postoperative EEG and longer preoperative duration of epilepsy predicted seizure recurrence, while early postoperative seizures and presence of gliosis or dysplasia were additional predictors on univariate analysis. At mean follow-up duration of 4.6 years, 63 (59.4%) patients were seizure-free. The cumulative probability of achieving complete AED-free status was 20% at fourth year, 34% at sixth year, 40% at eighth year, and 52% at 10th year after surgery.

Conclusions.—Following resective extratemporal epilepsy surgery, AED can be successfully discontinued in only in a minority of patients. One-third of patients who recur fail to regain seizure control upon AED reintroduction. Longer duration of epilepsy prior to surgery, abnormal postoperative EEG, early postoperative seizures, and focal gliosis or dysplasia as substrate predispose to seizure recurrence. This information will be helpful in making rational decisions on AED withdrawal following extratemporal resective epilepsy surgery.

▶ One of the dilemmas facing physicians treating patients with medically intractable epilepsy is the issue of the ideal time to taper off antiepileptic drugs (AEDs) after surgical treatment. Menon et al described the predictors of seizure recurrence using retrospective analysis of 106 consecutive patients 2 years or more after respective surgery for seizures. Forty-four patients (41.5%) had seizure recurrence while on AED taper. Fourteen (31.8%) did not become seizure free subsequently. Abnormal postoperative electroencephalogram, longer preoperative duration of epilepsy, early postoperative seizures, and the presence of gliosis or dysplasia predicted seizure recurrence. The sobering take-home message from this article is that a substantial number of patients tapered off AED after surgery did not subsequently become seizure free. The probability of achieving complete

AED-free status increases the further along a patient is after surgery, with 52% probability 10 years after surgery.

R. Riel-Romero, MD

Clinical outcomes, quality of life, and costs associated with implantation of vagus nerve stimulation therapy in pediatric patients with drug-resistant epilepsy

Helmers SL, Duh MS, Guérin A, et al (Emory Univ School of Medicine, Atlanta, GA; Analysis Group, Inc, Boston, MA; et al)

Eur J Paediatr Neurol 16:449-458, 2012

Background.—VNS (Vagus Nerve Stimulation Therapy) is approved in the USA to treat refractory epilepsy as adjunctive to antiepileptic drugs (AEDs) in patients ≥12 years with complex partial seizures.

Aims.—To evaluate clinical outcomes, quality-adjusted life years (QALY), and costs associated with VNS in pediatric patients with drug-resistant epilepsy in a real-world setting.

Methods.—A retrospective analysis was conducted using Medicaid data (USA). Patients had ≥1 neurologist visits with epilepsy diagnosis (ICD-9 345.xx, 780.3x), ≥1 procedure claims for VNS implantation, ≥1 AEDs, ≥6-months of Pre- and Post-VNS continuous enrollment. Pre-VNS period was 6-months and Post-VNS period extended from implantation until device removal, death, Medicaid disenrollment, or study end (up to 3 years). Incidence rate ratios (IRR) and costs ($2010) were estimated. QALYs were estimated using number of seizure-related events.

Results.—For patients 1–11 years old ($N = 238$), hospitalizations and emergency room visits were reduced Post-VNS vs. Pre-VNS (adjusted IRR = 0.73 [95% CI: 0.61–0.88] and 0.74 [95% CI: 0.65–0.83], respectively). Average total healthcare costs were lower Post-VNS vs. Pre-VNS ($18,437 vs. $18,839 quarterly [adjusted $p = 0.052$]). For patients 12–17 years old ($N = 207$), hospitalizations and status epilepticus events were reduced Post-VNS vs. Pre-VNS (adjusted IRR = 0.43 [95% CI: 0.34–0.54] and 0.25 [95% CI: 0.16–0.39], respectively). Average total healthcare costs were lower Post-VNS vs. Pre-VNS period ($14,546 vs. $19,695 quarterly [adjusted $p = 0.002$]). Lifetime QALY gain after VNS was 5.96 (patients 1–11 years) and 4.82 years (patients 12–17 years).

Conclusions.—VNS in pediatric patients is associated with decreased resource use and epilepsy-related events, cost savings, and QALY gain.

► The prevalence of medically intractable epilepsy has been reported to be between 9% and 24% in several studies done in different countries. In 1997, the US Food and Drug Administration approved the use of the vagus nerve stimulator (VNS) device as a tool in the adjunctive treatment for patients 12 years of age and older with medically refractory complex partial seizures. This is a retrospective study done to evaluate the clinical outcomes in patients implanted with the VNS using the quality-adjusted life years (QALY) and the health care costs before and after VNS implantation. The authors concluded that there was significant gain in QALY after VNS implantation over a lifetime and that health care costs related to resource use and epilepsy-related events (ie, seizure-related hospitalizations, emergency room visits, and outpatient neurology visits) as well as the occurrence of status epilepticus were reduced in pediatric patients after VNS implantation.

R. Riel-Romero, MD

Aggressive behavior and epilepsy: A multicenter study

Piazzini A, Bravi F, Edefonti V, et al (St Paolo Hosp, Milan, Italy; Univ of Milan, Italy)

Epilepsia 53:e174-e179, 2012

The aim of this study is to describe aggressiveness in the epilepsy population and to identify possible relationships between this type of behavior and clinical and sociodemographic variables. Aggressive responses were measured by the Aggression Questionnaire (AQ), a standardized and validated instrument, which was administered to 503 patients from nine Italian centers for the care of epilepsy. Aggressive behavior in patients with epilepsy was different from that in the normal Italian population. After adjustment for age and sex, when appropriate, the following variables significantly affected aggressiveness: presence of compromised intellectual functioning, psychiatric disturbances, disability status, number of medications, geographic distribution, education, chronologic age, and disease duration. Our study offers a starting point for further investigations aimed at better understanding the mechanisms connecting aggression and epilepsy.

▶ Aggressive behavior is a common comorbidity seen in epilepsy. The article reports a multicenter study describing characteristics of aggressive behavior during the interictal phase in adult patients (18 and older) with epilepsy as measured by the Aggression Questionnaire as well as the sociodemographic and clinical variables. As can be predicted, the variables significantly correlated with increased aggression include level of education/degree of intellectual disability, younger age, and disease duration. The other factors that impact aggression are disability status, geographic location (degree of social stigma attached to having seizures varied by region), and polytherapy. A drawback to the study included the lack of clear delineation of the psychiatric comorbidities present in the patients. Additionally, it would also be interesting to know how seizure freedom impacts aggressive behavior in patients with epilepsy.

R. Riel-Romero, MD

2 Headache

Thunderclap headache

Ducros A, Bousser M-G (Lariboisière Hosp, Paris, France)

BMJ 346:e8557, 2013

Background.—The term *thunderclap headache* refers to a severe headache with an instantaneous onset and progression to maximum pain within 1 minute. About 43 per 100,000 adults per year experience thunderclap headache, which is considered a secondary syndrome, most often to subarachnoid hemorrhage. The diagnosis can be tricky, since brain computed tomography (CT) and lumbar puncture may be normal. Because the underlying cause can be serious, including cervical artery dissection, cerebral venous thrombosis, and reversible cerebral vasoconstriction syndrome (RCVS), further investigation is warranted. The causes of thunderclap headache, investigations useful with normal CT and lumbar puncture results, and diagnostic guidelines were reviewed.

Definition and Etiology.—A detailed history is needed to identify thunderclap headache, noting how long the headache takes to peak and what the maximum severity is on an 11-point scale (0 to 10, with 10 being the worst pain ever experienced). Headaches that reach a 7 or more within less than 1 minute qualify. Thunderclap headaches may last minutes to several days, show no specific location or type of pain, and can be single or recurrent over a few days. They may begin spontaneously or be preceded by the Valsalva maneuver, exertion, sexual activity, emotional stress, bathing, or showering. General practitioners should refer patients with these headaches urgently to the emergency department of a hospital with a neurology department when possible. If the neurologic or physical examination reveals associated neurologic symptoms or abnormalities, urgent evaluation is advised.

Subarachnoid hemorrhage is the most common cause, followed by RCVS. Some causes of these headaches are revealed on plain CT or lumbar puncture, including ischemic stroke, hydrocephalus, brain tumors, acute sinusitis, and bacterial or viral meningitis. Causes that can be missed include cervical artery dissection, cerebral venous thrombosis, posterior reversible leukoencephalopathy syndrome (PRES), intracranial hypotension, pituitary apoplexy, spontaneous retroclival hematoma, myocardial infarction, aortic dissection, and temporal arteritis.

Diagnostic Investigations.—Plain head CT is always needed, but if it is normal, lumbar puncture is also required. Because patients with thunderclap headache may have a mass lesion, brain imaging is mandatory before doing the lumbar puncture. If the cerebrospinal fluid (CSF) is clear, opening pressure is measured to rule out cerebral venous thrombosis and intracranial hypotension. White and red blood cell counts, Gram staining, protein and glucose concentrations, visual inspection for xanthochromia, and spectrophotometry should also be done on CSF samples. Although some authors recommend waiting 12 hours to do the lumbar puncture, the possible adverse effects of this outweigh the benefits.

In subarachnoid hemorrhage, angiography is required to identify ruptured aneurysm. With a normal CT and normal, near-normal, or blood-stained CSF result, cervical and cerebral angiography is needed to find alternative diagnoses. A multidisciplinary neurovascular team can determine whether the aneurysm requires treatment. Brain magnetic resonance imaging (MRI) may show cortical cerebral venous thrombosis, pituitary apoplexy, PRES, or intracranial hypotension. The availability of CT angiography (CTA) and MR angiography (MRA) makes imaging of the cervical and cerebral vessels easier and more acceptable to patients than previously. Conventional angiography is indicated when no aneurysm is found on non-diagnostic CTA or MRA. Some patients with thunderclap headaches and non-diagnostic MRI, MRA, and CTA but persistent or worsening headache or other symptoms may need four-vessel cerebral angiography to find occult intracranial arterial dissection, cerebral vasoconstriction syndrome, or vasculitis.

Diagnostic Guidelines.—"Primary thunderclap headache" has been listed in the International Classification of Headache Disorders as a distinct entity, but there is doubt that this actually exists. Physicians should always look for an underlying cause in patients with thunderclap headache. When the onset is abrupt or related to cough, exertion, or sexual activity, diagnosing a primary headache disorder can be a dangerous choice. Patients with no history of a similar headache should be investigated to exclude a secondary cause, especially a carotid dissection. If the results of all noninvasive investigations are normal and the patient has no recurrence over several weeks of follow-up, the diagnosis can be "thunderclap headache of undefined origin."

▶ This review article on thunderclap headache discusses the bedside approach to this important entity quite lucidly. It is a useful and comprehensive review for the emergency physicians and the ward doctors.

A careful history has to be taken to label a headache as "thunderclap," because it is a type of headache that peaks in severity within a minute of onset, and very often this history is not clearly obtained in the emergency department. For all practical purposes, thunderclap headaches should be considered medical emergencies and should be completely investigated for underlying secondary causes because they only very rarely are manifestations of primary headaches.

In case of normal computed tomography (CT) scan of the brain, there should not be any doubt regarding whether or not to do a lumbar puncture, and it should be done promptly to rule out a subarachnoid hemorrhage or rarely central nervous system bacterial or viral infections. A magnetic resonance imaging scan of the brain must be done if the above are unrevealing of any significant information to look for important treatable causes such as cerebral venous thrombosis, pituitary apoplexy, posterior reversible leukoencephalopathy, and so on.

Intracranial hypotension from a dural tear is also one of the often overlooked diagnostic possibilities in case of thunderclap headaches and should be considered, especially so when there has been history of a trivial trauma and a positional (orthostatic) nature of headache. History of trauma may also suggest arterial dissection.

Magnetic resonance or CT angiography should be the next step to identify cervical carotid dissection or reversible cerebral vasoconstriction syndrome (RCVS). A repeat angiography at 3 weeks may be required in case of suspected RCVS to establish the diagnosis as initial angiograms may be normal at times. A conventional 4-vessel angiogram is only indicated in cases that have worsening or persistent headache or have appearance of new symptoms since the onset of the thunderclap headache to rule out possibilities of occult intracranial arterial dissection or vasculitis.

A. Panagariya, MD

Advances in Drug Development for Acute Migraine

Cady RJ, Shade CL, Cady RK (Missouri State Univ, Springfield; Banyan Group, Inc, Springfield, MO)
Drugs 72:2187-2205, 2012

Triptans revolutionized medical recognition and the acute treatment of migraine. Yet, throughout a lifetime, millions of patients who live with migraine endure hundreds of days of disability due to their disease. Most migraine attacks respond to migraine-specific interventions, but attack response does not predict patient response. Generally, migraine patients respond to acute treatment for some, but not necessarily all, attacks of migraine. Consequently, there remains a substantial unmet clinical need for better acute treatment of migraine.

Numerous avenues of research and clinical observation provide insight into potential advances in acute treatment of migraine. These include better delivery systems for existing drugs, as well as the development of potential new therapeutic agents. In addition, new changes in migraine taxonomy and clinical observations of migraine suggest additional important therapeutic opportunities. Based on clinical observations, this article explores future acute treatment needs, drugs in development for acute migraine, and new products that deliver established drugs to improve treatment response.

▶ Every neurologist realizes that the current armamentarium of drugs used for migraine attacks is indeed insufficient. What do we have practically, apart from nonsteroidal anti-inflammatory drugs and a few triptans in oral and intranasal forms? There is a need to develop more drugs to abort acute migraine attacks. Calcitonin gene-related peptide and AMPA/kainate receptor antagonists seem to offer new hopes in acute migraine treatment. Orally inhaled dihydroergotamine with the possibility of decreased side effects, sumatriptan transdermal patch, and needle-free injections are other modes of administration of well-known effective medications, which may turn out to be more useful during acute attacks.

This is an excellent review of the current status of advances in acute treatment of migraine; it is well written and informative and gives one a comprehensive overview of the ongoing developments in acute migraine therapy.

The authors beautifully summarized the process of migraine chronification when stating, "As migraine transforms from episodic to chronic, it becomes a more pervasive neurological assault," which also signifies the importance and the need for the development of newer drugs that abort the attacks without significant side effects, thus, preventing chronification while helping to avoid medication overuse headaches. Developing newer drugs for acute attacks may go a long way in significantly improving quality of life in chronic migraineurs.

A. Panagariya, MD

Improvement in Headaches With Continuous Positive Airway Pressure for Obstructive Sleep Apnea: A Retrospective Analysis

Johnson KG, Ziemba AM, Garb JL (Baystate Med Ctr, Springfield, MA; Smith College, Northampton, MA)

Headache 53:333-343, 2013

Objective.—We aimed to identify clinical features in patients with severe headaches that predicted obstructive sleep apnea (OSA) and determine clinical and sleep study characteristics that predicted headache improvement with continuous positive airway pressure (CPAP).

Background.—Many patients with headaches complain of sleep symptoms and have OSA. There is often improvement of headaches with CPAP treatment.

Methods.—We conducted a retrospective chart review of all patients referred to adult neurology clinic for headaches and sent for polysomnography between January 2008 and December 2009. Follow-up ranged from 18 to 42 months.

Results.—Eighty-two headache patients (70 females, 12 males) were studied. Mean age was 45 ± 13 years (females 45 ± 13, males 43 ± 11) and mean body mass index was 32 ± 9. Headache types included 17% chronic migraine without aura, 22% episodic migraine without aura, 32% migraine with aura, 21% tension-type headache, 6% chronic post-traumatic headache, 11% medication overuse headache, and 7% other types. All patients were receiving standard treatment for their headaches by their neurologist. Fifty-two patients (63%) had OSA. Increasing age, female gender, and chronic migraine without aura were predictive of OSA. Of the patients with OSA, 33 (63%) used CPAP and 27 (82%) were adherent to CPAP. Headache improvement was reported by 40 patients (49%) due to either standard medical therapy or CPAP. Patients with OSA who were CPAP adherent (21/27) were more likely to have improvement in headaches than patients intolerant of CPAP (2/6), those that did not try CPAP (8/19), and those who did not have OSA (16/30) (P =.045). Of the 33 patients who used CPAP, 13 reported improvement in headaches specifically due to CPAP therapy and 10 additional patients noted benefit in sleep symptoms. The presence of witnessed apneas (P =.045) and male gender (P =.021) predicted improvement in headaches due to CPAP.

Conclusions.—Headache patients should be evaluated for the presence of OSA. Treating OSA improves headaches in some patients.

▶ Management of chronic headaches is always a challenging task. Although sleep is one of the most important aspects of life, it is also one of the least inquired areas of history taking, especially in the busy neurology clinic. Despite the knowledge about the impact of quality of sleep on the overall health of an individual, very few physicians practically address sleep adequately in the diagnosis and treatment of chronic headaches.

This study has concluded that a large number of primary headache patients referred for polysomnography indeed had upper airway resistance syndrome, and many of them responded to continuous positive airway pressure, which, in fact, is a very important observation when it comes to the difficult to treat headache patients because it is one of the modifiable and treatable aspects.

The clinically important point to emphasize is that a detailed sleep history should be routinely obtained in the headache clinic, and appropriately selected patients should undergo polysomnography to identify any contribution of sleep disturbances in the genesis and perpetuation of chronic daily headaches. Also in general, it should be a practice to advise all headache patients to maintain a regular and healthy sleep schedule and to recognize the importance of sleep hygiene. A good night's sleep can prevent many headache attacks and may bring about an overall improvement in quality of life.

A. Panagariya, MD

Treatment of Pediatric Migraine in the Emergency Room

Gelfand AA, Goadsby PJ (Univ of California, San Francisco)

Pediatr Neurol 47:233-241, 2012

Migraine constitutes a relatively common reason for pediatric emergency room visits. Given the paucity of randomized trials involving pediatric migraineurs in the emergency department setting compared with adults, recommendations for managing these children are largely extrapolated from adult migraine emergency room studies and trials involving outpatient home pediatric migraine therapy. We review current knowledge about pediatric migraineurs presenting at the emergency room and their management, and summarize the best evidence available to guide clinical decision-making.

▶ This review gives insight into the prevalent practices of management of pediatric migraine in the emergency room. It is useful information for emergency room physicians because very often one is confused about the strategy of managing acute migraine attacks in a child who presents in the emergency room.

Of course, the first and foremost task is to establish the diagnosis of migraine, lest one overlook a secondary cause. Therefore, even in a rushed emergency room a thorough headache history must be obtained. There is a tendency to get a computed tomography scan done even in cases with recurrent headaches with acute episodic worsening so as not to miss a diagnosis. As a result, young children are often exposed to unjustified radiation repeatedly, which is avoidable if an additional 5 minutes were spent on the history.

Children with migraine attacks need to be rested in quiet surroundings, which is most often not possible in a bustling emergency room setting, and taking this point into account and ensuring a dimly lit, quieter space for the child with acute headache, as highlighted in this article, would improve the overall treatment outcome.

Most emergency room physicians are still not comfortable using triptans and dihydroergotamine in children or adults when treating migraine, which could be very helpful in providing relief when administered to appropriately selected patients. Use of nasal spray triptans is also rewarding. Sodium valproate in injectable form can be a good choice for acute migraine headaches in the emergency room setting.

The practice of giving opioids and steroids for acute headaches, especially in children, should be discouraged, as rightly pointed out in the article, which suggests that opioids are not very efficacious in migraine and steroids do not reduce the chances of recurrence of headache attacks.

It is important that the emergency room physicians take time to explain the benign nature of the condition to the parents and advise them to follow-up regularly in a headache clinic for comprehensive management of migraine. This will help prevent further emergency room visits, which add to their overall financial burden.

This review is important for pediatricians and emergency room doctors as it clearly states evidence-based recommendations for treating migraine in children and adolescents.

A. Panagariya, MD

Resident and Fellow Section

Levin M (Dartmouth Hitchcock Med Ctr, Lebanon, NH)
Headache 53:181-185, 2013

Background.—With rising incidences of obesity, type 2 diabetes, and vascular disease plus people living longer, cases of renal failure and resulting dialysis will also increase. Patients with end-stage renal disease (ESRD) are likely to suffer adverse effects associated with treatment, including headache disorders.

> *Case Report.*—Woman, 61, complained of intractable headache of 3 weeks' duration. Her medical history included type 2 diabetes, hypertension, obstructive sleep apnea, rheumatoid arthritis, psoriatic arthritis, nonalcoholic steatohepatitis, chronic anemia, nephrolithiasis, pyelonephritis with recent right nephrectomy, and ESRD,

for which she had recently begun hemodialysis. The patient reported that the headaches began about 3 months previously, near the time she began hemodialysis. She had no family or personal history of migraine. The headaches were bifrontal, throbbing, and lasted all day. They were accompanied by nausea and vomiting, photophobia, and phonophobia, but no aura or focal neurologic complaint. Two previous hospital admissions for the problem had resulting in treatments using high-dose opiates, which caused excessive sedation, encephalopathy, and respiratory depression. The most common secondary causes of headache were ruled out during these previous work-ups. The only notable findings were a slightly elevated protein level of 69 and atrial fibrillation on electrocardiogram. The patient had received 2 g intravenous (IV) magnesium and 5 days of high-dose methylprednisolone that gave no relief. She had tried numerous medications and was currently taking aspirin 81 mg, fluticasone, metoprolol tartrate 25 mg twice a day, nortriptyline 25/25/50 mg, gabapentin 100 mg three times a day, hydromorphone, and lorazepam. She also had a low-grade fever on admission and appeared uncomfortable sitting in a darkened room. Neurologic and fundoscopic evaluations were unrevealing. Her only abnormal laboratory results were elevated blood urea nitrogen and creatinine levels. She was started on a modified Raskin protocol of diphenhydramine 25 mg, metoclopramide 10 mg IV, and dihydroergotamine (DHE) 1 mg IV three times a day. Her headache worsened during dialysis the second day in the hospital but improved otherwise. Hydromorphone and lorazepam were gradually discontinued to avoid medication overuse headache, as was gabapentin. Topiramate 25 mg at bedtime was begun, with plans to increase by 25 mg weekly to a final dose of 200 mg at bedtime. She was also given chlorpromazine (CPZ) 50 mg orally before dialysis to reduce the intensity of the headaches. Even though she developed atrial fibrillation with rapid ventricular response, pulmonary edema, and hypoxia, the headaches were responding to the medication regimen. Topiramate was discontinued when she developed leukopenia. On discharge after 2 weeks in the hospital she was taking nortriptyline 50 mg at night and magnesium oxide 200 mg twice a day to prevent headaches, along with CPZ 50 mg before dialysis. Six months later her headaches were well controlled with magnesium oxide and CPZ premedication.

Conclusions.—Dialysis-related headache was diagnosed and was likely accompanied by probable migraine. The treatment chosen is typical for migraine prevention. The magnesium proved effective, but if headache symptoms return, the patient could be given onabotuliniumtoxin A, which would avoid systemic side effects or medication interactions.

▶ Neurologists are often asked to evaluate patients admitted in nephrology wards for various reasons, and headache is one of the most common causes for a neurologic consultation. Patients with renal disease can have headaches from many causes and need to be evaluated in detail.

This report discusses the management of headache in a patient with chronic renal disease undergoing dialysis and who responded to chlorpromazine and preventive migraine medication in the form of magnesium. Dialysis may induce severe headache as a result of a large amount of water and electrolyte shifts. It is important to recognize it because changing dialysis parameters or methods can prevent it. Headaches caused by hypoglycemia, hypotension, or caffeine withdrawal also occur as a result of hemodialysis. Also, primary headaches, like migraine and tension-type headache, may be worsened by dialysis.

Chronic kidney disease usually leads to anemia, which causes tissue hypoxia and may cause headache. Polycystic kidney disease may present with headaches and may be associated with intracranial aneurysms as well. Accelerated hypertension with hypertensive encephalopathy may cause headache, so many drugs can induce acute headache, including nitroglycerin, antihypertensive agents (eg, β-blockers, calcium channel blockers, angiotensin-converting enzyme inhibitors, methyldopa), dipyridamole, histamine receptor antagonists (eg, cimetidine, ranitidine), and cyclosporine. Drug-induced aseptic meningitis may rarely occur as a result of use of antibiotics (eg, trimethoprim-sulfamethoxazole, sulfasalazine, cephalosporins, ciprofloxacin, isoniazid, and penicillin), intrathecal drugs, intraventricular chemotherapy, intravenous immunoglobulin, vaccines, and some other drugs, such as carbamazepine and ranitidine.

Long-term steroid use may induce idiopathic intracranial hypertension (IIH); moreover, steroids also can lead to headaches without causing IIH. Like nonrenal patients, central nervous system infections, vasculitis, and carbon dioxide retention as a result of obstructive sleep apnea can lead to headaches in patients with renal diseases as well.

Even though the list is long, there is no excuse for the neurologist not to know, because he or she has to appropriately advise as an expert to provide relief to the patient.

A. Panagariya, MD

Unusual Headache Syndromes

Queiroz LP (Universidade Federal de Santa Catarina, Florianópolis, Brazil)
Headache 53:12-22, 2013

Objective/Background.—Some headache syndromes have few cases reported in the literature. Their clinical characteristics, pathogenesis, and treatment may have not been completely defined. They may not actually be uncommon but rather under-recognized and/or underreported.

Methods.—A literature review of unusual headache syndromes, searching PubMed and ISI Web of Knowledge, was performed. After deciding which disorders to study, relevant publications in scientific journals, including original articles, reviews, meeting abstracts, and letters or correspondences to the editors were searched.

Findings.—This paper reviewed the clinical characteristics, the pathogenesis, the diagnosis, and the treatment of five interesting and unusual headache syndromes: exploding head syndrome, red ear syndrome, neck-tongue syndrome, nummular headache, and cardiac cephalgia.

Conclusions.—Recognizing some unusual headaches, either primary or secondary, may be a challenge for many non-headache specialist physicians. It is important to study them because the correct diagnosis may result in specific treatments that may improve the quality of life of these patients, and this can even be life saving.

▶ A neurologist has to deal with a variety of headache syndromes day in and day out. Although a large number of the patients do fit into the common International Classification of Headache Disorders II—based diagnoses, a smaller yet significant proportion of cases do not fall into the usual categories and are always a greater challenge to diagnosis and treatment. This article comprehensively reviews some unusual headache syndromes, such as exploding head syndrome, red ear syndrome, nummular headache, neck tongue syndrome, and cardiac cephalgia. A neurologist needs to have a clear understanding of these headaches, because such patients move from pillar to post, many times landing themselves at the psychologist's door.

Cardiac cephalgia is one of the particularly interesting and important entities because of its distinct pathomechanism that is related to the underlying cardiac dysfunction, and therefore should be treated differently from other headaches. It requires a high index of suspicion for diagnosing this entity, which usually occurs after 50 years of age when the incidence of classic migraine is declining. Clinically, it resembles a typical migraine attack that could be either unilateral or bilateral accompanied with photophobia and phonophobia. Unlike migraine, however, the pain is more often nonpulsatile and is otherwise constrictive and oppressive in character and gets precipitated by exertion as little as just walking. Different theories have been postulated to explain this entity that is a manifestation of coronary ischemia. Coronary evaluation is always a must, because use of triptans or other drugs considering it a migraine-like headache could have disastrous consequences. Nitrates abating the headache corroborates with the diagnosis of cardiac cephalalgia; conversely, nitrates would precipitate a migraine attack in migraineurs.

Most of the other headaches discussed in the article are chronic but benign, and adequately explaining to the patient about the possible mechanisms of their headaches and reassuring them about their nonserious nature facilitates the treatment.

Epicrania fugax (cephalgic seizure) is another unusual headache syndrome, which we have encountered in our OPDs, more often seen in school-going boys, complaining of a sudden, sharp unilateral headache in frontal, temporal, or parietal regions along a zigzag trajectory, lasting for a few seconds and occurring multiple times a day. This may be associated with epileptiform discharges in the electroencephalograph but without any clinical evidence of seizure apart from the episodic headaches. These headaches usually cluster over a period of weeks to months and are very responsive to low doses of carbamazepine. This headache type probably is one of those that represents a border zone of epilepsy and headache and is underrecognized in the OPDs because of lack of a proper understanding.

A. Panagariya, MD

Her versus his migraine: multiple sex differences in brain function and structure

Maleki N, Linnman C, Brawn J, et al (MGH and CHB, Boston, MA; et al)
Brain 135:2546-2559, 2012

Migraine is twice as common in females as in males, but the mechanisms behind this difference are still poorly understood. We used high-field magnetic resonance imaging in male and female age-matched interictal (migraine free) migraineurs and matched healthy controls to determine alterations in brain structure. Female migraineurs had thicker posterior insula and precuneus cortices compared with male migraineurs and healthy controls of both sexes. Furthermore, evaluation of functional responses to heat within the migraine groups indicated concurrent functional differences in male and female migraineurs and a sex-specific pattern of functional connectivity of these two regions with the rest of the brain. The results support the notion of a 'sex phenotype' in migraine and indicate that brains are differentially affected by migraine in females compared with males. Furthermore, the results also support the notion that sex differences involve both brain structure as well as functional circuits, in that emotional circuitry compared with sensory processing appears involved to a greater degree in female than male migraineurs.

▶ The differences in the characteristics of the male and the female brain have always been an interesting and intriguing area for neuropsychologists. It is common knowledge that males and females differ in their responses to similar situations, in their perception of environment, and in their decision-making capacities. The basis of these outward differences, of course, can be traced back to the differences in the structural and functional wiring of the neuronal circuits. These physiological aspects have been a focus of research for neuroscientists, but how and why the brain structure and function are differentially altered in pathological conditions that have a sex preponderance is still not an extensively studied area.

This study has interestingly found that disease-related structural changes in insula and precuneus regions were seen in female migraineurs, whereas in male migraineurs structural changes were seen in parahippocampal gyrus. Functional changes in response to noxious heat showed more pronounced responses in female migraineurs in the amygdala and parahippocampus. Furthermore, sex differences involve functional circuits as well; emotional circuitry compared with sensory processing appears more involved in female than male migraineurs. The reasons for this are not very clear but may be attributable to the hormonal effects or the differences in the neurotransmitter profile of men and women.

With the possibility of the scientists theorizing that most likely the differential impact could be a result of the way men and women process information, these differences incite the idea that the therapeutic aspects of migraine in males and females should be addressed differently as well.

A. Panagariya, MD

Bilateral acute angle-closure glaucoma in a migraine patient receiving topiramate: a case report

Cole KL, Wang EE, Aronwald RM (Northwestern Univ, Chicago, IL; NorthShore Univ HealthSystem, Evanston, IL)

J Emerg Med 43:e89-e91, 2012

Background.—Patients with migraine headaches are frequently prescribed topiramate to treat their condition.

Case Report.—We present a case of bilateral acute angle-closure glaucoma occurring 2 days after topiramate therapy was increased for symptoms related to migraine.

Conclusion.—Acute angle-closure glaucoma secondary to topiramate is an uncommon but serious adverse reaction that may result in severe morbidity such as permanent visual loss if not recognized in a timely manner. Treatment differs from primary acute angle-closure glaucoma in that discontinuation of topiramate is necessary for the glaucoma to resolve.

► Topiramate is a commonly used drug in migraine prophylaxis and seizures. This case report has a very important clinical message for emergency physicians to suspect and be able to diagnose a rare but important side effect of this drug: acute angle closure glaucoma.

Acute angle closure glaucoma, an ophthalmologic emergency, is known to present with a misleading clinical picture and can be confused with migraine, cluster headache, temporal arteritis, and subarachnoid hemorrhage. The diagnosis of glaucoma in a known case of migraine requires a high index of suspicion. The pattern of headache may not be helpful in identification of glaucoma because the headache may be periorbital rather than orbital. Marked severity of headache may be suggestive of a phenomenon different from the usual migraine headache of the patient, but maximum emphasis should be placed on significant and objective visual diminution in the affected eye. Usually this happens early on when the treatment with topiramate is initiated or its dose is increased; therefore, one must be more vigilant during the initial weeks of therapy to look for any such adverse event.

Most emergency rooms are not usually equipped with tonometry to measure intraocular pressure, so it is advisable to obtain an urgent ophthalmological opinion in suspected cases. Administering β-blockers, steroid eye drops, and intravenous mannitol may be eye-saving measures in the absence of access to an urgent intraocular pressure assessment.

It would not be out of place to mention here that many other drugs used in neurological practice also may cause acute angle closure glaucoma (eg, cholinergics, anticholinergics, antidepressants, antianxiety medications, acetazolamide, periocular botulinum toxin).[1] Emergency physicians should be aware of this potentially blinding side effect of commonly used medications.

It is worthwhile to provide a checklist of drugs causing visual problems in the emergency rooms and wards for ready reference. Emphasizing the significance of identifying drug-related visual adverse effects, such as loss of color vision from ethambutol; impairment of vision by chloroquine and isoniazid; yellow vision from digoxin; and field defects from vigabatrin during medical training programs is very important.

A. Panagariya, MD

Reference

1. Lachkar Y, Bouassida W. Drug-induced acute angle closure glaucoma. *Curr Opin Ophthalmol.* 2007;18:129-133.

Obese children suffer more often from migraine

Verrotti A, Di Fonzo A, Agostinelli S, et al (Univ of Chieti, Italy; et al)
Acta Paediatr 101:e416-e421, 2012

Aim.—To determine a possible relationship between migraine and body mass index.

Methods.—Migraine shows a wide spectrum of comorbidities, including cardiocerebral, vascular, psychiatric, metabolic, neurological as well as other pathologies. Recent researches suggest that obesity was significantly correlated with migraine frequency and disability in children, as well as in adult population studies. We reviewed data from the literature to clarify this possible relationship.

Results.—Translational and basic science research shows multiple areas of overlap between migraine pathophysiology and the central and peripheral pathways regulating feeding. Specifically, neurotransmittors such as serotonin, peptides such as orexin, and adipocytokines such as adiponectin and leptin have been suggested to have roles in both feeding and migraine. A relationship between migraine and body mass index exists, and therefore, interventions to modify body mass index may provide a useful treatment model for investigating whether modest weight loss reduces headache frequency and severity in obese migraineurs.

Conclusion.—The effect of obesity and weight change on headache outcomes may have important implications for clinical care.

▶ The electrical circuits and the chemical environment of the brain may account for a multitude of neurological disorders that have a functional basis, one of which is the ever-intriguing migraine. A handful of major neurotransmitters and their complex interplay form the basis of many neuropsychological dysfunctions—it is no wonder that the borderlands of neurology and psychology overlap widely.

It is quite a common observation in the clinic that obese females come with persistent and drug-refractory chronic headaches. Idiopathic intracranial hypertension is also a very well-known disorder of obese women.

Association of migraine with obesity is still not definitively proved, yet recent research in adults logically implies that a higher body mass index does have a link to chronic headaches. Migraine severity and frequency of attacks have been found to be associated with higher body mass index rather than its prevalence. Feeding behaviors are responsible for obesity, and migraine is a neurological disorder that is certainly known to be triggered by certain foods and may have an indirect association with feeding behaviors.

This article discusses the relationship of migraine and obesity and the complex interrelationship of inflammatory mediators and neurotransmitters in the pathogenesis of both conditions. Interestingly, on the one hand, obesity has some association with migraine, indicating a common biochemical linkage; on the other hand, drugs such as flunarizine and valproate used for preventing migraine also have a side effect of weight gain. This fact should also be taken as a lead in further analyzing the biochemical theories of causation and prevention of migraine.

Obesity in children may be a harbinger of a variety of metabolic disorders and also may be a predisposing factor for migraine. Apart from the genetic reasons, obesity in children has a lot to do with environmental factors such as diet, exercise habits, and behavior. Chronic headaches have, in fact, emerged more as lifestyle-based disorders in recent times and may be amenable to behavioral and lifestyle changes. The foundation of a healthy lifestyle developed in childhood would mean a healthy adulthood with a reduced burden of headache and other diseases.

A. Panagariya, MD

Frequency and Burden of Headache-Related Nausea: Results From the American Migraine Prevalence and Prevention (AMPP) Study

Lipton RB, Buse DC, Saiers J, et al (Albert Einstein College of Medicine, Bronx, NY; The WriteMedicine, Inc, Chapel Hill, NC; et al)

Headache 53:93-103, 2013

Background.—While nausea is a defining feature of migraine, the association of nausea with other headache features and its influence on the burden of migraine have not been quantified. Population-based data were used to elucidate the relative frequency and burden of migraine-associated nausea in persons with migraine.

Methods.—Participants with episodic migraine who completed the 2009 American Migraine Prevalence and Prevention survey rated their headache-related nausea as occurring none of the time, rarely, < half the time, or ≥ half the time with their headaches. They also completed headache symptom severity and occupation/work status questions, the Headache Impact Test-6, and treatment attitude items that were part of the 2009 survey. Regression models that adjusted for both sociodemographic characteristics and symptom severity were used to assess the influence of nausea frequency on outcome measures. Partial and semipartial correlational analyses were used to estimate the influence of nausea alone and in combination with other headache symptoms on headache-related impact.

Results.—Among the 6488 respondents with episodic migraine, approximately half (49.5%) reported high-frequency nausea (ie, ≥ half the time) with headache. High-frequency nausea was more common in females than males (adjusted odds ratio 1.35, 95% confidence interval 1.26-1.44). Persons with high-frequency nausea, compared with the no/rare or less than half the time nausea groups, reported significantly more headache symptoms and more headache-related impact as measured by the Headache Impact Test-6. High-frequency nausea was also associated with being occupationally disabled or on medical leave, and more self-reported financial burden of headache medications, worry about running out of headache medication(s), and that headache medications interfered with work or school work, household work, and family/leisure activities. Regression-based correlational analyses indicated that nausea contributes significantly and independently to headache-related impact.

Conclusions.—High-frequency migraine-associated nausea is common and is a marker for severe, debilitating migraine. Nausea makes an independent contribution to migraine-associated disability and impact. Management strategies that take nausea into account could reduce the burden of migraine. Nausea is an important target for monitoring and treatment.

▶ Nausea is one of the characteristic features and a very common accompaniment of migraine headaches. It is stating the obvious that nausea contributes to a significant functional disability associated with migraine; yet, in a busy clinic, one tends to overlook the need to address this associated symptom of migraine. This study highlights this very basic aspect of management of migraine.

Gastroparesis occurs as part of migraine often and is reported by most patients as an uncomfortable feeling that significantly adds to the disability and interferes with the timely ingestion of prescribed medications early in the attack, which is the time when the drugs are known to be most effective. Also, gastroparesis contributes to poorer absorption of the oral drugs. Above all, even when the patient takes his or her prescribed pills, more often than not they are vomited out before they can act. Not many patients take another analgesic pill when the first one is regurgitated, so the full-fledged debilitating attack of migraine sets in and follows its natural course. The idea of aborting the attack at the onset by taking medications early on, before the headache reaches its peak, is itself defeated. It is also not practically possible for these outpatients to have immediate access to any parenteral medications at headache onset.

The clinical point to emphasize is that those patients who do report considerable nausea and vomiting as part of their migraine attack need to be advised to take a prokinetic agent before their analgesic medication, which can substantially improve the efficacy of the prescribed medications and reduce overall disability associated with the attack.

A. Panagariya, MD

The syndrome of transient headache and neurological deficits with cerebrospinal fluid lymphocytosis (HaNDL) as an acute ischemic stroke mimic leading to systemic thrombolysis: A case report

Krause T, Nolte CH (Charité - Universitätsmedizin Berlin, Germany)

Clin Neurol Neurosurg 114:689-690, 2012

Background.—The diagnosis of acute ischemic stroke (AIS) must be made properly within a very short time to initiate systemic thrombolysis, which is effective just within 4.5 hours of symptom onset. Stroke-like conditions such as the syndrome of transient headache and neurologic deficits with cerebrospinal fluid lymphocytosis (HaNDL) must be quickly identified. This rare, benign, and self-limited disorder is usually seen in young adults and is characterized by an initial presentation with severe headache. An uncommon initial presentation without headache was documented.

Case Report.—Man, 39, suffered a sudden right-sided hemiparesis and expressive aphasia at 3 AM while in a taxi. In the emergency department his National Institute of Health Stroke Scale (NIHSS) score was 4 points, but he had normal vital signs, echocardiogram (ECG), and blood samples and no previous history of neurologic problems. Computed tomography (CT) scan of his brain was normal also. Systemic thrombolytic therapy was begun 1 hour 45 minutes after the onset of symptoms and was well tolerated. The neurologic symptoms resolved within 2 hours and remained absent for 2 days. On the third day after admission, the patient had an abrupt onset of left-sided hemihypesthesia. CT scan was unremarkable, and symptoms resolved in a few hours. The following day he developed severe holocephalic headache, nausea, and vomiting, along with mild signs of meningeal irritation. A magnetic resonance imaging (MRI) scan with diffusion and perfusion weighted imaging and arterial and venous angiography was unrevealing, and the headache and nausea disappeared within a few hours. Cerebrospinal fluid (CSF) analysis revealed lymphopleocytosis, but no other abnormalities. Similar episodes of nausea, vomiting, and headache with meningeal irritation recurred over the next several days, usually lasting a few hours. Most episodes were accompanied by transient left-sided hemihypesthesia. CSF cell counts fell eventually to 109/mm^3. Bilateral and frontotemporal mild slowing was noted in the electroencephalogram (EEG), but no epileptiform discharge was seen. The patient suffered no recurrence after 14 days and was discharged.

Conclusions.—The patient's first episode included no headache, thus prompting a diagnosis of AIS and treatment with systemic thrombolytic therapy. Neurologic signs then developed, with headache seen 2 days later, leading to the correct diagnosis of HaNDL. Only normal findings in diffusion-weighted MRI can differentiate between ischemic etiology and other causes of this symptom complex. HaNDL should be considered in the differential diagnosis for younger, otherwise healthy persons who have acute neurologic deficits. Treatment with systemic thrombolysis in such patients generally has no adverse effects.

▶ Syndrome of transient headache with neurological deficits and cerebrospinal fluid (CSF) lymphocytosis (HaNDL) is a relatively newly identified and, therefore, unfamiliar entity. It has been classified by the International Health Service in the category of "headache attributable to nonvascular intracranial disorders." HaNDL is an uncommon disorder and is a diagnosis of exclusion, yet it is important for physicians to be aware of this entity from the clinical standpoint.

There can be rare instances of mistaking the clinical presentation of HaNDL for stroke, as presented in this case report. Clinical history of an acute-onset neurological deficit and occasional CSF pleocytosis that may occur even in stroke also makes the issue challenging for the clinician who has to make appropriate decisions to optimize the line of treatment.

The diagnostic criteria of HaNDL mention that headache may sometimes follow the neurological deficits. It is this fact that accounted for the confusion in diagnosis in this particular patient. This patient was diagnosed with an ischemic stroke in view of acute presentation of hemiparesis and aphasia without any history of headache and a normal computed tomography (CT) scan and was, therefore, thrombolyzed. This once again highlights the often discussed deficiency in the criteria for thrombolysis in ischemic stroke, which requires only a CT scan of the brain and may sometimes miss such stroke mimics.

The clinical message from this case report is that an entity such as HaNDL should also be taken into consideration in such cases. Moreover, because HaNDL has a self-limited and benign course, patients and caregivers can be reassured once the correct diagnosis is established.

When a patient presents with a transient headache followed by neurological deficits and an extensive workup reveals a normal neuroimaging, focal slowing on electroencephalogram, CSF lymphocytosis along with increased proteins, negative viral markers in CSF, and a negative vasculitic profile, one is bound to think in terms of an aseptic meningitis caused by some hitherto unknown virus or some autoimmune or vasculitic process.

In fact, this is actually the case because the pathophysiology of HaNDL syndrome is still considered to be a result of some viral infection inciting an autoimmune phenomenon against neural and vascular antigens and, subsequently, a leptomeningeal vasculitic process and migraine-like cortical spreading depression leading to headache and neurological deficits. This may be extrapolated to assume that most neurological diseases do represent a continuum and that it is a complex interplay of the basic pathomechanisms that determines the profile of a disease. Whether the cortical spreading depression in migraine is also triggered by some unknown inciting virus may be a question for researchers to probe further.

A. Panagariya, MD

LASH Syndrome: A Third Reported Case Twelve Years After the First

Rozen TD (Geisinger Health System, Wilkes-Barre, PA)

Headache 52:1433-1438, 2012

Background.—The spectrum of headaches with associated cranial autonomic symptoms ranges from trigeminal autonomic cephalalgias (TACs), including paroxysmal hemicranias (PH), to migraine with autonomic features and hemicranias continua (HC). Long-lasting autonomic symptoms with hemicranias (LASH) is an indomethacin-responsive headache variant reported in two patients that may bridge the span between PH and HC. A third patient with LASH was identified, helping to establish this as a distinct headache syndrome.

Case Report.—Woman, 36, had a history of 5 to 6 headache days per month over the previous 3 years. These represented an average of two distinct headaches that each lasted 2 to 3 days. Usually the headaches occurred every month, but sometimes she had 2 or 3 months free of headaches. The occurrence of the headaches did not correlate with any time of the month or year or menses. The current headaches differed completely from migraines she had in her teens and twenties and had not had for many years. The symptoms occurred only on her left side. Two to 8 hours before the onset of head pain she developed cranial autonomic symptoms, including eye swelling, left nasal congestion, and rhinorrhea. Eyelid ptosis, conjunctival injection, lacrimation, and eyelid twitching occurred before or during the headache. Several hours after the cranial autonomic symptoms, the headache phase began with severe (10 on a 10-point scale) sharp pain in the left retro-orbital, periorbital, and left temple areas. The peak intensity occurred in about 20 minutes. Autonomic symptoms continued and were sometimes associated with migrainous symptoms, including photophobia, osmophobia, and worsening of head pain with movement, and some lightheadedness. The patient also reported agitation and restlessness, but denied focal motor or sensory disturbances or visual symptoms. After 2 or 3 days the pain resolved, but cranial autonomic symptoms continued for several hours, gradually subsiding. Nothing appeared to provoke the attacks. Examination between headache attacks revealed mild left greater occipital nerve tenderness to palpation but no pain over the supraorbital, temple, or trochlear areas. Magnetic resonance imaging (MRI) tests with pituitary cuts suggested bilateral pituitary microadenomas versus artifact, but further imaging suggested these were pituitary cysts. Neurohormonal tests were negative. LASH was diagnosed, and the patient was given indomethacin 25 mg three times a day (TID) for 1 month. The patient's pain was minimized but not removed until the dose was increased to 50 mg TID daily. At this point the patient was free of headaches and cranial autonomic symptoms, but she had to discontinue the indomethacin because of gastrointestinal discomfort. When it was discontinued, the LASH episodes recurred at pre-indomethacin frequency. High-flow oxygen helped to reduce the head pain to mild intensity but did not ameliorate cranial autonomic symptoms. With the indomethacin, she no longer needed the high-flow oxygen. After 2 years of follow-up, the indomethacin continues to work well when the patient uses it preventively rather than just when she has attacks.

Conclusions.—LASH is the rarest of the TACs, but responds to indomethacin administration. If the diagnosis is missed and indomethacin is not given, patients suffer undue morbidity and reduced quality of life.

▶ Trigeminal autonomic cephalalgias (TACs) are an interesting group of disorders in terms of their distinct clinical picture and their response to treatment. Whereas cluster headache (CH) and short-lasting unilateral neuralgiform headache attacks with conjunctival injection and tearing belong to the non—indomethacin-responsive group, paroxysmal hemicrania (PH) and hemicrania continua (HC) are the indomethacin-responsive headaches. Long-lasting autonomic symptoms with hemicrania (LASH syndrome) are a suggested addition to this category of indomethacin-responsive TACs.

What differentiates it from PH is its longer duration and precedence of autonomic symptoms over headache and what differentiates it from HC is its episodic nature and predominance of autonomic symptoms over headache. The connecting link among the 3 entities is good response to indomethacin.

Just 3 case reports in more than a decade is actually too little evidence to suggest such a separate category; still, it is noteworthy that such cases do suggest that a continuum of distinct clinical phenotypes exists in most neurological diseases and may emerge from common pathophysiological mechanisms coming into play in graded severity.

Here I would like to mention that the onset of the episode of LASH being marked by autonomic features may quite possibly be missed and overlooked by the patient who might not be forthcoming with the history of autonomic symptoms unless specifically asked. Physicians need to be on the lookout for autonomic phenomena in association with headache and the actual temporal course of events in order to be able to distinctly classify patients into varieties of TACs.

Identification of LASH as a separate group may increase its rate of diagnosis in the community. Probably, in the absence of a categorization, many such patients are being dismissed as migraine with autonomic features or some nonspecific headache diagnosis. The therapeutic implication is that an indomethacin trial should more often be considered for such patients.

It may be interesting to watch out for the diagnosis of LASH in headache clinics and try to determine what percentage of headache cases can be given this diagnosis.

A. Panagariya, MD

Does Health Information Exchange Reduce Unnecessary Neuroimaging and Improve Quality of Headache Care in the Emergency Department?

Bailey JE, Wan JY, Mabry LM, et al (Univ of Tennessee Health Science Ctr, Memphis; et al)

J Gen Intern Med 28:176-183, 2013

Background.—Health information exchange (HIE) is advocated as an approach to reduce unnecessary testing and improve quality of emergency department (ED) care, but little evidence supports its use. Headache is a specific condition for which HIE has theoretical benefits.

Objective.—To determine whether health information exchange (HIE) reduces potentially unnecessary neuroimaging, increases adherence with evidence-based guidelines, and decreases costs in the emergency department (ED) evaluation of headache.

Design.—Longitudinal data analysis.

Subjects.—All repeat patient-visits (N = 2,102) by all 1,252 adults presenting with headache to a Memphis metropolitan area ED two or more times between August 1, 2007 and July 31, 2009.

Intervention.—Use of a regional HIE connecting the 15 major adult hospitals and two regional clinic systems by authorized ED personnel to access the patient's record during the time period in which the patient was being seen in the ED.

Main Measures.—Diagnostic neuroimaging (CT, CT angiography, MRI or MRI angiography), evidence-based guideline adherence, and total patient-visit estimated cost.

Key Results.—HIE data were accessed for 21.8% of ED patient-visits for headache. 69.8% received neuroimaging. HIE was associated with decreased odds of diagnostic neuroimaging (odds ratio [OR] 0.38, confidence interval [CI] 0.29–0.50) and increased adherence with evidence-based guidelines (OR 1.33, CI 1.02–1.73). Administrative/nursing staff HIE use (OR 0.24, CI 0.17–0.34) was also associated with decreased neuroimaging after adjustment for confounding factors. Overall HIE use was not associated with significant changes in costs.

Conclusions.—HIE is associated with decreased diagnostic imaging and increased evidence-based guideline adherence in the emergency evaluation of headache, but was not associated with improvements in overall costs. Controlled trials are needed to test whether specific HIE enhancements to increase HIE use can further reduce potentially unnecessary diagnostic imaging and improve adherence with guidelines while decreasing costs of care.

▶ With the advent of electronic communication, revolutionary changes have taken place in the field of health care, and health information exchange (HIE) is one of the exciting areas with a vast scope of improving and upgrading health services.

HIE involves reliable, secure, authorized, and interoperable electronic sharing of medical data within a health organization or regionally among aligned health care centers to improve and facilitate patient care. Electronic medical records are being used by most hospitals, and formal electronic health data exchange has actually become a reality.

This study is on HIE being used in the emergency department (ED) to reduce the number of unnecessary imaging in the patients presenting with recurrent headache, and it is important from a clinical standpoint. Emergency physicians are under stress to rule out serious causes of headache, such as subarachnoid or intracranial hemorrhage, meningitis, and cerebral venous thrombosis, and they tend to overdo neuroimaging for fear of missing an important diagnosis. Although this aggressive approach is justified in patients presenting with a first or worst-ever headache, patients with recurrent and chronic headaches who come to the ED might not be the right candidates to undergo repeated imaging. This not only increases the cost of health care but also exposes the patients to the risk of excessive radiation.

The HIE, when used for decision making for such patients, can be a useful option for the ED physician to rationalize investigations and treatment. The traditional concept of teamwork, leading to increased efficiency and accuracy, stands true in every situation, and in the era of electronic media, this is especially possible even in the ED. Even when the experts are not immediately present, their expert opinion is just a few clicks away.

In the years to come, technology is surely bound to expand the scope of medical care much more than is conceivable presently. Inevitably a majority of physicians' diagnostic and presentation work could be replaced with smart hardware and software, and health care will become better, more consistent, and more scientific across physicians all over the world.

A. Panagariya, MD

Dry Eyes and Migraines: Is There Really a Correlation?

Koktekir BE, Celik G, Karalezli A, et al (Selçuk Univ, Konya, Turkey; Baskent Univ, Ankara, Turkey)

Cornea 31:1414-1416, 2012

Purpose.—The purpose of this study was to evaluate the tear film functions and clinical symptoms of patients with migraines.

Methods.—This observational comparative study consisted of 33 migraine (26 women and 7 men) patients referred from neurology clinics and 33 (22 women and 11 men) control subjects referred from ophthalmology outpatient clinics. The control subjects had neither systemic nor ocular disease nor any type of headache. All 66 patients underwent a complete ophthalmic examination and diagnostic tests for dry eye, including tear break-up time, Schirmer test with topical anesthesia, lissamine green staining, and an ocular surface disease score. Patients with migraine were classified as migraine with an aura, migraine without an aura, and basilar migraine; a pain score from 1 to 4 was determined for each patient, based on the American Headache Society's Migraine Disability Assessment Test.

Results.—Of the 33 patients who participated in the migraine group, 17 (51%) suffered from migraine with aura, 11 (33%) suffered from migraine without aura, and 5 (15%) suffered from basilar migraine. Significant differences in dry eye scores were found between the patients with migraine and the control subjects. In the migraine group, the mean tear break-up time was 7.75 ± 2.37 seconds, whereas in the control group it was 9.15 ± 1.93 seconds. For the Schirmer test, the migraine group had a mean value of 12.09 ± 4.95 mm/5 minutes, whereas the control group had a mean value of 14.90 ± 4.26 mm/5 minutes. Testing with lissamine green staining resulted in a mean value of 1.00 ± 0.16 in the migraine group and 0.30 ± 0.46 in the control group. In the migraine group, the mean for the ocular surface disease index scoring was 36.27 ± 17.54. In the control group, it was 28.42 ± 9.0. A significant difference ($P < 0.05$) was found in the dry eye syndrome testing results between the 2 groups in this study.

Conclusions.—An increased frequency of dry eye disease was found to occur in patients with migraine, which might suggest that migraine headaches are related to dry eye disease. Some migraine attacks may be aggravated in the presence of dry eye syndrome.

▶ Migraine treatment is not just about prescribing medications, but it is also a great deal about making the patient aware about its pathogenesis, the importance of identification of triggers and consciously avoiding them. It is always important to impress on patients the significance of general lifestyle measures on each visit to the clinic if fruitful outcome of treatment is expected. Preventing dry eyes also may be an important advice on the prescription of migraine medication.

We do always counsel our patients suffering from migraine to avoid dehydration, protect themselves from bright sunlight, avoid missing meals, have a regular sleep schedule, regular bowel habits, moderate physical activity, avoid stress, practice deep breathing exercises, and to avoid their own triggers.

This article interests me because of the simple practice implication it holds when treating patients with migraine. Dry eyes are not a classical migraine trigger and not routinely enquired about in migraineurs. It is probably an association that can be found in many patients with headache. Prolonged use of computer screens, cell phone screens, and prolonged reading and writing also cause eye fatigue and dryness and may precipitate a migraine headache.

Objective assessment of association of dry eyes with migraine and whether dry eyes are part of the migraine syndrome or occur only when migraine is associated with some connective tissue or inflammatory disorder needs to be evaluated further in structured studies. In the meantime, however, a routine enquiry about dry eyes and advising patients to adequately treat it may, in fact, be a simple and good idea to reduce the discomfort and may possibly prevent migraine attacks.

A. Panagariya, MD

Pediatric Posttraumatic Headache: Two Cases Using Steroids as Abortive Therapy

Bramley H, Melinosky C, Silvis M, et al (Penn State Milton S. Hershey Med Ctr, PA; Univ of Maryland Med Ctr, Baltimore)

Pediatr Emerg Care 28:1081-1084, 2012

Pediatric traumatic brain injury is a common occurrence, and even an ostensibly mild injury may result in disabling posttraumatic headaches. The headache may result in a number of subsequent unremitting symptoms refractory to many standard headache therapies. Current treatment recommendations are sparse because there is a lack of clinical trial data recommendations and outcomes. From these 2 cases, we report the effectiveness of steroids for severe posttraumatic headache, along with recommended treatment strategies for acute pain management and prevention.

▶ Posttraumatic headaches are quite commonly encountered in neurology practice and are an important health problem. They are more often associated with minor head injuries but can occur as a consequence of moderate and severe head injuries as well. The International Classification of Headache Disorders II classifies posttraumatic headaches into acute (that resolve within 3 months) and chronic (persistent beyond 3 months) categories.

In fact, the post–head concussion symptomatology does not include just headaches but a variety of subtle changes in the form of behavioral problems, difficulties with memory and concentration, language and verbal fluency, decreased working capacity, balance problems, and sleep disturbances. Some of the postulated reasons of head and neck pain after trauma are musculoskeletal pain, pain in scalp scars, occipital or supraorbital neuralgia, precipitation of migraine in predisposed individuals, and rarely serious intracranial complications. But certainly the underlying mechanisms are far more diffuse and complicated to account for the varied and multiple symptoms occurring after concussion, which are yet to be elucidated.

Patients are very often anxious and apprehensive about the headaches appearing after a head injury. A normal brain imaging does rule out any significant structural brain lesion or injury, which allays their worries to some extent, but the persistent headache is quite bothersome. Other investigations, such as cerebrospinal fluid studies, electroencephalograms, evoked potentials, and neuropsychological testing, may or may not show abnormalities. Another challenge is to distinguish malingerers who may be targeting a better compensation.

The treatment approach for the posttraumatic headache group has to be individualized according to the headache characteristics and the associated features. Most of the time these patients respond to nonsteroidal anti-inflammatory agents and reassurance, but those who develop a chronic headache need to be treated with antidepressants.

The use of steroids in headache is always a debatable issue. Steroids probably act by reducing perivascular neurogenic inflammation and also modulating the peripheral and central sensitization processes leading to chronicity of headaches. Steroid use as a rescue medication in acute and chronic severe headaches not responding to analgesics may help in breaking the vicious pain cycle by interfering with the inflammatory and sensitization mechanisms and may be justified for short-term use in problematic headaches.

This article has reported 2 pediatric posttraumatic headache cases that did benefit substantially with a short course of steroids. It is a useful documentation for practicing clinicians, which may increase confidence regarding short-term steroid use in appropriately selected cases.

Our own experience with traumatic frontotemporal hemorrhagic and nonhemorrhagic contusions causing headache favors the use of tapering dexamethasone therapy for 10 days. Not only does it reduce long-term morbidity, but it also shortens recovery time.

A. Panagariya, MD

3 Infectious Diseases of the Nervous System

Ultrasound study shows nerve atrophy in post herpetic neuralgia
Renna R, Erra C, Almeida V, et al (Università Cattolica del Sacro Cuore, Rome, Italy; Don Carlo Gnocchi Onlus, Milan, Italy; Hosp de Santa Maria - CHLN, Lisbon, Portugal)
Clin Neurol Neurosurg 114:1343-1344, 2012

Background.—Herpes zoster (HZ) results when the latent varicella zoster virus (VZV) in the dorsal root of trigeminal ganglia is reactivated. HZ is seen most often in persons over age 50 years and usually appears as a unilateral dermatomal vesicular rash and severe pain. Usually the painful rash occurs along the thoracic nerves or ophthalmic division of the trigeminal nerve distribution. About 25% of people who have had chickenpox suffer this reactivation. A common and debilitating accompaniment to HZ is post-herpetic neuralgia (PHN), the term for pain persisting more than 3 months after the rash has resolved. The diagnosis of HZ and PHN is made clinically based on the characteristic rash and other symptoms. An ultrasonographic study was done of a patient with gangionopathy caused by VZV reactivation that was followed by PHN.

> *Case Report.*—Man, 69, had neuropathic pain of 12 months' duration in the right sole that began after HZ rash on the lateral surface of his right leg resolved. He did not receive antiviral agents to manage the acute phase of HZ. Nerve conduction studies found reduced sural and superficial peroneal nerve sensory action potential amplitudes (SAP) on the right side but normal ones on the left side. Sensory production velocities (SCV) were normal bilaterally. Clinical and neurophysiologic findings overall were consistent with L5-S1 right gangionopathy caused by the reactivation of VZV. An ultrasound (US) study of the sural and superficial peroneal nerves was done, revealing the cross-sectional areas of the right sural and superficial peroneal nerves were significantly smaller than those on the left.

Conclusions.—Studies of autopsy tissue from patients with and without PHN have found that patients with PHN have spinal cord dorsal horn degeneration. The virus or inflammation may spread from the sensory ganglion to the roots or peripheral nerves. Epidermal innervation is lost, and there may be reduced or missing SAP in nerves originating from roots corresponding to the involved dermatomes. Apparently the sensory fibers are damaged at ganglionic or postganglionic levels. Even in patients with normal responses, amplitudes are markedly reduced compared to the uninvolved contralateral nerve. US allows the assessment of nerve disease and offers the advantages of low cost, noninvasive nature, and good acceptance by patients. It may be able to show abnormalities that are characteristic of PHN.

▶ The use of ultrasound scaning to image peripheral nerve and muscle has emerged as a diagnostic subspecialty field. Continuous improvements in technology have increased our ability to study peripheral nerves and muscles noninvasively. While neuromuscular ultrasound scan has been used primarily to diagnose conditions like carpal tunnel syndrome, it may also be useful in identifying nerve tumors, traumatic injuries to nerves, inflammatory neuropathies, and to guide both diagnostic and therapeutic procedures (such as injections of botulinum toxin). The procedure may complement findings from other electrodiagnostic studies such as measurement of nerve conduction studies (NCS) and electromyography (EMG). This report describes findings in a patient with postherpetic neuralgia that developed after herpes zoster infection in the L5 dermatome of his right leg. The NCS and EMG findings were nonrevealing, but ultrasound imaging of the right superficial peroneal and sural nerves showed atrophy compared with normal nerve size on the left side, suggesting a sensory ganglionopathy. This apparently is the first study to report these changes in postherpetic neuralgia. Whether the future use of neuromuscular ultrasound scan will be helpful in identifying involvement of individual nerves remains to be seen.

R. Schwendimann, MD

Case 1-2013: A 63-Year-Old Man with Paresthesias and Difficulty Swallowing

Greer DM, Robbins GK, Lijewski V, et al (Yale Univ School of Medicine, New Haven, CT; Massachusetts General Hosp, Boston; Massachusetts Dept of Public Health, Boston)

N Engl J Med 368:172-180, 2013

Background.—Determining the diagnosis is particularly challenging with fairly rare disorders. For patients with a myriad of symptoms, various disorders must be considered, including bacterial toxins such as tetanus, diphtheria, and botulism; substance issues such as alcohol withdrawal and drug reactions; and infections.

Case Report.—Man, 63, was admitted to the hospital with paresthesias, difficulty drinking liquids, and anxiety. Over the previous 4 days he progressively developed aching in his elbows, decreased appetite, difficulty forming words, mild light-headedness, gagging sensation and difficulty breathing when given water to drink, increasing anxiety, intermittent decreased fluency in speech, and pruritus at the nape of his neck. He was very anxious, hyperventilating, had dry mucous membranes, and could not drink water, although he could eat solids, when admitted. He was given lorazepam and intravenous fluids, which reduced the anxiety. His history included hypertension, chronic ptosis of the right eyelid, and a tick bite 6 months previously, for which he received doxycycline. He also took hydrochlorothiazide and low-dose aspirin daily and had received influenza and tetanus vaccinations within the previous year. He reported no animal bites, but bats were seen in his home and in a barn where he had worked. He and his wife were awakened by a bat in their bedroom one night.

His blood pressure was 171/80 mm Hg, pulse 86 beats per minute, temperature 36.4°C, respiratory rate 16 breaths per minute, and oxygen saturation of 98% on ambient air. In addition to his ptosis, he had mild facial twitching, postural hand tremors, dysmetria on finger-nose-finger and heel-shin testing, no truncal ataxia, symmetrically hyperactive deep tendon reflexes, flexor plantar reflexes, and mild difficulty tandem walking. His speech was rushed but fluent, with occasional slurred words and pauses to search for words. Magnetic resonance imaging (MRI) of the brain without contrast and MR angiography (MRA) of the head and neck found abnormal signal hyperintensity scattered in the periventricular and subcortical white matter on T_2-weighted and fluid-attenuated inversion recovery (FLAIR) imaging. The patient became increasingly anxious and suffered discomfort from ambient noises and severe anxiety related to swallowing liquids. The second day his temperature rose to 38.2°C and he became tremulous, agitated, oriented but confused, and could not relate a clear history. On lumbar puncture, the opening pressure was 33 cm H_2O, but cerebrospinal fluid (CSF) studies were normal. The patient then developed cyanosis, with a systolic blood pressure of 240 mm Hg, pulse 160 beats per minute, respiratory rate 40 breaths per minute, and oxygen saturation 40% to 49%. He had supraventricular tachycardia at 150 beats per minute, but his pulse suddenly fell to 60 then rose again to 150 beats per minute. He was given metoprolol and furosemide intravenously, followed by diltiazem. Signs indicative of pulmonary edema were found on a chest radiograph. The patient was intubated and admitted to the cardiac care unit, where an electroencephalogram (EEG) showed moderate generalized background slowing without focal features, epileptiform activity, or correlation to arm tremors and twitching.

The diagnostic process identified rabies as the probable cause of the patient's symptoms, which formed a classic rabies prodrome of malaise and irritability, paresthesia, pain, and pruritus. Imaging findings were consistent with the diagnosis of rabies. The abnormal signal enhancement indicated a poor prognosis, occurring late in the disease course. The patient appeared to be in the encephalitis phase of rabies and exhibited classic autonomic dysfunction. Death typically follows within 5 days of developing acute neurologic signs. Once rabies encephalitis has begun, no treatment has proved efficacious and the death rate is nearly 100%. Standard care is palliation, but a more aggressive treatment approach was chosen, called the Milwaukee protocol. The patient was intubated and sedated to minimize brain injury and allow his immune response to eradicate the virus. After 27 days of hospitalization, CSF showed no neutralizing antibodies, and interferon was given to stimulate antibody development. After 3 days, the patient had fixed pupils, progressive multisystem organ failure, and a flat EEG when not sedated. Care was withdrawn and the patient died after 30 days in the hospital. The autopsy was consistent with a diagnosis of rabies. Several care workers and close contacts of the patient underwent postexposure prophylaxis.

Conclusions.—The Milwaukee protocol was used successfully for a 15-year-old girl, but is not supported by the current evidence. It should only be considered for patients early in the disease course who are otherwise healthy. Even then, patients and family members should be cautioned it is unlikely to be successful.

▶ This article is from an excellent clinical pathologic conference from Massachusetts General Hospital published in the *New England Journal of Medicine*. If you read the case from beginning to end instead of looking at the final diagnosis first, you will be able to use all of the clinical information to arrive at the diagnosis. This is a case of rabies encephalitis, which is rare but should still be considered in the differential of patients with clinical evidence of encephalitis. This article is an excellent review of the presenting symptoms of rabies and diagnostic studies that may lead to the diagnosis. It mentions that treatment for rabies is highly efficacious, although once rabies encephalitis has begun, the mortality rate approaches 100%. The article reviews the pathologic findings with photomicrographs of the pathognomonic Negri body.

This article made me recall seeing a rabid dog that was finally shot down in the streets of a small Arkansas town, much like Old Yeller was shot down in the Walt Disney film of the same name. The patient's exposure to the rabies virus was through a rabid bat. This brought back memories of how the dog in Stephen King's horror story *Cujo* became rabid after being bitten by a bat. Rabies is a very scary infection, and this study helps us remember that the virus still lives in bats, raccoons, foxes, and skunks and can still be transmitted to humans.

R. Schwendimann, MD

Varicella-zoster virus encephalitis and vasculopathy in a patient treated with fingolimod

Ratchford JN, Costello K, Reich DS, et al (Johns Hopkins Univ School of Medicine, Baltimore, MD)
Neurology 79:2002-2004, 2012

Background.—Fingolimod, given to treat multiple sclerosis (MS), has the effect of diminishing the egress of lymphocytes from lymph nodes and can reduce the number of circulating lymphocytes by 70%. This immunosuppression can open the door for infection, as shown in this patient who developed herpes zoster.

Case Report.—Man, 50, with MS was admitted to the hospital with a seizure and coma after taking fingolimod for 4 months. Although clinically stable, the patient was essentially wheelchair-bound with relatively preserved upper extremity function. A brain magnetic resonance imaging (MRI) scan done before beginning fingolimod showed the MS was stable. The patient had chickenpox in his history but had not received the shingles vaccine. Herpes zoster developed 3 months after he began taking fingolimod. The patient started on oral valacyclovir 4 days after he noticed the rash, then suffered a generalized seizure and was hospitalized. He was deeply comatose and required intubation. Significant laboratory results included an absolute lymphocyte count of 190 cells/μL and a low-level positive cerebrospinal fluid (CSF) JC virus PCR test result. There was no clinical or radiographic evidence of progressive multifocal leukoencephalopathy (PML), and the acute onset of disease and presence of erythrocytes in the CSF argued against PML.

The patient was diagnosed with varicella zoster virus (VZV) encephalitis, seizures, and a brainstem infarct believed to be caused by VZV vasculitis. Treatment consisted of levetiracetam, intravenous acyclovir for 21 days, and prednisone 1 mg/kg daily for 7 days for the vasculitis. Over the course of a complex hospitalization the patient slowly improved. After 1 month he was awake and oriented with significant psychomotor slowing and persistent quadriparesis. He was moved to a rehabilitation facility to continue ventilator weaning.

Conclusions.—Generally months elapse between the rash and the onset of neurologic symptoms in VZV vasculitis, but these symptoms can occur simultaneously, as shown in this case. Neurologists should be aware that patients receiving fingolimod or other immunosuppressant agents can develop serious herpesvirus family infections. Patients should be instructed to contact the clinician urgently if any new rashes or neurologic symptoms develop. Antiviral treatment is begun at the first sign of herpes zoster in patients taking fingolimod; parenteral antiviral agents may also be needed. All patients should have VZV immunization before beginning fingolimod, but whether the vaccine decreases the risk of reactivating VZV in fingolimod-treated patients is not known. If the vaccine is given, it should be scheduled at least 1 month before beginning fingolimod.

▶ Fingolimod is one of the new immune-modulating drugs available for the treatment of multiple sclerosis (MS). Unlike most of the other drugs indicated for the treatment of MS, fingolimod is an oral formulation and does not require delivery by subcutaneous, intramuscular, or intravenous injection. This drug effectively decreases egress of lymphocytes from lymph nodes, reducing the number of circulating lymphocytes by 70%. The patient described in this case had herpes zoster. Valacyclovir was given for treatment, but within days the patient had a generalized seizure and became comatose. Cerebrospinal fluid examination results were polymerase chain reaction–positive for varicella-zoster virus (VZV). There was evidence of vasculopathy that occurred in association with the encephalitis. The patient survived but remained significantly impaired neurologically. There were reports of increased incidence of herpes zoster infections in several of the clinical trials assessing the effectiveness of fingolimod, but the incidence was not statistically significant. The patient had not received vaccination against herpes zoster before starting treatment with fingolimod, although there was a history of chickenpox. Neurologists should be aware of the possibility of severe herpesvirus family infections and should consider vaccination against the VZV before treatment with fingolimod.

R. Schwendimann, MD

Steroids and Childhood Encephalitis

Esposito S, Picciolli I, Semino M, et al (Università degli Studi di Milano, Italy)
Pediatr Infect Dis J 31:759-760, 2012

Background.—Glucocorticosteroids (GS) offer both anti-inflammatory and immunosuppressive effects, making them a common choice for pediatric clinical conditions believed to have disease signs and symptoms caused by inflammation and/or autoimmunity. However, GS have not been proved to be efficacious through controlled trials, and the risk for adverse events associated with high-dose or prolonged GS administration has not been well studied. GS are given for encephalitis, which covers a wide range of clinical conditions with varying etiology, pathogenesis, clinical presentation, and spontaneous evolution. The impact of GS treatment in children with acute infectious encephalitis (AIE) and acute disseminated encephalomyelitis (ADEM) was noted.

AIE.—Viruses are the most common cause of central nervous system (CNS) involvement in AIE. Vaccination programs have significantly reduced many viral diseases, including measles, mumps, and rubella in industrialized nations, but herpes simplex virus (HSV) and virus varicella zoster (VZV) remain the most common causes of AIE. The available data are too limited to officially recommend the systematic use of GS to treat HSV AIE. However, GS may be useful when antiviral therapy does not appear to control the clinical symptoms and CNS damage is clearly increasing. AIE associated with VZV reactivation, especially if nuclear magnetic resonance imaging (MRI) suggests a stroke secondary to large vessel vasculitis, may also respond to GS. The suggested dose is 60 to 80 mg of prednisolone (2 mg/kg/day for children) once a day for 3 to 5 days. GS appear ineffective against Japanese encephalitis virus infection.

ADEM.—ADEM, which affects mainly children, is a demyelinating disease of the CNS, with clinical features and history that complicate the diagnosis. Recurrent ADEM tends to occur days or weeks after an infection or vaccination. GS are useful for children with ADEM. Methylprednisolone 10 to 20 mg/kg/day intravenously for 3 to 5 days is followed by a tapered course of oral prednisolone. A few children with ADEM appear to be refractory to steroid therapy, requiring the addition of immunoglobulins or the use of plasmapheresis. The possible relationship between ADEM and multiple sclerosis further supports the use of GS, even with the lack of sufficient evidence to conclusively link the two.

Conclusions.—Although the systematic use of GS for all children with HSV AIE cannot be supported at the present time, GS is proving useful for the treatment of some children with HSV and VZV AIE. The use of GS is recommended for children with ADEM.

▶ The use of steroids in meningitis and encephalitis has been a topic of controversy for many years. This very brief article discusses the use of steroids in the treatment of acute infectious encephalitis and acute disseminated encephalomyelitis in childhood. The article points out that herpes simplex virus (HSV) is the most common type of encephalitis encountered, particularly with effective vaccines against rubella, measles, and mumps available. There is inconclusive evidence that the use of steroids is beneficial in HSV encephalitis or any of the other viral encephalitides. In HSV, use of steroids is indicated only when there has been no response to treatment with antiviral agents, such as acyclovir. Acute disseminated encephalomyelitis, on the other hand, is a childhood inflammatory process that appears to be responsive to the use of steroids acutely. My suspicion is that steroids will continue to be used for treating both of these conditions, particularly if the patient seems to be doing poorly.

R. Schwendimann, MD

Iatrogenic prion diseases in humans: an update

Barrenetxea G (Universidad del País Vasco/Euskal Herriko Unibertsitatea, Bilbao, Spain)

Eur J Obstet Gynecol Reprod Biol 165:165-169, 2012

Although Creutzfeldt–Jakob disease (CJD) was first identified in 1920, prevention of transmission raised particular concern all over the world when a new variant of the disease was first described in 1996. There is good evidence of iatrogenic transmission of this new variant among human beings through blood, blood components, tissues and growth hormone. Furthermore, four cases of iatrogenic transmission of CJD through fertility treatment with human pituitary-derived gonadotrophins have been reported.

It is important to distinguish the categories of infectivity and categories of risk, which require consideration not only of the level of infectivity of a given tissue or fluid, but also the amount of tissue/fluid to which a person is exposed, the duration of exposure and the route by which infection is transmitted.

The potential presence and infectivity of prion proteins in human urinary gonadotrophin preparations is a matter of debate. Differences in the sensitivity of bioassay methods are of paramount importance when considering the infectivity of a tissue. Some new methods might detect small amounts of agent in some tissues currently thought to be free of infectivity.

No cases of human prion disease due to the use of urinary gonadotrophins have been recognized to date. However, the detection of prions in the urine of experimental animals and in some urine-based preparations, and the young age of fertility drug recipients, require the application of the precautionary principle to urinary preparations.

▶ It is hard for me to believe that it has been 25 years since bovine spongiform encephalopathy in cows was first identified. This, of course, led to the almost worldwide scare that eating beef from these infected cattle was a risk for developing a spongiform encephalopathy. Ten years later the first descriptions of variant Creutzfeldt-Jakob disease (CJD) were reported in humans. Earlier, classic CJD was known to be transmitted by various routes that affected patients and medical professionals alike. There were reports of transmission from contaminated surgical instruments, contaminated human growth hormone, and corneal and dural grafts. We have had instances where neurosurgeons have been quite reluctant to perform needed surgery or biopsies on patients suspected of having CJD.

Because safety is a major concern in hospitals today, it is important to be aware of the other ways these prion diseases can be transmitted iatrogenically. These concerns have led to development of guidelines for handling surgical instruments, pathologic specimens, and other tissues as well as handling bodies of those who have died with the disease. The laboratory markers of this disease are not always present, and tissue diagnosis is still sometimes needed. This article discusses other possible ways that variant CJD can be transmitted, including by way of blood, blood components, tissues, and growth hormones.

R. Schwendimann, MD

Seizures and encephalitis: Clinical features, management, and potential pathophysiologic mechanisms
Michael BD, Solomon T (Univ of Liverpool, United Kingdom)
Epilepsia 53:63-71, 2012

Encephalitis is an inflammation and swelling of the brain, which is often caused by a viral infection; it is an important cause of acute symptomatic seizures as well as subsequent epilepsy. Herein we describe the definition, epidemiology, and etiology of encephalitis as a cause of seizures. We then focus on encephalitis due to herpes simplex virus (the most common sporadic viral cause of encephalitis) and Japanese encephalitis virus (the most common epidemic viral cause). We also discuss the evidence for seizures occurring in the context of antibody-associated encephalitis, an increasingly important condition. Finally, we describe the acute and longer-term management of encephalitis-related seizures and their potential pathophysiologic mechanisms, concluding with the emerging etiologic role of human herpesvirus 6.

▶ This is a review article discussing the association of seizures with various types of encephalitis. It includes information about the most common type of infectious encephalitis, Herpes simplex, as well as other viral encephalitis and more recently described autoimmune encephalitis. I was interested in the article because it is a nice review of the likelihood of seizures in various types of encephalitis. It also caused me to recall the importance of electroencephalography (EEG) in the diagnosis of herpes simplex encephalitis. Prior to magnetic resonance imaging of the brain that may show patterns strongly suggestive of herpes simplex encephalitis, the EEG was an important diagnostic tool. The presence of periodic epileptiform discharges, although not specific, was thought to be very indicative of the type of focal inflammatory process produced by the herpes simplex virus. Even today, the EEG may add diagnostic evidence of this inflammation. The presence of these discharges along with the clinical picture might influence decisions to start antiviral agents such as acyclovir earlier rather than later in the course of the disease. In addition, continuous EEG monitoring with video recording is a procedure that may also be helpful in identifying those patients with encephalitis who become poorly responsive but show no outward signs of having convulsive seizures. Continuous EEG monitoring may show patterns indicative of nonconvulsive status epilepticus and help change the management of this clinical problem.

R. Schwendimann, MD

The Index Case for the Fungal Meningitis Outbreak in the United States
Pettit AC, Kropski JA, Castilho JL, et al (Vanderbilt Univ School of Medicine, Nashville, TN)
N Engl J Med 367:2119-2125, 2012

Persistent neutrophilic meningitis presents a diagnostic challenge, because the differential diagnosis is broad and includes atypical infectious causes.

We describe a case of persistent neutrophilic meningitis due to *Aspergillus fumigatus* in an immunocompetent man who had no evidence of sinopulmonary or cutaneous disease. An epidural glucocorticoid injection was identified as a potential route of entry for this organism into the central nervous system, and the case was reported to the state health department.

▶ One of the biggest medical stories of 2012 involved the cases of fungal meningitis that were proved to be related to contaminated steroids produced by a compounding pharmacy in New England. This report published in the *New England Journal of Medicine* was the index case that led to the identification of the contaminated drugs, most of which were being injected into the epidural space for the management of chronic back pain. The patient's clinical course described in this case report was complicated, and the infection that he acquired led to his ultimate demise. The case itself is interesting as far as the initial management and continued diagnostic studies that led to the identification of the fungus are concerned. Fortunately, autopsy findings revealed leptomeningeal of the spinal cord close to the sites where epidural steroids had been given. This led the physicians involved to report their findings to the state health department.

There were numerous other reports of fungal meningitis subsequently reported to the Centers for Disease Control and Prevention (CDC). All of these events led to the identification of contaminated lots of methylprednisolone from the New England Compounding Center. Cases of fungal meningitis were subsequently reported in 18 states, and as of late October 2012 there were 323 cases of meningitis reported to the CDC along with 24 deaths. All of this led to national surveillance and further efforts to identify facilities that may have supplies of the contaminated drug. The whole story is fascinating and unfolds like a good mystery novel.

This case and others like it will likely lead to increased oversight of the estimated 7500 compounding pharmacies in the United States. It further helps to point out that better protection for our patients is needed. We need to know what medications, supplements, herbals, and so forth our patients may be taking on their own. We need to know more about how these items are produced and the deleterious effects they may have.

R. Schwendimann, MD

Nationwide survey of patients in Japan with Bickerstaff brainstem encephalitis: epidemiological and clinical characteristics

Koga M, Kusunoki S, Kaida K, et al (Yamaguchi Univ Graduate School of Medicine, Japan; Kinki Univ School of Medicine, Osaka, Japan; Natl Defense Med College, Tokorozawa, Saitama, Japan; et al)

J Neurol Neurosurg Psychiatry 83:1210-1215, 2012

Background.—Information regarding the epidemiological background of Bickerstaff brainstem encephalitis (BBE) is limited.

Methods.—We conducted a nationwide survey of BBE in the Japanese population in two steps: the first aimed to identify patients with brainstem encephalitis for the specified 3 year period and the second to evaluate whether the clinical picture met our diagnostic criteria for BBE.

Results.—The number of patients with brainstem encephalitis was estimated as 704 (95% CI 478 to 930) over the 3 years. The annual onset of BBE was roughly estimated as 100 cases, which accounted for 43% of brainstem encephalitis. BBE was slightly male predominant and often young onset. Among brainstem encephalitis patients, BBE was characterised by antecedent infectious symptoms, oropharyngeal palsy and sensory disturbance at the distal extremities with absent or decreased tendon reflexes, in addition to a triad of symptoms (external ophthalmoplegia, ataxia and impaired level of consciousness) and shorter duration to the peak, with good outcome. Anti-GQ1b antibodies were present in 75% of cases. Several BBE patients with atypical clinical features or without anti-GQ1b antibodies were also identified. These cases often had marked CSF pleocytosis, abnormal brain MRI findings and a longer duration to peak symptoms, sometimes with considerable residual deficits.

Conclusions.—BBE is a rare disorder but accounts for a major proportion of brainstem encephalitis. BBE consists of typical and atypical cases. Typical BBE has similar neurological and serological features to Fisher syndrome and shows good recovery whereas atypical BBE is characterised by delayed recovery, negative anti-GQ1b antibodies, and abnormal CSF and brain MRI findings with other possible pathogeneses.

▶ Bickerstaff brainstem encephalitis (BBE) is a condition that has been heard about more often over the past 10 years or so. The clinical picture for this encephalitis was described initially in 1951 and was thought to be related to a viral illness that produced a clinical picture resembling encephalitis, often associated with ophthalmoparesis and ataxia. Bickerstaff described a monophasic type of illness and reported that cases had an excellent prognosis for acute recovery. The disease is much more common in Japan, and this article reports on 704 diagnosed cases of BBE. In nearly 40 years of neurologic practice, I have seen only 1 patient who appeared to have BBE. Nevertheless, it is important to recognize the clinical picture and the similarity to another uncommon neurologic condition, Miller Fisher syndrome (MFS). There is definitely an overlap between these 2 clinical entities as both may be associated with positive anti-GQ1b antibodies in the serum of affected patients. To date there is no evidence of an effective treatment for either of these conditions, although various treatments, such as intravenous immunoglobulin (IVIG) and plasma exchange, have been tried.

Part of my interest in BBE comes from a medical–legal case that alleged malpractice when a patient who possibly had BBE or MFS was not treated with IVIG. This article is a very nice review of the diagnostic criteria and clinical features of this condition that is rare in Western countries.

R. Schwendimann, MD

Locally acquired West Nile encephalitis

Martindale JL, Macias Konstantopoulos WL (Harvard-Affiliated Emergency Medicine Residency, Boston, MA; Massachusetts General Hosp, Boston)

J Emerg Med 43:e435-e438, 2012

Background.—West Nile virus (WNV) has spread rapidly across the United States since 1999, causing epidemics of neurologic illnesses including meningitis, encephalitis, and acute flaccid paralysis. West Nile encephalitis can be fatal; recovery can be incomplete; and constitutional and neurological symptoms can persist for months to years.

Objectives.—To raise awareness of an important epidemiologic cause of febrile illness with neurologic involvement in the United States.

Case Report.—We report the case of a 46-year-old woman who presented with fever, altered mental status, and maculopapular rash, who was diagnosed with locally acquired WNV encephalitis.

Conclusion.—Infection with WNV should be considered in patients presenting to emergency departments with fever and neurologic symptoms. Recommended evaluation includes serologic testing of cerebrospinal fluid and serum.

▶ I selected this case report because it points out that West Nile virus (WNV) infection can be quite devastating in a small number of patients. Most commonly, WNV causes a self-limited febrile illness from which patients recover completely. There are cases, as in the one presented, of severe central nervous system involvement. A high index of suspicion of WNV will lead to proper laboratory studies that may confirm the diagnosis. WNV can infect neurons in the cerebral cortex, basal ganglia, and spinal cord. Signs and symptoms of meningitis and encephalitis commonly occur. Flaccid paralysis secondary to involvement of anterior horn cells in the spinal cord is not uncommon. In our hospital this season, we evaluated patients presenting with paraplegia, monoparesis of a lower limb, and an acute Parkinson type of picture. There has definitely been a resurgence of WNV infections in our area of the country where mild winters do not help eliminate the mosquito population. Although no effective treatments are available, accurate diagnosis can be helpful in the management of the disease and in alerting communities that the virus is present, and measures to prevent its spread may be necessary.

R. Schwendimann, MD

Advances in treatment of bacterial meningitis

van de Beek D, Brouwer MC, Thwaites GE, et al (Univ of Amsterdam, Netherlands; Kings College London, UK; et al)

Lancet 380:1693-1702, 2012

Bacterial meningitis kills or maims about a fifth of people with the disease. Early antibiotic treatment improves outcomes, but the effectiveness of widely available antibiotics is threatened by global emergence of multidrug-resistant bacteria. New antibiotics, such as fluoroquinolones, could have a role in these circumstances, but clinical data to support this notion are scarce. Additionally, whether or not adjunctive anti-inflammatory therapies (eg, dexamethasone) improve outcomes in patients with bacterial meningitis remains controversial; in resource-poor regions, where the disease burden is highest, dexamethasone is ineffective. Other adjunctive therapeutic strategies, such as glycerol, paracetamol, and induction of hypothermia, are being tested further. Therefore, bacterial meningitis is a substantial and evolving therapeutic challenge. We review this challenge, with a focus on strategies to optimise antibiotic efficacy in view of increasingly drug-resistant bacteria, and discuss the role of current and future adjunctive therapies.

► This is the second of 3 articles about bacterial meningitis published in *Lancet Neurology*. This article discusses the most common types of bacterial meningitis as well as current treatments and antibacterial drugs that may be effective in the management of these bacterial infections. The article reviews newer antibiotics available for treatment of meningitis along with recommendations for their use. Selection of appropriate antibiotic therapies is becoming more difficult because of drug-resistant bacterial strains. This article discusses the best therapies for the most common types of bacterial meningitis. Much of the information is presented in the form of tables that are helpful for quick reference.

The use of dexamethasone in treating acute bacterial meningitis remains a controversy. There is a review of recent studies regarding recommendations for the use of dexamethasone in the treatment of acute bacterial meningitis. The use of dexamethasone appears to be efficacious only in high-income countries. The article includes a review of other adjunctive therapies such as glycerol and hypothermia.

A third article appeared in *Lancet* on November 10, 2012, on the effect of vaccines on bacterial meningitis worldwide that I did not choose to feature but would recommend highly as well.

R. Schwendimann, MD

Acute meningitis prognosis using cerebrospinal fluid interleukin-6 levels

Vázquez JA, Adducci MdC, Coll C, et al (Hospital Italiano de San Justo, Buenos Aires, Argentina; Univ of Buenos Aires, Argentina; et al)

J Emerg Med 43:322-327, 2012

Background.—Improved diagnostic tests would aid in diagnosing and treating community-acquired meningitis.

Objective.—To analyze the diagnostic value of interleukin-6 (IL-6) in the cerebrospinal fluid (CSF) of patients presenting with symptoms of acute meningitis.

Material and Methods.—In a 6-month prospective, observational, cross-sectional emergency department (ED) study, serum and CSF samples were obtained from all patients with a headache and fever in whom the physician suspected meningitis. Patients were excluded if computed tomography findings contraindicated a lumbar puncture, if they had bleeding disorders, or if their serum indicated bleeding. IL-6 levels were measured and compared in patients with (Group A) and without (Group B) bacterial meningitis.

Results.—Samples were obtained from 53 patients, of whom 40 were ultimately found to have meningitis. These 40 patients averaged 49.6 ± 21.9 years, with number of men 18 (45%), hospitalizations 21 (52%), mortality 3 (.07%), and IL-6 average rating 491 (median: 14.5; range 0000–6000). Findings in the two groups were: Group A (with meningitis): n = 13, average IL-6 level: 1495 (median: 604; 25/75 percentiles: 232.5–2030; 95% confidence interval [CI] 371.7–2618.6; range 64–6000). Group B (with aseptic meningitis): n = 27, average IL-6 level: 7.34 (median: 5; 25/75 percentiles: 0.0/15.1; 95% CI 3.94–10.73; range 0–23.6). Mann-Whitney rank sum test: $p < 0.0001$.

Conclusions.—In patients with acute bacterial meningitis, CSF cytokine concentrations are elevated. Measuring CSF inflammatory cytokine levels in patients with acute meningitis could be a valuable ED diagnostic tool. Using this tool could improve the prognosis of patients with bacterial meningitis by allowing more rapid initiation of antibiotic treatment.

▶ Community-acquired bacterial meningitis occurring in adults may be difficult to diagnose because of a lack of typical presenting symptoms and signs. Analysis of the cerebrospinal fluid can, at times, be confusing as well. It is very important to diagnose bacterial meningitis early in the course of the infection in order to initiate proper treatment and to identify those cases that seem to be most severe. This small study shows that measurement of the inflammatory cytokine interleukin 6 (IL-6) can be performed rapidly and can be helpful in identifying cases of bacterial meningitis that may be more severe and may require more aggressive therapy. Elevated IL-6 levels of greater than 90 ng/dL showed a 100% sensitivity and 95% specificity in the identification of bacterial meningitis. Levels even higher than this correlated well with the most severe infections and led to aggressive therapy with antibiotics and corticosteroids. This test can be performed in about 70 minutes and requires only 100 μL of cerebrospinal fluid for analysis.

R. Schwendimann, MD

Dilemmas in the diagnosis of acute community-acquired bacterial meningitis

Brouwer MC, Thwaites GE, Tunkel AR, et al (Univ of Amsterdam, Netherlands; Kings College London, UK; Monmouth Med Ctr, Long Branch, NJ)

Lancet 380:1684-1692, 2012

Rapid diagnosis and treatment of acute community-acquired bacterial meningitis reduces mortality and neurological sequelae, but can be delayed by atypical presentation, assessment of lumbar puncture safety, and poor sensitivity of standard diagnostic microbiology. Thus, diagnostic dilemmas are common in patients with suspected acute community-acquired bacterial meningitis. History and physical examination alone are sometimes not sufficient to confirm or exclude the diagnosis. Lumbar puncture is an essential investigation, but can be delayed by brain imaging. Results of cerebrospinal fluid (CSF) examination should be interpreted carefully, because CSF abnormalities vary according to the cause, patient's age and immune status, and previous treatment. Diagnostic prediction models that use a combination of clinical findings, with or without test results, can help to distinguish acute bacterial meningitis from other causes, but these models are not infallible. We review the dilemmas in the diagnosis of acute community-acquired bacterial meningitis, and focus on the roles of clinical assessment and CSF examination.

▶ This article is the first of 3 published in *Lancet* about bacterial meningitis. This article reviews the typical clinical presentation (headache, fever, and stiff neck) of meningitis and includes the differential diagnosis of other central nervous system infections as well as subarachnoid hemorrhage that might mimic meningitis. Barriers to diagnosis include delays in waiting for imaging studies, even in the absence of focal deficits, papilledema, or other signs of reduced consciousness. The article discusses typical changes in the cerebrospinal fluid that are strongly suggestive of bacterial meningitis as well as other diagnostic markers, such as lactate, C-reactive protein, and various molecular studies that may aid in the early diagnosis and treatment of acute bacterial meningitis. There is a discussion of various prediction models that can be useful in determining a bacterial etiology of meningitis in children. Elevation of C-reactive protein and procalcitonin may be quite helpful in differentiating pediatric bacterial meningitis from viral meningitis, and the sensitivities and specificities of these elevated values approach 100%. Costs of some of the newer molecular tests may restrict their use worldwide, particularly in resource-poor settings. This points out that bacterial meningitis is a medical emergency whose early identification is essential.

R. Schwendimann, MD

A comparison of tau and 14-3-3 protein in the diagnosis of Creutzfeldt-Jakob disease

Hamlin C, Puoti G, Berri S, et al (Case Western Reserve Univ, Cleveland, OH; et al)

Neurology 79:547-552, 2012

Objective.—To compare the respective efficiency of CSF tau (quantitative) and CSF 14-3-3 protein (qualitative) in the diagnosis of prion disease.

Methods.—We made measurements on 420 live subjects, who subsequently underwent a postmortem neuropathology examination, including protein chemistry, immunohistochemistry, and histology. We performed tau by ELISA. We detected 14-3-3 protein by Western blot. Both assays were optimized for maximum efficiency (accuracy).

Results.—We found tau and 14-3-3 proteins to be closely correlated, but tau had a significantly better ability to predict disease status than 14-3-3 protein. Also, tau distinguished disease status at least as well as when both assays' results are combined in a variety of ways. Importantly, the area under the receiver operating characteristic curve for tau (0.82) was significantly larger than that for 14-3-3 protein (0.68) ($p < 0.001$). Diagnostic test statistics are provided for the study subjects with 58.3% prevalence, and for a more typical, nonselected, 7.5% prevalence as received by our center.

Conclusion.—In this study, tau is superior to 14-3-3 protein as a marker in the diagnosis of Creutzfeldt-Jakob disease, and is as efficient singly compared to a variety of combinations with 14-3-3 protein. This is the first study of this magnitude to examine prion disease diagnostic tests in a carefully characterized patient population with detailed statistical evaluation.

▶ The 14-3-3 diagnostic test for prion diseases was adopted by the World Health Organization in 1998. This is a less-than-perfect test with a sensitivity ranging from 43% to 100% and a specificity ranging from 47% to 97%. This study compares 14-3-3 to measurements of the tau protein. The tau protein in this study was found to be superior to 14-3-3 as a marker in the diagnosis of Creutzfeldt-Jakob disease (CJD). A comment published within this article by Dr David Drachman relates the need for accurate diagnosis to ensure adequate precautions to avoid the spread of disease by transmissible material and to eliminate the diagnosis of CJD in non-CJD subacute dementing disorders for which treatments might be available. Drachman further points out that neither test is appropriate as a screening test. The typical clinical picture of CJD—rapidly progressive dementia with ataxia, visual disturbances, extrapyramidal features, startle myoclonus, basal ganglia abnormalities on magnetic resonance imaging, and periodic sharp-wave discharges on electroencephalogram—most often establishes the diagnosis before laboratory studies have been completed.

R. Schwendimann, MD

Extreme delta brush: A unique EEG pattern in adults with anti-NMDA receptor encephalitis

Schmitt SE, Pargeon K, Frechette ES, et al (Hosp of the Univ of Pennsylvania, Philadelphia; Columbia Univ, NY; Stanford Univ, Palo Alto, CA; et al)
Neurology 79:1094-1100, 2012

Objectives.—To determine continuous EEG (cEEG) patterns that may be unique to anti-NMDA receptor (NMDAR) encephalitis in a series of adult patients with this disorder.

Methods.—We evaluated the clinical and EEG data of 23 hospitalized adult patients with anti-NMDAR encephalitis who underwent cEEG monitoring between January 2005 and February 2011 at 2 large academic medical centers.

Results.—Twenty-three patients with anti-NMDAR encephalitis underwent a median of 7 (range 1–123) days of cEEG monitoring. The median length of hospitalization was 44 (range 2–200) days. Personality or behavioral changes (100%), movement disorders (82.6%), and seizures (78.3%) were the most common symptoms. Seven of 23 patients (30.4%) had a unique electrographic pattern, which we named "extreme delta brush" because of its resemblance to waveforms seen in premature infants. The presence of extreme delta brush was associated with a more prolonged hospitalization (mean 128.3 ± 47.5 vs 43.2 ± 39.0 days, $p = 0.008$) and increased days of cEEG monitoring (mean 27.6 ± 42.3 vs 6.2 ± 5.6 days, $p = 0.012$). The modified Rankin Scale score showed a trend toward worse scores in patients with the extreme delta brush pattern (mean 4.0 ± 0.8 vs 3.1 ± 1.1, $p = 0.089$).

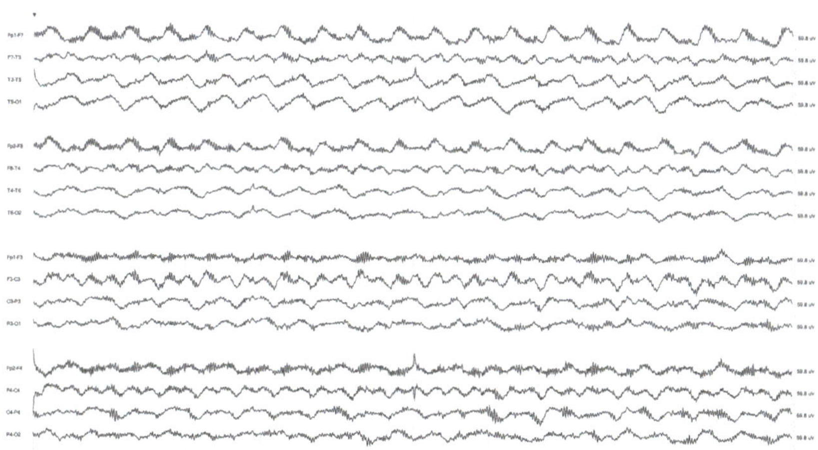

FIGURE 2.—Continuous EEG recording in a 19-year-old man with anti-NMDA receptor encephalitis associated with dyskinesias, seizures, and coma. The initial EEG demonstrates generalized rhythmic delta frequency activity at 2–2.5 Hz with superimposed rhythmic beta frequency activity. (Reprinted from Schmitt SE, Pargeon K, Frechette ES, et al. Extreme delta brush: a unique EEG pattern in adults with anti-NMDA receptor encephalitis. *Neurology.* 2012;79:1094-1100, with permission from AAN Enterprises, Inc.)

Conclusions.—Extreme delta brush is a novel EEG finding seen in many patients with anti-NMDAR encephalitis. The presence of this pattern is associated with a more prolonged illness. Although the specificity of this pattern is unclear, its presence should raise consideration of this syndrome (Fig 2).

▶ Encephalographic patterns occur in several infectious diseases and may be indicators of the underlying pathology. In herpes simplex encephalitis and in Jakob-Creutzfeldt disease, periodic epileptiform patterns may occur early in the course of the disease. In the past, electroencephalographic (EEG) abnormalities were a clue to a diagnosis of subacute sclerosing panencephalitis. This article describes a pattern termed "extreme delta brushes" that may be seen with continuous EEG monitoring of patterns with *N*-methyl-D-aspartate (NMDA)-receptor encephalitis.

The delta brush pattern is well known to neurologists who interpret neonatal EEGs. These are delta waves (1-3 Hz) with superimposed fast activity and are a pattern of prematurity that gradually disappear as the brain develops.

The delta brush activity described in 7 of 23 patients with NMDA-receptor encephalitis was associated with a more severe and prolonged illness and hospitalization. The authors suggest that the presence of this EEG pattern in patients who have evidence of an unexplained encephalopathy or encephalitis should alert the neurologist to the possibility of NMDA-receptor encephalitis, possibly leading to an earlier diagnosis.

R. Schwendimann, MD

A Life-Threatening Central Nervous System–Tuberculosis Inflammatory Reaction Nonresponsive to Corticosteroids and Successfully Controlled by Infliximab in a Young Patient With a Variant of Juvenile Idiopathic Arthritis

Jorge J-H, Graciela C, Pablo A-P, et al (Centro Médico ISSEMYM, Toluca, México; Instituto Nacional de Neurología y Neurocirugía, Secretaria de Salud, México)
J Clin Rheumatol 18:189-191, 2012

We report a young patient with a variant of juvenile idiopathic arthritis, who, after 4 years of infliximab treatment, developed miliary tuberculosis (TB) with central nervous system involvement (meningitis and multiple tuberculomas). After anti-TB treatment, clinical and radiologic responses were observed, but severe cerebrospinal fluid and brain inflammatory reaction, nonresponsive to corticosteroids, persisted. It was considered a life-threatening paradoxical reaction based on initial cerebrospinal fluid isolation of *Mycobacterium tuberculosis* fully sensitive to primary anti-TB drugs. After 4 months in the hospital, infliximab was administered considering that infliximab is a potent tumor necrosis factor α inhibiting agent that participates in the formation and preservation of granulomas and may help to modulate the exaggerated cell-mediated immune response against mycobacterial antigens. Clinical complications associated to brain

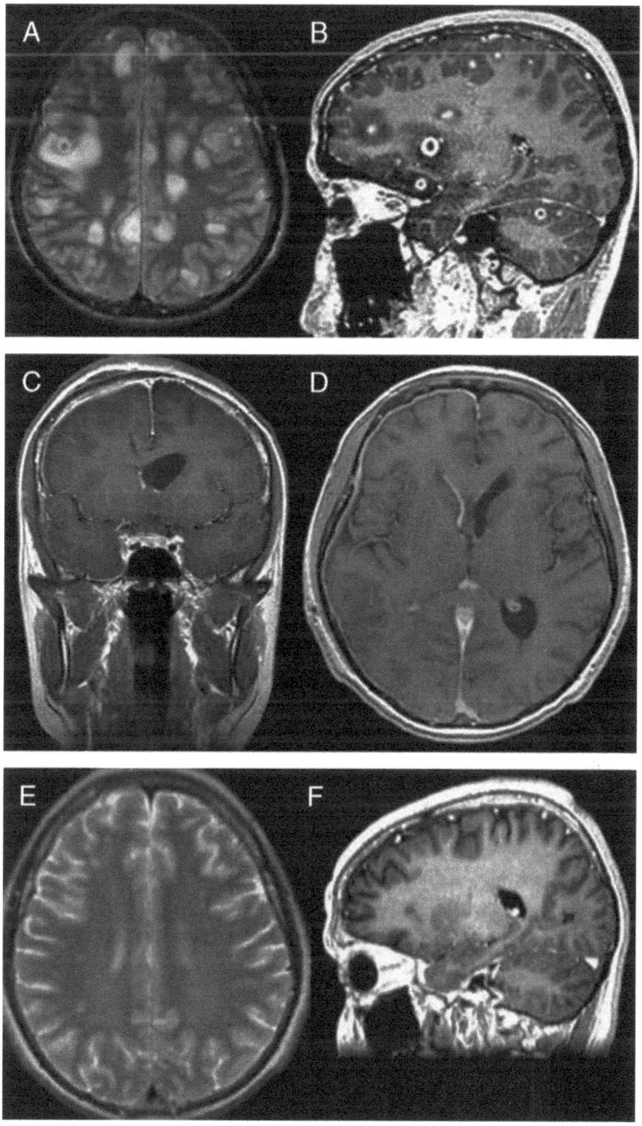

FIGURE 2.—A and B, Axial and sagittal gadolinium-enhanced MR images on admission at a neurology center showing multiple ring-enhanced lesions compatible with brain tuberculomas. C and D, Coronal and axial gadolinium-enhanced MR images showing diffuse abnormal meningeal enhancement with a right side predominance. E and F, Axial and sagittal gadolinium-enhanced MR images after 20 months of ATT showing resolution of tuberculomas and reduction of meningeal enhancement. (Reprinted from Jorge J-H, Graciela C, Pablo A-P, et al. A life-threatening central nervous system—tuberculosis inflammatory reaction nonresponsive to corticosteroids and successfully controlled by infliximab in a young patient with a variant of juvenile idiopathic arthritis. *J Clin Rheumatol.* 2012;18:189-191, with permission from Lippincott Williams & Wilkins.)

inflammation resolved, and after 3 years of follow-up, the patient remains self-sufficient without neurologic sequels (Fig 2).

▶ Tumor necrosis factor-α inhibitors are in wide use in the treatment of various rheumatological diseases. As with most drugs, they have both good and bad effects. One of the deleterious effects of these drugs is the risk of developing tuberculosis (TB). This is a case report of a patient with juvenile idiopathic arthritis treated with infliximab for 4 years who developed miliary TB with central nervous system involvement. This patient had a rather protracted clinical course as evidenced by magnetic resonance imaging findings. The patient developed cerebral vasculitis and subsequent hydrocephalus that required placement of a ventriculoperitoneal shunt. A brief discussion of this complication and possible avenues to successful treatment, including the reinstitution of treatment with infliximab, is given. Most clinical neurologists may have little experience with this class of medications. Complications with these drugs may be life threatening and neurologists should be aware of such complications.

There are other medications that are reported to be beneficial in the treatment of various neurological diseases. An example is the use of rituximab in the treatment of myasthenia gravis. This drug has been associated with progressive multifocal leukoencephalopathy. It is important to be familiar with the deleterious effects of such medications as well as the positive effects.

R. Schwendimann, MD

4 Movement Disorders

Clinical features of dopamine agonist withdrawal syndrome in a movement disorders clinic

Pondal M, Marras C, Miyasaki J, et al (Univ Health Network and Univ of Toronto, Ontario, Canada)

J Neurol Neurosurg Psychiatry 84:130-135, 2013

Background.—Recently, symptoms similar to addictive drug withdrawal have been reported in a structured longitudinal study of patients with idiopathic Parkinson's Disease (PD) withdrawing from dopamine agonists (DA): the dopamine agonist withdrawal syndrome (DAWS).

Objectives.—The objective of this study was to establish the frequency, predictors, and outcomes of DAWS in a movement disorders clinic.

Methods.—We conducted a retrospective chart review of a sample of patients with a clinical diagnosis of PD treated with DA in whom withdrawal or attempted withdrawal of DA was carried out because of adverse effects, or for any other reason. Out of 487 PD patient charts reviewed, 84 were withdrawn from the agonists and were evaluable.

Results.—Thirteen patients (15.5%) met criteria for DAWS (DAWS+) and 71 did not (DAWS−). DAWS developed upon withdrawal from pergolide, pramipexole and ropinirole, and did not respond to levodopa. DAWS outcomes included recovery in less than 6 months in 61%, in more than a year in 23%, and an inability to discontinue DA in 15% of patients. Development of impulse control disorders was the reason for DA withdrawal in all DAWS+, but only in 41% of DAWS− patients ($p < 0.0001$). DAWS+ and DAWS− patients did not differ in other variables.

Conclusion.—DAWS is a disabling complication of DA use. Critical features of the syndrome are the strong link with impulse control disorders, possibly the independence of DA dosage and type, and the resistance to treatment, including levodopa. Further studies are required to characterise those at risk as well as to define an effective treatment.

► Dopamine agonist withdrawal syndrome (DAWS) is a recently described syndrome with symptoms similar to that seen during withdrawal from drugs of abuse, such as cocaine and amphetamine. The proposed cause of DAWS is withdrawal of dopaminergic stimulation from relatively intact mesocorticolimbic circuits. The syndrome consists of a number of psychiatric symptoms, such as anxiety, panic attacks, depression, agitation, irritability, dysphoria, insomnia, fatigue, and generalized pain, as well as autonomic symptoms, such as orthostatic hypotension, dizziness, nausea, and diaphoresis. Interestingly, the authors of the original description of DAWS as well as those who wrote this article link DAWS to patients with impulse control disorders (ICD) secondary to dopamine agonist use. This is perhaps not surprising because patients who are vulnerable to symptoms from overstimulation of mesocorticolimbic circuits would likely be affected by withdrawal of the stimulant as well. The type or complexity of the ICD does not appear to be related to the risk of developing DAWS. Unfortunately, the authors are unable to provide any recommendations for management of DAWS, though, understandably, this was not their focus. The emergence of DAWS and ICD should lead to a reexamination of the standard therapeutic approach of starting dopamine agonists as the first-line therapy of choice for younger patients with Parkinson disease, especially when one considers that DAWS is more common in younger patients. Though this will not dramatically change my practice, I may be more reluctant to push dopamine agonists to high doses and instead combine low-dose agonists with levodopa or other anti-Parkinson medications.

B. Robottom, MD

Clinical subtypes of anterocollis in parkinsonian syndromes

Revuelta GJ, Benatar M, Freeman A, et al (Med Univ of South Carolina, Charleston; Univ of Miami School of Medicine, FL; Emory Univ School of Medicine, Atlanta, GA)
J Neurol Sci 315:100-103, 2012

Background.—Disproportionate anterocollis is a debilitating condition which occurs in the later stages of parkinsonian syndromes and for which there is no effective therapy. Multiple hypotheses have been proposed to explain its underlying etiology, including myopathy of the cervical extensors, and dystonia of the cervical flexors.

Methods.—We examined the records of 39 patients (8 prospectively) with anterocollis and parkinsonian syndromes to explore demographics, historical and clinical data, findings from electromyography and response to therapies. We classified our patients based on whether or not they were weak on neck extension and also based on primary diagnosis (PD vs atypical parkinsonian syndrome). Demographic, clinical, historical and EMG features are reported for each group.

Results.—There were no significant demographic differences between clinical subtypes, or primary diagnosis. Electromyographic (EMG) findings demonstrated myopathic changes in both groups, although they were more prominent in the group which was weak in extension. Historical features were similar between groups except for dopamine agonist use, which was more common in the myopathic subgroup ($p = 0.02$). There were no other significant clinical differences between clinical subtypes or primary diagnosis with the exception that patients with atypical parkinsonian syndromes had more advanced motor symptoms.

Conclusions.—We conclude that anterocollis is a heterogeneous condition in which at least two distinct subtypes exist. Recognizing these subtypes may help guide therapy and future research.

▶ The nature of anterocollis in Parkinson disease has been an area of recent intense interest and controversy. The debate is centered around the etiology of anterocollis. There are currently 2 leading hypotheses: the dystonia hypothesis and the myopathy hypothesis.

Briefly, the proponents of dystonia suggest that anterocollis is simply a form of cervical dystonia commonly seen in parkinsonism. The myopathy camp suggests that there is a primary, focal myopathy affecting neck extensors leading to anterocollis. Ultimately, there may be some truth to both arguments. This cohort study collected patients with anterocollis in the setting of Parkinson disease and atypical parkinsonism (progressive supranuclear palsy, multiple system atrophy, corticobasal degeneration) and further defines the clinical syndrome through detailed physical examination and electromyography.

The results of the study suggest that there are at least 2 distinct subtypes of anterocollis. One subtype is characterized by neck extensor weakness (with or without pseudohypertrophy of the neck musculature) and electromyography (EMG) evidence of myopathy. The other subtype is patients without weakness or EMG abnormalities and with a clinical phenotype more suggestive of dystonia. This group may or may not have accompanying torticollis or laterocollis. Surprisingly, the subtype of anterocollis is not suggestive of the underlying neurodegenerative diagnosis, although there was a trend toward myopathic anterocollis being more common in atypical parkinsonism. Practically speaking, the data presented here are difficult to translate into clinical practice.

However, defining the clinical subtypes is an important first step to moving beyond the debate surrounding etiology and moving toward treatment paradigms.

B. Robottom, MD

Accuracy of a Panel of 5 Cerebrospinal Fluid Biomarkers in the Differential Diagnosis of Patients With Dementia and/or Parkinsonian Disorders

Hall S, Öhrfelt A, Constantinescu R, et al (Lund Univ, Sweden; The Sahlgrenska Academy at Univ of Gothenburg, Sweden; Sahlgrenska Univ Hosp, Gothenburg, Sweden; et al)

Arch Neurol 69:1445-1452, 2012

Objective.—To assess the ability of 5 cerebrospinal fluid (CSF) biomarkers to differentiate between common dementia and parkinsonian disorders.

Design.—A cross-sectional, clinic-based study.

Participants.—Cerebrospinal fluid samples (N = 453) were obtained from healthy individuals serving as controls and from patients with Parkinson disease (PD), PD with dementia (PDD), dementia with Lewy bodies (DLB), Alzheimer disease (AD), progressive supranuclear palsy (PSP), multiple system atrophy (MSA), or corticobasal degeneration (CBD).

Setting.—Neurology and memory disorder clinics.

Main Outcome Measures.—Cerebrospinal fluid biomarker levels in relation to clinical diagnosis.

Results.—Cerebrospinal fluid levels of α-synuclein were decreased in patients with PD, PDD, DLB, and MSA but increased in patients with AD. Cerebrospinal fluid levels of β-amyloid 1-42 were decreased in DLB and even further decreased in AD. Cerebrospinal fluid levels of total tau and hyperphosphorylated tau were increased in AD. Multivariate analysis revealed that these biomarkers could differentiate AD from DLB and PDD with an area under the curve of 0.90, with α-synuclein and total tau contributing most to the model. Cerebrospinal fluid levels of neurofilament light chain were substantially increased in atypical parkinsonian disorders (ie, PSP, MSA, and CBD), and multivariate analysis revealed that the level of neurofilament light chain alone could differentiate PD from atypical parkinsonian disorders, with an area under the curve of 0.93.

Conclusions.—Ascertainment of the α-synuclein level in CSF somewhat improves the differential diagnosis of AD vs DLB and PDD when combined with established AD biomarkers. The level of neurofilament light chain alone may differentiate PD from atypical parkinsonian disorders.

▶ The diagnosis of Parkinson disease is clinical, based on a careful physical examination and history. Today, there are no specific imaging or laboratory markers that make a diagnosis of Parkinson disease, although the DaTscan may be useful as supportive evidence for a diagnosis in the appropriate clinical setting. Surrogate biomarkers for Parkinson disease diagnosis and progression would be very helpful in the context of clinical trials and potentially could be applied to clinical care as well.

The current study examines 5 different cerebrospinal fluid biomarkers in patients with Parkinson disease, other Parkinson syndromes, and Alzheimer disease. A few findings are of particular interest. One finding that should be of interest in clinical research is that neurofilament light chain levels in the cerebrospinal fluid correlate with disease severity in patients with Parkinson disease, progressive supranuclear palsy, and Alzheimer disease. Although this has little impact on clinical care, it might be useful as a surrogate measure for disease modification (or neuroprotection) in neurodegenerative disease trials. Unfortunately, no specific marker had high enough sensitivity and specificity to be useful in the diagnosis of Parkinson disease. Another downfall of this type of study is that it requires all patients to have lumbar punctures, which is not a reasonable strategy for clinical practice. However, I could certainly envision the time when these analyses could be performed in a noninvasive manner—for instance, using modified spectroscopy to aid in the diagnosis of clinically uncertain or early cases of Parkinson disease.

B. Robottom, MD

Cerebral pathological and compensatory mechanisms in the premotor phase of leucine-rich repeat kinase 2 parkinsonism

Van Nuenen BFL, on behalf of the LRRK2 Ashkenazi Jewish Consortium (Radboud Univ Nijmegen Med Centre, The Netherlands; et al)

Brain 135:3687-3698, 2012

Compensatory cerebral mechanisms can delay motor symptom onset in Parkinson's disease. We aim to characterize these compensatory mechanisms and early disease-related changes by quantifying movement-related cerebral function in subjects at significantly increased risk of developing Parkinson's disease, namely carriers of a leucine-rich repeat kinase 2-G2019S mutation associated with dominantly inherited parkinsonism. Functional magnetic resonance imaging was used to examine cerebral activity evoked during internal selection of motor representations, a core motor deficit in clinically overt Parkinson's disease. Thirty-nine healthy first-degree relatives of Ashkenazi Jewish patients with Parkinson's disease, who carry the leucine-rich repeat kinase 2-G2019S mutation, participated in this study. Twenty-one carriers of the leucine-rich repeat kinase 2-G2019S mutation and 18 non-carriers of this mutation were engaged in a motor imagery task (laterality judgements of left or right hands) known to be sensitive to motor control parameters. Behavioural performance of both groups was matched. Mutation carriers and non-carriers were equally sensitive to the extent and biomechanical constraints of the imagined movements in relation to the current posture of the participants' hands. Cerebral activity differed between groups, such that leucine-rich repeat kinase 2-G2019S carriers had reduced imagery-related activity in the right caudate nucleus and increased activity in the right dorsal premotor cortex. More severe striatal impairment was associated with stronger effective connectivity between the right dorsal premotor cortex and the right extrastriate body area. These findings suggest that altered movement-related activity in the caudate nuclei of leucine-rich repeat kinase 2-G2019S carriers might remain behaviourally latent by virtue of cortical compensatory mechanisms involving long-range connectivity between the dorsal premotor cortex and posterior sensory regions. These functional cerebral changes open the possibility to use a prospective study to test their relevance as early markers of Parkinson's disease.

▶ Leucine-rich repeat kinase-2 (*LRRK2*) is the most frequent genetic disease of Parkinson disease (PD) worldwide, and is quite interesting in that it is one of the few genetic causes of PD that has a predilection for late-onset cases, which results in a pattern that mimics autosomal dominant diseases with reduced penetrance.

This study recruited subjects who were at risk for the *LRRK2* mutation and, using functional MRI, examined cerebral organization during motor imagery tasks. In this cohort of relatively young, asymptomatic *LRRK2* carriers, there is clear impairment in the caudate nucleus. This certainly suggests that subclinical pathology is present before any clinical symptoms of PD, although on the basis of these data alone one cannot determine if the abnormality on functional MRI actually indicates a premotor phase of PD. As with other surrogate markers for PD, these data will be most useful in the clinical arena only after disease-modifying therapies have been developed. Another piece of data that was of particular interest is the comparison between the functional MRI abnormality seen in this *LRRK2* population and the abnormalities seen in asymptomatic carriers of *Parkin* and *PINK1* mutations. Abnormalities arose in different areas of the striatum, indicating different underlying pathological mechanisms. These differences simply underscore the enormity of the challenge facing researchers who are attempting to develop a broadly applicable disease-modifying therapy.

B. Robottom, MD

Neurologist-associated reduction in PD-related hospitalizations and health care expenditures

Willis AW, Schootman M, Tran R, et al (Washington Univ School of Medicine, St Louis, MO)

Neurology 79:1774-1780, 2012

Objective.—To investigate the impact of neurologist care on Parkinson disease (PD)–related hospitalizations. Recent data indicate that neurologist treatment in PD may be associated with improved survival, yet is underutilized. Factors contributing to this improved survival remain unknown, but may be due in part to optimal disease treatment or avoidance of disease-related complications.

Methods.—This was a retrospective cohort study of Medicare beneficiaries diagnosed with PD in 2002 and still living in 2006. Hospitalization for PD-related (neurodegenerative disease, psychosis, depression, urinary tract infection, and traumatic injury) and general medical (hypertension, diabetes, congestive heart failure, angina, and gastrointestinal obstruction) illnesses was compared by PD treating physician specialty using Cox proportional hazard models, adjusting for confounders. Secondary analyses included PD-related rehospitalization and cost stratified by frequency of neurologist care.

Results.—We identified 24,929 eligible incident PD cases; 13,489 had neurologist care. There were 9,112 PD-related hospitalizations, and these occurred and recurred less often among neurologist-treated patients. Neurologist PD care was associated with lower adjusted odds of both initial and repeat hospitalization for psychosis (hazard ratio [HR] 0.71, 95% confidence interval [CI] 0.59–0.86), urinary tract infection (HR 0.74, 0.63–0.87), and traumatic injury (HR 0.56, 0.40–0.78). PD-related outcomes improved with frequency of neurologist care in a stepwise manner. Odds of general illness hospitalization or hospitalization did not differ by neurologist involvement.

Conclusions.—Regular neurologist care in PD is specifically associated with lower risk of hospitalization and rehospitalization for several

PD-related illnesses. This may reflect an improved ability of neurologists to prevent, recognize, or treat PD complications.

► This article builds on previous research performed by the same group. In an earlier retrospective cohort, the authors found a decreased risk of hip fracture and improved survival in Parkinson patients treated by neurologists rather than primary care physicians. In this article, they again examine a retrospective cohort and compare specialist care with primary care and outcomes in Parkinson disease. The degree of specialist care was further stratified by the frequency of visits over the first 4 years after the diagnosis of Parkinsonism. There was an interesting and clear correlation between frequency of neurology visits and improved outcome. Patients who saw neurologists once or more per year had fewer hospitalizations for psychosis, urinary tract infection, or traumatic injury. This association remained after controlling for relevant or economic and general medical factors and the frequency of medical visits. In an environment where specialty care is being vigorously attacked as costly or unnecessary, it is important for neurology advocates to use these data. Additionally, it would be helpful to learn how neurologists are providing higher-quality care. Are there factors related to Parkinson care that can be expanded to include other disease states to improve outcomes? Can we use Parkinson care to develop complex care coordination strategies for the Accountable Care Organization model? At minimum, the data suggest that neurologists should always be involved in ongoing care of Parkinson disease and similar disease states.

B. Robottom, MD

Risk factors for freezing of gait in Parkinson's disease

Contreras A, Grandas F (Hospital General Universitario Gregorio Marañón, Madrid, Spain)

J Neurol Sci 320:66-71, 2012

Freezing of gait is an episodic gait disorder that may occur in patients with Parkinson's disease. The risk factors for this disorder are poorly understood.

To determine the relevant risk factors for this condition, we screened 160 consecutive patients with Parkinson's disease for freezing of gait and assessed 36 potentially related variables.

Freezers and non-freezers were compared using statistical univariate analysis, followed by bivariate and multivariate logistic regression, receiver operating characteristics curves and Kaplan–Meier estimates.

Seventy-one patients (44.4%) reported freezing of gait. At onset, the mean disease duration was 8.1 ± 6.3 years. Freezers experienced falls more frequently than non-freezers (57.7% vs 23.6%, $p < 0.001$). Disease duration was the independent variable most associated with freezing of gait (OR = 1.10, 95% CI = 1.01–1.19, $p = 0.020$). Its specificity was 77%, but its sensitivity was low, and Hoehn and Yahr staging and the UPDRS (part III) score showed similar accuracy to that of disease duration in predicting freezers. Previous antiparkinsonian treatments and predominant motor signs (tremor/akinesia-rigidity subtypes) at the onset of Parkinson's disease were not related to freezing of gait. Patients who developed Parkinson's disease before the age of 60 years experienced freezing of gait earlier than older patients (log-rank, $p < 0.005$).

Freezing of gait is a common and disabling motor complication of Parkinson's disease that is related to the progression of the disease. It is not primarily associated with dopamine replacement therapy and may occur early in young patients.

▶ Freezing of gait (FOG) in Parkinson disease (PD) is an interesting phenomenon characterized by the episodic inability to initiate normal gait. Although it is quite common, the pathophysiology has not been elucidated. FOG is reportedly more common in advanced stages of disease and in patients with the akinetic-rigid subtype of PD. The authors of this article performed a cross-sectional analysis of a group of unselected PD patients to determine risk factors for FOG. In general, patients with FOG had more advanced PD with longer disease duration, more hallucinations, and poorer cognition. These findings are in line with previous studies. Of more interest is that patients with younger onset of PD were more likely to have FOG, and that FOG was observed even in treatment-naive patients with early disease. These findings suggest that the etiology of FOG may relate more to disruption of nondopaminergic pathways. There are several tantalizing small studies looking at treatment of FOG using novel agents such as methylphenidate, and further work like this that elucidates risk factors for FOG may improve our understanding, ultimately leading to better treatment options.

B. Robottom, MD

Treatment patterns and associated costs with Parkinson's disease levodopa induced dyskinesia

Suh D-C, Pahwa R, Mallya U (Chung-Ang Univ, Seoul, South Korea; Univ of Kansas Med Ctr, Kansas City; Novartis Pharmaceuticals Corporation, East Hanover, NJ)

J Neurol Sci 319:24-31, 2012

Objectives.—This study examined the treatment patterns, direct healthcare costs and predictors of treatment costs associated with levodopa-induced dyskinesia (LID) in Parkinson's disease (PD).

Methods.—This retrospective cohort study followed PD patients for 1-year pre- and post-onset of LID, using a large US health insurance claims database from January 1, 2004 to December 31, 2008. Patients with LID were matched to patients without LID based on propensity scores to control for potential selection bias. Descriptive statistics and bootstrap techniques were employed to assess patient demographic and clinical characteristics and costs incurred. Factors influencing treatment costs were analyzed using a generalized linear model with log-link function and gamma distribution. Costs were adjusted to 2009 prices.

Results.—After patients developed LID, their total treatment costs were increased from $18,645 during the 12 months preceding LID onset to $26,439 for the 12-month period subsequent to LID onset (incremental costs of $7795: $P < 0.001$). PD-related costs increased from $3917 to $8110 (incremental costs of $4194: $p < 0.001$) LID events, medical resource utilization, higher levodopa dosage, and use of alternative PD medications were associated with increases in total treatment costs. Few changes in medication treatment patterns were noted following the initial LID, with only slight increases in levodopa dosage and few additions of alternative agents.

Conclusions.—In the United States, PD patients with LID impose a significant economic burden when compared to patients without LID. Currently available, treatment strategies for dyskinesia should be used more frequently in PD management, and new treatment strategies should be considered as they may lower healthcare costs.

▶ Levodopa-induced dyskinesias (LID) are a common side effect of long-term use of levodopa, the most efficacious medication for the treatment of Parkinson disease (PD). LID are generally mild and are not of great consequence; however, they can be disabling, leading to further loss of function and quality of life. Young-onset PD patients are at highest risk of developing LID, leading to a particular conundrum in treatment, as young-onset PD patients may also see the most benefit from aggressive therapy so that they may continue to work and maintain the highest quality of life possible. Previous studies pitting levodopa vs dopamine agonists such as monotherapy have consistently favored levodopa when examining disease severity, tolerability, and quality of life. This is despite the typical emergence of LID and motor fluctuations.[1,2] The typical practice in managing PD has been to initiate treatment with levodopa in older patients, who are less likely to develop dyskinesia, and to start dopamine agonists and then augment with levodopa when necessary in younger patients. Instead of simply looking at incidence of LID and related complications, the authors attempt to quantify the medical costs associated with LID. Interestingly, a substantial increase in medical costs was identified in the 12-month period following the diagnosis of LID. The costs were attributed to a number of different factors, but the majority of the costs were PD-related. Better strategies to manage LID would certainly be welcomed.

B. Robottom, MD

References

1. Parkinson Study Group. Pramipexole vs levodopa as initial treatment for Parkinson disease: a randomized controlled trial. Parkinson Study Group. *JAMA.* 2000; 284:1931-1938.
2. Rascol O, Brooks DJ, Korczyn AD, De Deyn PP, Clarke CE, Lang AE. A five-year study of the incidence of dyskinesia in patients with early Parkinson's disease who were treated with ropinirole or levodopa. 056 Study Group. *N Engl J Med.* 2000; 342:1484-1491.

Anti-cholinergics for axial symptoms in Parkinson's disease after subthalamic stimulation

Baba Y, Higuchi M-A, Abe H, et al (International Univ of Health and Welfare School of Rehabilitation, Fukuoka, Japan; Fukuoka Univ School of Medicine, Japan; et al)

Clin Neurol Neurosurg 114:1308-1311, 2012

Objective.—We studied the effect of anti-cholinergic therapy on axial symptoms that show a tendency to worsen over time after deep brain stimulation of the subthalamic nucleus (STN-DBS) in patients with Parkinson's disease (PD).

Patients and Methods.—We conducted a prospective study of 20 consecutive patients treated with the anti-cholinergic agent trihexyphenidyl after bilateral STN-DBS and assessed the effect of anti-cholinergic therapy on parkinsonism 1 month after its initiation using the Unified Parkinson's Disease Rating Scale (UPDRS).

Results.—After a mean post-operative follow-up period of 22.3 months, the scores of axial symptoms on UPDRS part II (ADL score) and part III (motor score) deteriorated by 87% and 54% (baseline), respectively, compared with the pre-operative scores ($P < 0.001$ for both comparisons). After adding trihexyphenidyl to dopaminergic medication with stimulation, the scores of axial symptoms on UPDRS part II and part III improved from baseline by 33% and 39%, respectively ($P < 0.001$ for both comparisons).

Conclusions.—Our findings demonstrated that the anti-cholinergic agent trihexyphenidyl shows positive effect for a patient population developing deterioration of axial symptoms after STN-DBS. The results in the present study may provide insights into the mechanism of emergence or progression of axial symptoms in patients with PD after STN-DBS.

▶ Deep brain stimulation (DBS) has become standard of care for treatment of advanced Parkinson disease (PD) characterized by motor fluctuations. Most centers target the subthalamic nucleus (STN-DBS), although that may change as relatively recent results from a head-to-head trial comparing STN and globus pallidus interna demonstrated similar outcomes. Stimulation of STN generally provides very effective relief of motor fluctuations, but it has been linked to psychiatric complications, dysarthria, and increasing axial symptom burden. Increased falls and postural instability after STN-DBS have been speculated to be secondary to accumulation of adenosine, leading to activation of adenosine A_{2A} receptors. In this open-label prospective study, the authors use trihexyphenidyl, an anticholinergic agent that is also an adenosine A_{2A} antagonist, in an attempt to improve axial symptoms after STN-DBS. In my practice, trihexyphenidyl is usually one of the first agents removed after STN-DBS because it is generally thought of as a mild agent that is predominately helpful for tremor rather than other cardinal symptoms of PD. Because tremor is generally responsive to stimulation, this medication is often decreased or stopped after surgery. An additional reason to stop trihexyphenidyl is that it is often poorly tolerated secondary to side effects, such as constipation, dry mouth, or cognitive impairment. In this study, the authors add relatively low-dose trihexyphenidyl (2–6 mg/day) and prospectively assess axial symptoms. Their results show small but clear improvement in parts II and III of the Unified Parkinson's Disease Rating Scale (UPDRS). Any improvement in axial symptoms is potentially very meaningful, even if the total change on the UPDRS is numerically small. The authors' approach is certainly of interest, and it personally excites me to see what will come of the ongoing phase III trials of other adenosine A_{2A} antagonists such as Preladenant. At this point, the results of a single, small, open-label trial will not substantially change practice, but I will be more likely to assess for emergence of axial symptoms after withdrawing trihexyphenidyl and may use it for patients with troublesome axial symptoms.

B. Robottom, MD

Musculoskeletal problems as an initial manifestation of Parkinson's disease: A retrospective study

Farnikova K, Krobot A, Kanovsky P (Univ Hosp, Olomouc, Czech Republic)
J Neurol Sci 319:102-104, 2012

Objective.—The purpose of this study was to review the prevalence of musculoskeletal pain in the prodromal phase of PD, before the PD diagnosis is made.

Methods.—A retrospective review of 82 PD patients was performed. Hospital inpatient notes and outpatient clinic admission notes were reviewed. The initial complaints prompting patients to seek medical attention were noted, as were the initial diagnoses. The symptoms were considered retrospectively to be associated with PD.

Results.—Musculoskeletal pain was present as a prodromal PD symptom in 27 (33%) cases initially diagnosed with osteoarthritis, degenerative spinal disease, and frozen shoulder. The mean time from the initial symptom appearance to dopaminergic treatment was 6.6 years in the musculoskeletal pain group and 2.3 years in the group with typical PD signs. Significant improvement of musculoskeletal pain after the initiation of dopaminergic treatment was present in 23 (85%) cases.

Conclusions.—Of the PD patients who went on to develop motor features of PD, one third manifested musculoskeletal pain as the initial symptom. A good response to L-DOPA therapy was seen in 85% of cases presenting with musculoskeletal pain. Our findings suggest that musculoskeletal pain may be a significant feature in earlier PD stages.

▶ Nonmotor symptoms have been an area of increasing research focus in Parkinson disease (PD). One of the most interesting aspects of nonmotor Parkinson symptoms is that they may occur many years before the appearance of cardinal features of PD. This has been demonstrated in longitudinal cohort studies, with the most common features preceding PD, including constipation, rapid eye movement-sleep behavioral disorder, and anosmia/hyposmia. Another underrecognized nonmotor symptom is that of chronic pain. Although the connection between frozen shoulder and PD was first reported more than 20 years ago,[1] the incidence of frozen shoulder and similar musculoskeletal complaints preceding PD is not well established. The authors of this article show in a retrospective series that musculoskeletal and sensory complaints are quite common, occurring in almost half of PD patients before the development of typical Parkinson symptoms. As the quest continues to develop disease-modifying or neuroprotective medications for PD, a greater understanding of premotor symptoms will become increasingly important. In addition to improving recognition of early PD, it is also important to note that many musculoskeletal complaints identified by the authors improved with dopaminergic therapy, indicating that these are treatable symptoms that should be addressed to improve quality of life.

B. Robottom, MD

Reference

1. Riley D, Lang AE, Blair RD, Birnbaum A, Reid B. Frozen shoulder and other shoulder disturbances in Parkinson's disease. *J Neurol Neurosurg Psychiatry.* 1989;52:63-66.

Randomized clinical trial of fipamezole for dyskinesia in Parkinson disease (FJORD study)

LeWitt PA, Hauser RA, Lu M, et al (Henry Ford Hosp, Detroit, MI; Univ of South Florida, Tampa; et al)
Neurology 79:163-169, 2012

Objective.—Fipamezole, a selective α_2-adrenergic receptor antagonist, reduced levodopa-induced dyskinesias (LID) in 1-methyl-4-phenyl-1,2,3,6-tetrahydropyridine-lesioned monkeys. In 10 dyskinetic subjects with Parkinson disease (PD), a proof-of-concept study showed beneficial effects at single doses of 60 and 90 mg. The primary study objective was to assess suppression of LID by fipamezole at day 28, as measured by the Levodopa-Induced Dyskinesia Scale (LIDS), a modification of the Abnormal Involuntary Movement Scale.

Methods.—This was a double-blind, randomized, placebo-controlled, dose-escalating 28-day study in levodopa-treated patients with PD experiencing LID, conducted at 25 centers in the United States (115 subjects) and 7 centers in India (64 subjects). Dyskinesias were evaluated 3 times after subjects became "on" from levodopa. Outcome assessment was performed with analysis of variance, which evaluated fipamezole dose-effects in a hierarchical stepwise manner and the Jonckheere test for dose responsiveness.

Results.—The total study population showed no statistically significant primary endpoint difference. However, because of inhomogeneity recognized between US and Indian study populations, a prespecified subgroup analysis of US subjects was conducted, showing fipamezole at 90 mg reduced LID (mean, 95% CI, LID rating improvement vs placebo −1.9 [0.0 to −3.8; $p = 0.047$]). Dose responsiveness was demonstrated ($p = 0.014$ for placebo, 30, 60, and 90 mg fipamezole). Fipamezole induced mild, transient blood pressure elevation and was associated with an acceptable profile of adverse effects.

Conclusions.—The evidence of efficacy in the US subgroup suggested that fipamezole at 90 mg TID may be useful to treat LID in PD without exacerbating parkinsonism.

Classification of Evidence.—This study provides Class III evidence that fipamezole is well-tolerated and, in the US subpopulation, lessens LID at 90 mg TID.

▶ Levodopa-induced dyskinesias (LID) have become a popular target for drug development, as there is currently only one Parkinson agent with proven antidyskinetic benefit, amantadine. Fipamezole is an α_2-adrenoreceptor antagonist that has shown some promise for reducing LID. The FJORD study was a phase II study conducted at sites in the United States and India designed to evaluate safety and efficacy of fipamezole in 3 doses: 30 mg, 60 mg, and 90 mg. The lower doses did not show efficacy; however, the 90-mg dose did show benefit in the US subjects, and the US subjects did show a dose-response effect. The authors conclude that the trials were promising enough that the compound should move to phase III trials. Although the development of new classes of anti-Parkinson medications is always of interest, the mixed results of this trial call into question the routine practice of conducting international, multicenter trials. The study authors were unable to explain the markedly different results seen in the US and Indian sites. The study populations were clearly different: disease duration, duration of dyskinesias, total levodopa dose, weight, age. Using the same inclusion criteria and study protocol, each geographic region produced a unique study population. The reasons are unclear for this discrepancy, but the implications are clear. Sponsors need well-defined study populations to conduct successful trials, and recruiting from multiple countries may impede their ability to recruit a cohesive trial population.

B. Robottom, MD

Comparison of patient rated treatment response with measured improvement in Parkinson's disease

Davidson MB, McGhee DJM, Counsell CE (Univ of Aberdeen, UK)

J Neurol Neurosurg Psychiatry 83:1001-1005, 2012

Background.—A marked response to dopamine replacement therapy is important in supporting a diagnosis of idiopathic Parkinson's disease (PD). The aim of the study was to compare PD patients' subjective rating of improvement with measured improvement on a number of scales.

Methods.—People with clinically defined PD were identified from a prospective long term follow-up study of incident parkinsonian patients. Changes in the Unified Parkinson's Disease Rating Scale (UPDRS) (activities of daily living and motor subsections), timed tests and Parkinson's Disease Questionnaire, full version, between assessments immediately before starting adequate dopamine replacement and the two subsequent follow-up assessments (mean 6 and 12 months after baseline) were calculated. These were compared with the patients' own subjective ratings of improvement (nil, slight, moderate, good, excellent).

Results.—133 patients were included (mean age 71 years, 56% men). Thirty-eight patients were treated with a dopamine agonist and 95 with L-dopa (median L-dopa equivalent dose 300 mg). Most patients showed improvements in their measured scores but there was no statistically significant association between these scores and the patient subjective response, except for the motor UPDRS at the first follow-up. A third of those who showed no improvement in their motor UPDRS at the first follow-up rated their improvement as moderate or better, while 29% of those whose motor UPDRS improved by over 50% said they had no or slight improvement.

Conclusion.—PD patients' subjective ratings of their degree of improvement often do not accurately reflect the degree of objective change in parkinsonian impairment or disability. Clinicians should record a simple measure of motor impairment before and after treatment to assess treatment response more accurately.

▶ This research article addresses an area of particular interest. The problem highlighted is the discrepancy between the patient's perception of treatment and the physician's perception. This is a particularly important concept in the treatment of a disease such as Parkinson disease (PD), where the treatment is aimed at improving quality of life and symptoms of disease rather than stopping or slowing the progression of disease. Few practicing neurologists routinely include objective measurements of patient's response to treatment in a clinical visit. Instead, the patient's perception often plays a large role. The results of this study indicate that there is a surprisingly large discrepancy between the 2 perceptions. Perhaps unsurprisingly, patients who were started on levodopa (rather than dopamine agonists), which is the most robust treatment for PD motor symptoms, had a slightly better correlation between their subjective response to treatment and the patient's physician's objective rating of their disease. However, even with the most robust treatment available, there was still a sizable discrepancy between patient report and physician assessment. This difference suggests that physicians should routinely use reproducible, measurable scales to assess response to Parkinson treatment because patient report alone is likely unreliable.

B. Robottom, MD

A randomized, double-blind, placebo-controlled trial of antidepressants in Parkinson disease

Richard IH, For the SAD-PD Study Group (Univ of Rochester, NY; et al)

Neurology 78:1229-1236, 2012

Objective.—To evaluate the efficacy and safety of a selective serotonin reuptake inhibitor (SSRI) and a serotonin and norepinephrine reuptake inhibitor (SNRI) in the treatment of depression in Parkinson disease (PD).

Methods.—A total of 115 subjects with PD were enrolled at 20 sites. Subjects were randomized to receive an SSRI (paroxetine; n = 42), an SNRI (venlafaxine extended release [XR]; n = 34), or placebo (n = 39). Subjects met *DSM-IV* criteria for a depressive disorder, or operationally defined subsyndromal depression, and scored >12 on the first 17 items of the Hamilton Rating Scale for Depression (HAM-D). Subjects were followed for 12 weeks (6-week dosage adjustment, 6-week maintenance). Maximum daily dosages were 40 mg for paroxetine and 225 mg for venlafaxine XR. The primary outcome measure was change in the HAM-D score from baseline to week 12.

Results.—Treatment effects (relative to placebo), expressed as mean 12-week reductions in HAM-D score, were 6.2 points (97.5% confidence interval [CI] 2.2 to 10.3, $p = 0.0007$) in the paroxetine group and 4.2 points (97.5% CI 0.1 to 8.4, $p = 0.02$) in the venlafaxine XR group. No treatment effects were seen on motor function.

Conclusions.—Both paroxetine and venlafaxine XR significantly improved depression in subjects with PD. Both medications were generally safe and well tolerated and did not worsen motor function.

Classification of Evidence.—This study provides Class I evidence that paroxetine and venlafaxine XR are effective in treating depression in patients with PD.

► Increased focus on nonmotor symptoms of Parkinson disease (PD) has been an ongoing theme in recent publications. This is the largest randomized, placebo-controlled trial of a selective serotonin reuptake inhibitor (SSRI) for PD-related depression and the first to evaluate a serotonin and norepinephrine reuptake inhibitor (SNRI). There are several interesting findings from this trial that are of practical importance. Previous smaller studies have suggested that paroxetine is ineffective for PD depression. This trial proves otherwise, helping validate the common practice of using SSRI as first-line therapy. Additionally, SNRIs are also proven to be effective, giving clinicians additional options for patients who cannot tolerate or who do not respond to therapy with SSRIs. Unfortunately, as is often the case with depression trials, only a minority of patients met remission criteria (44% for paroxetine and 37% for venlafaxine extended release), although a higher percentage were responders (68% vs 53%). With the introduction of new American Academy of Neurology quality measures suggesting that neurologists screen for depression and other mood disorders, trials such as this that provide an evidence-based medicine basis for treatment are certainly welcome.

B. Robottom, MD

Randomized trial of deep brain stimulation for Parkinson disease: Thirty-six-month outcomes

Weaver FM, For the CSP 468 Study Group (Hines VA Hosp, IL; et al)

Neurology 79:55-65, 2012

Objectives.—Our objective was to compare long-term outcomes of deep brain stimulation (DBS) of the globus pallidus interna (GPi) and subthalamic nucleus (STN) for patients with Parkinson disease (PD) in a multicenter randomized controlled trial.

Methods.—Patients randomly assigned to GPi (n = 89) or STN DBS (n = 70) were followed for 36 months. The primary outcome was motor function on stimulation/off medication using the Unified Parkinson's Disease Rating Scale motor subscale. Secondary outcomes included quality of life and neurocognitive function.

Results.—Motor function improved between baseline and 36 months for GPi (41.1 to 27.1; 95% confidence interval [CI] −16.4 to −10.8; $p < 0.001$) and STN (42.5 to 29.7; 95% CI −15.8 to −9.4; $p < 0.001$); improvements were similar between targets and stable over time ($p = 0.59$). Health-related quality of life improved at 6 months on all subscales (all p values significant), but improvement diminished over time. Mattis Dementia Rating Scale scores declined faster for STN than GPi patients ($p = 0.01$); other neurocognitive measures showed gradual decline overall.

Conclusions.—The beneficial effect of DBS on motor function was stable and comparable by target over 36 months. Slight declines in quality of life following initial gains and gradual decline in neurocognitive function likely reflect underlying disease progression and highlight the importance of non-motor symptoms in determining quality of life.

Classification of Evidence.—This study provides Class III evidence that improvement of motor symptoms of PD by DBS remains stable over 3 years and does not differ by surgical target.

▶ Deep brain stimulation (DBS) is increasingly performed as standard of care rather than being restricted to academic centers as a "last-ditch" effort to provide symptomatic treatment for patients with advanced Parkinson disease.

The representatives from Medtronics, currently the only approved device manufacturer in the United States, boast that more than 100 000 Medtronics DBS devices have been implanted worldwide for the treatment of Parkinson disease and essential tremor. Amazingly, until the publication of this trial, there had been no long-term studies (> 24 months) examining the utility of 2 commonly used implantation sites—the globus pallidus interna (GPi) and the subthalamic nucleus (STN). This trial randomized Parkinson disease patients to bilateral GPi versus STN implants for treatment of motor fluctuations secondary to Parkinson disease. This trial showed that clinical equipoise exists between the 2 surgical locations though some potentially important differences emerge. After 3 years, patients who received GPi DBS had better motor function (as scored on the Unified Parkinson's Disease Rating Scale) in the fully off state (off medication, off stimulation) and the fully on state (on medication, on stimulation).

Balancing this potential benefit of GPi stimulation is the marked reduction in medication usage in the STN group with a mean reduction of almost 400 mg of levodopa, which for many patients could help substantially by reducing dopaminergic side effects of therapy such as dyskinesia and hallucinosis. Ultimately, I believe that this study is certainly of interest and will generate discussion as to the proper target for treatment of Parkinson disease, but most centers will continue to perform STN implants because there is simply a greater level of comfort with the surgical site and the programming parameters.

B. Robottom, MD

Placebo-controlled trial of lubiprostone for constipation associated with Parkinson disease

Ondo WG, Kenney C, Sullivan K, et al (Univ of Texas Health Science Ctr—Houston; Univ of South Florida, Tampa; et al)

Neurology 78:1650-1654, 2012

Objective.—To evaluate the efficacy and tolerability of lubiprostone (Amitiza) for constipation in Parkinson disease (PD) in a double-blind, randomized, controlled study.

Methods.—Patients with PD and clinically meaningful constipation (constipation rating scale score >10 [range: 0–28]) were recruited from 2 academic movement disorder centers to participate in the study. After enrollment, patients were initially followed for 2 weeks and then were randomly assigned 1:1 to lubiprostone, and the dose was titrated up to 48 μg/day. They returned 4 weeks later for a final assessment. Data included stool diaries and global impressions (coprimary endpoints), demographics, Unified Parkinson's Disease Rating Scale scores, constipation scale scores, visual analog scale (VAS) scores, a stool diary, and adverse events.

Results.—Fifty-four subjects (39 male, mean age 67.0 ± 10.1 years, and mean duration of PD 8.3 ± 5.4 years) were randomly assigned to lubiprostone or placebo. One patient in the drug group discontinued the study because of logistics, and one patient in the placebo group discontinued the study because of lack of efficacy. A marked or very marked clinical global improvement was reported by 16 of 25 (64.0%) subjects receiving drug vs 5 of 27 (18.5%) subjects receiving placebo ($p = 0.001$). The constipation rating scale ($p < 0.05$), VAS ($p = 0.001$), and stools per day in the diary ($p < 0.001$) all improved with drug compared with placebo. Adverse events with drug were mild, most commonly intermittent loose stools.

Conclusion.—In this randomized controlled trial, lubiprostone seemed to be well tolerated and effective for the short-term treatment of constipation in PD.

► Historically, the treatment of Parkinson disease (PD) has focused on motor symptom improvement. Although nonmotor symptoms, such as constipation are well recognized, there is a dearth of treatment trials. Constipation in particular is a vexing problem because many patients have already tried over-the-counter remedies from supplements such as Colace and senna to home remedies such as mineral oil and prune juice. Lubiprostone (Amitiza) is a prescription medication that is approved for the treatment of idiopathic chronic constipation in adults. Its mechanism of action is based on activation of the chloride channel type 2 leading to enhancement of chloride-rich intestinal fluid secretion.

It had not previously been studied for PD-related constipation. In this trial, a majority of subjects (64%) reported either a marked or very marked clinical global improvement. This is a welcome addition to the PD armamentarium. Personally, I have found this to be effective for my patients, although a word of caution is in order. Lubiprostone is an expensive medication, and as such many Medicare patients will be unable to afford this as it will quickly place them in the "doughnut hole" when combined with other name brand medications.

B. Robottom, MD

Worsening essential tremor following deep brain stimulation: disease progression versus tolerance

Favilla CG, Ullman D, Wagle Shukla A, et al (Univ of Florida College of Medicine, Gainesville)

Brain 135:1455-1462, 2012

A major concern regarding ventralis intermedius nucleus deep brain stimulation for essential tremor has been the loss of surgical efficacy over time in a minority of patients. Some experts have ascribed the worsening tremor to tolerance, while other evidence has suggested that disease progression may play a role. Suboptimal lead placement has also been reported to be a factor in worsening tremor following deep-brain stimulation; however, most authors consider this phenomenon to manifest within a few months of the actual surgery. We aimed to dissect the tolerance versus disease progression issue by analysing preoperative versus long-term post-surgical Fahn–Tolosa–Marin Tremor Rating Scale scores both on and off stimulation among 28 patients who underwent ventralis intermedius nucleus deep brain stimulation and 21 age-matched controls. Of the 28 patients in the treatment arm of the cohort, seven (25) demonstrated evidence of tremor progression, and had a 34 increase in the tremor score off stimulation at the 36 month follow-up compared with a 32 increase among controls ($P = 0.67$). In one of the seven patients there was evidence of suboptimal lead placement given the lateral position of the lead, and the motor side effects during threshold testing. This patient demonstrated a loss of stimulation benefit between 24 and 36 months, which may have been more indicative of tolerance. The other six subjects (86) maintained stimulation benefit throughout the follow-up period, despite worsening tremor off stimulation (at a comparable rate to that of controls), making disease progression the most likely explanation. The data suggest that deep brain stimulation tolerance may be over-reported in the literature, and that a tolerance versus disease progression work-up should include: examining the trend in off stimulation scores, accounting for image based lead locations, and during programming sessions checking for thresholds which may elicit clinical benefits and side effects.

▶ Essential tremor (ET), despite being an extremely common problem, is somewhat of an orphan disease. With one notable exception (Louis Elan), there are very few researchers who are pursuing meaningful research into the etiology and pathophysiology of the disease. Likewise, there is a dearth of new therapeutic options for ET. The most effective therapy for ET, deep brain stimulation (DBS) of the ventralis intermedius nucleus of the thalamus, is much more efficacious than medication but is, in my opinion, underutilized. One potential reason for underutilization has been an ongoing controversy regarding long-term efficacy of DBS for ET. Some investigators have attributed loss of efficacy to disease progression; whereas others report loss of efficacy is caused by development of tolerance to stimulation. In this article, the authors report longitudinal data from the University of Florida Center for Movement Disorders and Neurorestoration to examine the tolerance versus disease progression controversy. The study design was elegant in its simplicity. The Fahn-Tolosa-Marin tremor rating scale was documented at each visit in the on and off stimulation state. Approximately 25% of patients had worsening of tremor rating scales over a 3-year follow-up period. Of these patients, most (6 of 7) still had a clear response to stimulation, as seen by the persistent separation of the on and off scores. The continued response to stimulation should indicate that the decline in tremor control over time can be attributed to disease progression rather than development of tolerance to stimulation. These data are of great interest to clinicians who are counseling patients about the potential benefits of DBS surgery. If a large percentage of patients develop true tolerance to stimulation, then recommending elective neurosurgery for a few years of tremor control may not be a worthwhile proposition. On the other hand, knowing that DBS remains helpful despite disease progression substantially changes the risk/benefit calculation, and this allows the clinician to recommend DBS with few reservations.

B. Robottom, MD

5 Multiple Sclerosis and Other Demyelinating Diseases

"Undiagnosing" multiple sclerosis: the challenge of misdiagnosis in MS

Solomon AJ, Klein EP, Bourdette D (Univ of Vermont College of Medicine, Burlington)

Neurology 78:1986-1991, 2012

Objective.—To describe the clinical characteristics of encounters with patients misdiagnosed with multiple sclerosis (MS).

Methods.—A cross-sectional Internet-based physician survey of MS specialists was performed.

Results.—The response rate for the survey was 50.4%. Of those who responded, the majority (95%) reported having evaluated 1 or more patients who had been diagnosed with MS, but who they strongly felt did not have MS, within the last year. The majority of respondents (>90%) also reported the use of disease-modifying therapy in a proportion of these patients. Most respondents (94%) found clinical encounters with these patients equally or more challenging than giving a new diagnosis of MS. Fourteen percent of respondents reported that they did not always inform such patients of their opinion that they did not have MS.

Conclusions.—The misdiagnosis of MS is common and has significant consequences for patient care and health care system costs. Caring for a patient with a misdiagnosis of MS is challenging, and at times honest disclosure of a misdiagnosis represents an important ethical concern for neurologists. More data are needed on this patient population to improve diagnostic acumen and the care of these patients.

► Multiple sclerosis (MS) is an immune-mediated demyelinating and degenerative disease of the human central nervous system that affects young adults and causes significant, irreversible neurological disability. Correct diagnosis of MS requires attention to a number of diagnostic criteria and exclusion of MS imitators. In the world of MS, we encounter both overdiagnosis and underdiagnosis of this devastating disease. Many clinicians periodically see patients who are misdiagnosed with MS and are even on some form of treatment. The treatments for MS are expensive and do have serious side effects. Currently, there are no data about what percentage of patients with MS, with or without treatment, are correctly diagnosed and treated and what percentage are misdiagnosed. The present article addresses this significant health issue and provides readers with some information about the percentage of misdiagnosed MS patients. Based on the results of this study, up to 95% of physicians who participated reported seeing 1 or more patients misdiagnosed with MS, and 14% of them did discuss the issue with the patients and informed them about the issue of misdiagnosis. It is very important to remind our readers that erroneous diagnosis of patients with MS and, worse than that, treating them with MS medications, carries serious health, financial, and legal consequences for the patient and for the clinician. A sincere discussion with the patients about the mistaken diagnosis and informing them of the truth is the best approach to this complicated issue.

A. Minagar, MD

Fatigue in multiple sclerosis – A brief review

Induruwa I, Constantinescu CS, Gran B (Univ of Nottingham, UK)

J Neurol Sci 323:9-15, 2012

Fatigue is the most common and debilitating symptom in multiple sclerosis (MS) and is believed to be distinctly different from fatigue seen in other chronic conditions. It can affect a patient's mood, sleep and have a detrimental effect on their quality of life. In the recent years much literature has emerged in an attempt to elucidate the potential causes and treatment of this common symptom. This review article aims to examine the most recent theories on the pathophysiology of fatigue in MS as well as its association with sleep and depression. We describe the pharmacological and non-pharmacological approaches to its treatment and propose a multidisciplinary, patient enabled and individualised manner to the management of fatigue in MS.

▶ Fatigue and lack of energy are among the most common complaints voiced by patients with multiple sclerosis (MS). Fatigue in MS is devastating and significantly restricts the patient's mental and physical activities, leading to functional disability. In addition, fatigue in MS affects a patient's mood, rest and sleep, and their overall quality of life. Fatigue in MS can originate from the underlying and progressive neuropathology, may be a side effect of disease-modifying agents or symptomatic treatments for MS, or may stem from depression, which commonly affects these patients. Fatigue is a serious therapeutic challenge for clinicians and imposes a significant financial burden on society. Identifying fatigue in this population and understanding the pathophysiology of fatigue can assist us in developing more potent medications to reduce fatigue and elevate patients' energy level and productivity. The present article is an excellent review for all neurologists who treat MS patients. The authors of this comprehensive review discuss the clinical features of fatigue in MS and discuss the existing hypotheses concerning its pathogenesis. The relationship between fatigue and sleep is presented in detail. Finally, the authors discuss potential pharmacological and nonpharmacological approaches to therapy of fatigue in MS patients and emphasize the fact that treatment of fatigue in MS is also an individualized process. I strongly recommend this interesting article to all our readers.

A. Minagar, MD

Low vitamin D and elevated immunoreactivity against Epstein–Barr virus before first clinical manifestation of multiple sclerosis

Décard BF, von Ahsen N, Grunwald T, et al (Ruhr-Univ Bochum, Germany; Univ Med Ctr Göttingen, Germany; et al)

J Neurol Neurosurg Psychiatry 83:1170-1173, 2012

Objective.—Vitamin D deficiency and Epstein–Barr virus (EBV) infection may be associated with the development of multiple sclerosis (MS). We investigated serum 25-hydroxyvitamin D (25-OH-D) levels and anti-EBV immunoreactivity in 25 individuals before the first clinical manifestation of MS.

Patients and Methods.—56 serum samples of 25 individuals who had donated blood prior to the first clinical MS manifestation (clinically isolated syndrome (CIS)) (four male subjects, 21 female subjects, mean age 31.5 years at time of pre-CIS blood sampling; mean age at disease onset 33.4 years) were available, covering an interval of 7.3 years–2 months (mean 31.5 months) before CIS. In 18 of 25 patients serum samples were also obtained after established diagnosis of MS. Longitudinal age- and gender-matched healthy blood donors (four male subjects, 21 female subjects, 39 samples, mean age 32.5 years) served as controls. Serum 25-OH-D was measured by isotope dilution-liquid chromatography-tandem mass spectrometry. 25-OH-D levels were deconvoluted using published seasonal coefficients from a German population. Immunoglobulin G (IgG) against Epstein–Barr virus nuclear antigen-1 (EBNA1) were assessed using commercially available ELISA.

Results.—Low 25-OH-D levels were observed during the 24-month pre-CIS interval (47.8 (32.5–77.2) nmol/l, median (IQR); healthy controls: 81.6 (57.7–98.5), $p = 0.004$, however, still higher than after established diagnosis (24.5 (13.7–47.7), $p < 0.0001$ compared with controls). IgG against EBNA1 during the 36-month pre-CIS interval was increased (185.9 (91.2–460.0) IU/ml, median (IQR); healthy controls 63.7 (29.5–121.6), $p = 0.002$).

Conclusions.—Low vitamin D and remote EBV infection may be associated with clinical MS breakthrough within 2–3 years.

► Multiple sclerosis (MS) is perceived as an immune-mediated disease of the central nervous system that leads to destruction of myelin/oligodendrocyte complex and axonal and neuronal loss. Presently, the etiology and cure for MS remain unrecognized. In addition, the initial triggers that turn on the immune system against autoantigens remain unknown. Recently, the role of 25-hydroxyvitamin D (25-OH-D), as well as exposure to or infection with Epstein-Barr virus

(EBV), has received much attention by various neuroimmunologists, and a number of epidemiologic observations have explored their role in the development and pathogenesis of MS. The present study is an attempt to assess the role of serum 25-OH-D levels and anti-EBV immunoreactivity in 25 individuals prior to the onset of the first clinical manifestation of MS. The investigators collected 56 serum specimens from 25 individuals who had donated blood prior to development of the clinically isolated syndrome (CIS). Of these, 21 subjects were female and 4 male. In 18 of 25 patients, serum specimens were also collected following a diagnosis of MS. Longitudinal age- and gender-matched healthy blood donors were collected as controls. Using isotope dilution-liquid chromatography-tandem mass spectrometry, serum levels of 25-OH-D were measured. In addition, they measured immunoglobulin G (IgG) against EBV nuclear antigen-1 (EBNA1) using a commercially available enzyme-linked immunosorbent assay. The investigators detected low serum 25-OH-D levels during the 24-month pre-CIS interval compared with the healthy controls; however, the serum levels were still higher than their serum levels after they were diagnosed with MS. IgG against EBNA1 during the 36-month pre-CIS interval was significantly elevated compared with the healthy controls. The authors concluded that low serum vitamin D levels and remote EBV infection may precede a clinical MS breakthrough within 2 to 3 years. In fact, the results of this significant study places more emphasis on the potential role of vitamin D in pathogenesis of MS and the need to replace it in our MS patients regularly.

A. Minagar, MD

Disease-modifying drugs for multiple sclerosis in pregnancy: A systematic review

Lu E, Wang BW, Guimond C, et al (Univ of British Columbia, Vancouver, Canada)
Neurology 79:1130-1135, 2012

Objective.—To systematically review the literature regarding safety of disease-modifying drug (DMD) use during pregnancy on perinatal and developmental outcomes in offspring of patients with multiple sclerosis (MS).

Methods.—A PubMed and EMBASE search up to February 2012 was conducted with a manual search of references from relevant articles. Selected studies were evaluated using internationally accepted criteria.

Results.—Fifteen studies identified 761 interferon β-, 97 glatiramer acetate-, and 35 natalizumabexposed pregnancies. Study quality ranged from poor to good; no study was rated excellent. Small sample sizes limited most studies. Compared with data for unexposed pregnancies, fair- to good-quality prospective cohort studies reported that interferon β exposure was associated with lower mean birth weight, shorter mean birth length, and preterm birth (<37 weeks), but not low birth weight (<2,500 g), cesarean delivery, congenital anomaly (including malformation), or spontaneous abortion. Fewer studies of fair quality were available for glatiramer acetate and natalizumab. Glatiramer acetate exposure was not associated with lower mean birth weight, congenital anomaly, preterm birth, or spontaneous abortion. Natalizumab exposure did not appear to be associated with shorter mean birth length, lower mean birth weight, or lower mean gestational age. No studies examined mitoxantrone or fingolimod exposure. One study of paternal DMD use during conception found no effect on gestational age or birth weight. Few studies examined longer-term developmental outcomes.

Conclusion.—Further studies are needed to determine the potential risks associated with preconceptional and in utero DMD exposure in patients with MS. Discontinuation of DMDs before conception is still recommended.

▶ Multiple sclerosis (MS) commonly affects women of childbearing age, and the issue of pregnancy is a frequently encountered therapeutic issue in this population. Despite clinicians' efforts to ensure a planned pregnancy with timely cessation of the disease-modifying drugs before conception, many of us see patients with unplanned pregnancy, and by the time we become aware of the situation, the unborn child had already been exposed to the MS-treating medication. Therefore, the question needs to be answered as to how the currently available disease-modifying agents affect the course of pregnancy and the unborn child. This systematic review by Lu et al, which is based on their extensive search of PubMed and EMBASE, is an excellent resource for practicing neurologists concerning how to address such an important issue for their pregnant MS patients who have been exposed to these medications. Based on their findings, exposure of pregnant MS patients to interferon-β was associated with lower mean birth weight, shorter mean birth length, and preterm birth (<37 weeks), but not low birth weight (<2500 g), cesarean delivery, congenital anomaly (including malformation), or spontaneous abortion. Exposure to glatiramer acetate was not associated with lower mean birth weight, congenital anomaly, preterm birth, or spontaneous abortion. Pregnancy while on natalizumab was not associated with shorter mean birth length, lower mean birth weight, or lower mean gestational age. Currently, there are no studies that have assessed the effects of mitoxantrone or fingolimod exposure on fetus. The authors of this significant report conclude that more studies are required to determine the potential risks associated with preconceptional and in utero exposure to disease-modifying agents in patients with MS. Cessation of disease-modifying drugs before conception is strongly recommended.

A. Minagar, MD

Distinct lesion morphology at 7-T MRI differentiates neuromyelitis optica from multiple sclerosis

Sinnecker T, Dörr J, Pfueller CF, et al (Charité-Universitaetsmedizin Berlin, Germany; et al)

Neurology 79:708-714, 2012

Objective.—To investigate distinct white matter and cortical gray matter pathology in neuromyelitis optica spectrum disorders (NMOSDs) and multiple sclerosis (MS) at 7-T MRI in a cross-sectional study.

Methods.—We included 10 patients with NMOSDs and 18 patients with MS in our 7-T MRI study. The imaging protocol comprised T2*-weighted fast low angle shot and turbo inversion recovery magnitude sequences. White matter and cortical gray matter lesions were assessed with special regard to their (perivascular) localization as well as the expression of a hypointense rim.

Results.—In total, we detected 140 white matter lesions in 7 of 10 patients with NMOSDs. In contrast to MS plaques, which were nearly exclusively centered by a small vein (92%) and showed a characteristic hypointense rim (23%), white matter changes in patients with NMOSDs were nonspecific in appearance and were only infrequently neighbored by a blood vessel (49 lesions [35%], $p = 0.003$). Hypointense rims were very rarely detectable (3 lesions [2%], $p < 0.001$). Cortical pathology was absent in NMOSDs. In our MS cohort, we detected 36 leukocortical, 8 intracortical, and 8 subpial cortical lesions in 7 of 18 patients.

Conclusion.—The MRI features of white matter and the absence of cortical gray matter findings substantially differentiate NMOSDs from MS and can be used as a potential marker to distinguish these 2 entities. The fact that cortical pathology is common in MS but is not present in patients with NMOSDs may reflect the difference in the underlying pathogenesis.

▶ This interesting research article by Sinnecker et al addresses the fundamental differences between white matter and cortical gray matter lesions in patients with neuromyelitis optica spectrum disorders (NMOSDs) and multiple sclerosis (MS). Based on our current knowledge about the pathogenesis of these neurological diseases, NMOSDs are regarded as different neuropathological conditions from MS and their treatment regimens are dissimilar to those of MS. However, despite such fundamental differences, in many cases, differentiation of these diseases from MS, at least at their early phases, poses a diagnostic challenge to treating neurologists. During this cross-sectional neuroradiological study, the investigators used a 7-T magnetic resonance imaging system to assess and compare white matter and cortical gray matter lesions in 10 patients with NMOSDs and 18 MS patients; the lesions were assessed with emphasis on their location as well as expression of a hypointense rim. Their neuroimaging protocol included T2*-weighted fast low-angle shot and turbo inversion recovery magnitude sequences. Based on their findings, the MS lesions were almost entirely perivenular with a typical hypointense rim. However, the white matter lesions in patients with NMOSDs demonstrated nonspecific appearance, did not occur commonly in the vicinity of a blood vessel, and rarely had a hypointense rim. In addition, cortical pathology was not detected in patients with NMOSDs. This neuroimaging study is one of the few studies that attempts to differentiate these 2 disease groups at their early stages, and this diagnostic methodology can be used as a biomarker to differentiate these 2 entities.

A. Minagar, MD

Alemtuzumab for patients with relapsing multiple sclerosis after disease-modifying therapy: a randomised controlled phase 3 trial

Coles AJ, for the CARE-MS II investigators (Univ of Cambridge, UK; et al)

Lancet 380:1829-1839, 2012

Background.—The anti-CD52 monoclonal antibody alemtuzumab reduces disease activity in previously untreated patients with relapsing-remitting multiple sclerosis. We aimed to assess efficacy and safety of alemtuzumab compared with interferon beta 1a in patients who have relapsed despite first-line treatment.

Methods.—In our 2 year, rater-masked, randomised controlled phase 3 trial, we enrolled adults aged 18–55 years with relapsing-remitting multiple sclerosis and at least one relapse on interferon beta or glatiramer. Eligible participants were randomly allocated in a 1:2:2 ratio by an interactive voice response system, stratified by site, to receive subcutaneous interferon beta 1a 44 μg, intravenous alemtuzumab 12 mg per day, or intravenous alemtuzumab 24 mg per day. Interferon beta 1a was given three-times per week and alemtuzumab was given once per day for 5 days at baseline and for 3 days at 12 months. The 24 mg per day group was discontinued to aid recruitment, but data are included for safety assessments. Coprimary endpoints were relapse rate and time to 6 month sustained accumulation of disability, comparing alemtuzumab 12 mg and interferon beta 1a in all patients who received at least one dose of study drug. This study is registered with ClinicalTrials.gov, number NCT00548405.

Findings.—202 (87%) of 231 patients randomly allocated interferon beta 1a and 426 (98%) of 436 patients randomly allocated alemtuzumab 12 mg were included in the primary analyses. 104 (51%) patients in the interferon beta 1a group relapsed (201 events) compared with 147 (35%) patients in the alemtuzumab group (236 events; rate ratio 0·51 [95% CI 0·39–0·65]; $p < 0 \cdot 0001$), corresponding to a 49·4% improvement with alemtuzumab. 94 (47%) patients in the interferon beta 1a group were relapse-free at 2 years compared with 278 (65%) patients in the alemtuzumab group ($p < 0 \cdot 0001$). 40 (20%) patients in the interferon beta 1a group had sustained accumulation of disability compared with 54 (13%) in the alemtuzumab group (hazard ratio 0·58 [95% CI 0·38–0·87]; $p = 0 \cdot 008$), corresponding to a 42% improvement in the alemtuzumab group. For 435 patients allocated alemtuzumab 12 mg, 393 (90%) had infusion-associated reactions, 334 (77%) had infections (compared with 134 [66%] of 202 patients in the interferon beta 1a group) that were mostly mild-moderate with none fatal, 69 (16%) had thyroid disorders, and three (1%) had immune thrombocytopenia.

Interpretation.—For patients with first-line treatment-refractory relapsing-remitting multiple sclerosis, alemtuzumab could be used to reduce relapse rates and sustained accumulation of disability. Suitable risk management strategies allow for early identification of alemtuzumab's main adverse effect of secondary autoimmunity.

▶ During the past 2 decades, treatment strategies for multiple sclerosis (MS) have evolved from immunomodulation and general immunosuppression with serious side effects to the introduction of very selective monoclonal antibodies aimed to block or inactivate specific molecules or antigen(s) on the cells that participate in MS inflammation. One such molecule is alemtuzumab, which is a humanized, immunoglobulin-G1 monoclonal antibody that targets the cell-surface molecule CD52. The CD52 molecule is expressed by a number of cells, including T and B lymphocytes, natural killer cells, thymocytes, monocytes, and macrophages.[1,2] Treatment of MS patients with alemtuzumab causes rapid elimination of cells that carry CD52 antigen via complement-dependent cytotoxicity and antibody-mediated cellular cytolysis. This, in turn, significantly reduces the number of autoreactive lymphocytes, which potentially reduces their attack on the antigen(s) within the human central nervous system. The massive depletion of the targeted cells by alemtuzumab is a prolonged process and may last from 3 months to 5 years, depending on the cell type affected. Based on such profound immunosuppressive effects, the efficacy and safety of alemtuzumab has been assessed for treatment of patients with relapsing-remitting MS.

In this randomized and controlled phase 3 clinical trial, the authors compared the safety and efficacy of alemtuzumab with interferon-β1a for treatment of treatment-naïve MS patients. Alemtuzumab was more effective than interferon-β1a in reducing relapse rate and increasing the relapse-free intervals in MS patients. However, adverse events, such as serious infections, and secondary autoimmune diseases, such as Graves disease, were more common in MS patients who were treated with alemtuzumab compared with those who were randomized to interferon-β1a. Alemtuzumab is currently under further investigation for treatment of MS patients.

A. Minagar, MD

References

1. Korniychuk E, Dempster JM, O'Connor E, et al. Evolving therapies for multiple sclerosis. *Int Rev Neurobiol.* 2007;79:571-588.
2. Buttmann M, Rieckmann P. Treating multiple sclerosis with monoclonal antibodies. *Expert Rev Neurother.* 2008;8:433-455.

The cervical spinal cord in neuromyelitis optica patients: A comparative study with multiple sclerosis using diffusion tensor imaging

Pessôa FMC, Lopes FCR, Costa JVA, et al (Federal Univ of Rio de Janeiro, Brazil; et al)

Eur J Radiol 81:2697-2701, 2012

Introduction.—This study aims to evaluate "in vivo" the integrity of the normal-appearing spinal cord in patients with neuromyelitis optica (NMO), using diffusion tensor MR imaging, comparing to controls and patients with multiple sclerosis (MS).

Materials and Methods.—We studied 8 patients with NMO and 17 without any neurologic disorder. Also, 32 MS patients were selected. Fractional anisotropy (FA), axial diffusivity (AD), radial diffusivity (RD) and mean diffusivity (MD) were calculated within regions of interest at C2 and C7 levels in the four columns of the spinal cord.

Results.—At C2, the FA value was decreased in NMO patients compared to MS and controls in the anterior column. Also in this column, RD value showed increase in NMO compared to MS and to controls. The FA value of the posterior column was decreased in NMO in comparison to controls. At C7, AD value was higher in NMO than in MS in the right column. At the same column, MD values were increased in NMO compared to MS and to controls.

Conclusions.—There is extensive NASC damage in NMO patients, including peripheral areas of the cervical spinal cord, affecting the white matter, mainly caused by demyelination. This suggests a new spinal cord lesion pattern in NMO in comparison to MS.

▶ For decades, neuromyelitis optica (NMO) was classified as a variant of multiple sclerosis (MS). However, with further neuropathologic and neuroimaging research into the nature of NMO, it is becoming clearer that these 2 diseases possess dissimilar pathologies and pathogenesis. With the introduction of the autoantibody anti–aquaporin-4 water channel as a significant immunodiagnostic feature of NMO, the diagnosis of NMO has become more accurate.[1] Anatomic locations of NMO differ from those of MS, and they usually affect optic nerve and spinal cord. In addition, NMO lesions of the spinal cord are extensive, and elongated (involving > 3) vertebral bodies strongly support the presence of NMO rather than MS.[2] This neuroimaging study is an excellent project to further differentiate these 2 diseases. Utilizing diffusion tensor magnetic resonance imaging, Pessôa et al aimed to assess in vivo the integrity of the normal-appearing spinal cord in patients with NMO, comparing the findings with those of patients with MS and healthy controls. The investigators examined 8 patients with NMO and 17 without any neurologic disorder. In addition, the study included 32 MS patients. The researchers calculated the fractional anisotropy (FA), axial diffusivity (AD), radial diffusivity (RD), and mean diffusivity (MD) within regions of interest at C2 and C7 levels in the 4 columns of the spinal cord. The study found that at C2 level, the FA value was decreased in NMO patients compared with the MS patients and controls in the anterior column. They also detected that in this column, RD value was increased in NMO compared with MS and with controls. The FA value of the posterior column was decreased in NMO patients compared with the controls. At C7 level, AD value was higher in patients with NMO than in MS in the right column, and, at the same column, MD values were increased in NMO compared with MS and with controls. The investigators concluded that extensive NASC damage in NMO patients, including peripheral areas of the cervical spinal cord, affecting the white matter, stemmed from demyelination. The findings of this study point toward a new pattern of spinal cord injury in NMO patients compared with MS patients and sheds more light on the underlying nature of this complex and devastating disease.

A. Minagar, MD

References

1. Lennon VA, Wingerchuk DM, Kryzer TJ, et al. A serum autoantibody marker of neuromyelitis optica: distinction from multiple sclerosis. *Lancet.* 2004;364: 2106-2112.
2. Wingerchuk DM, Lennon VA, Pittock SJ, Lucchinetti CF, Weinshenker BG. Revised diagnostic criteria for neuromyelitis optica. *Neurology.* 2006;66:1485-1489.

Decreased Frontal Lobe Gray Matter Perfusion in Cognitively Impaired Patients with Secondary-Progressive Multiple Sclerosis Detected by the Bookend Technique

Aviv RI, Francis PL, Tenenbein R, et al (Sunnybrook Health Sciences Centre, Toronto, Ontario, Canada; et al)
AJNR Am J Neuroradiol 33:1779-1785, 2012

Background and Purpose.—There is increasing evidence implicating microvascular impairment in MS pathogenesis. Perfusion imaging offers a unique opportunity to investigate the functional impact of GM pathology. We sought to quantify differences in MR imaging–based bookend-derived cerebral perfusion between cognitively impaired and nonimpaired patients with SPMS.

Materials and Methods.—Patients were prospectively recruited and assessed using MR imaging and the standard cognitive battery called the Minimal Assessment of Cognitive Function in MS. Patients exhibiting impairment on ≥2 individual tests were classified as cognitively impaired. Healthy controls were prospectively recruited and assessed using MR imaging to validate bookend assumptions. Structural and perfusion scans were coregistered and partitioned into anatomic brain regions and tissue compartments. Clinical and radiologic characteristics were compared between patients with and without impairment to identify potential confounders. A Bonferroni adjusted P value threshold ($P < .005$) was used for lobar and sublobar level analyses to correct for multiple comparisons.

Results.—Thirty-seven patients with SPMS (age 56 ± 9 years; 23 women, 14 men) and 10 age- and sex-matched healthy controls were recruited. Bookend assumptions were found to be valid in MS. GM and WM qCBV were all globally reduced in impaired patients. After adjusting for potential confounders while examining sublobar level perfusion, only GM qCBV was significantly different between cognitive groups, and this hypoperfusion localized to the bilateral medial superior frontal regions and left inferior, middle, and superior frontal regions ($P < .005$) of impaired patients compared with nonimpaired patients. GM qCBV accounted for 22.5% of the model variance compared with a model including only confounders ($P = .0007$).

Conclusions.—Bookend-derived GM qCBV was significantly reduced in cognitively impaired patients with SPMS in functionally relevant brain regions.

▶ Up to 65% of multiple sclerosis (MS) patients suffer from cognitive decline and neuropsychiatric abnormalities. Cognitive decline in MS leads to loss of social status and income, unemployment, significant compromise of activities of daily living, and serious disability. Patients with secondary progressive MS commonly suffer from cognitive decline stemming from both gray and white matter involvement and injury in pathogenesis of MS.[1,2] Neuropathologic studies of MS indicate microvascular injury in MS with perivenular formation of demyelinating lesions, lymphocyte cuffing, wall hyalinization, chronic ischemia, and microcirculation abnormalities.[3,4]

Currently, magnetic resonance imaging (MRI) of the brain and spinal cord is the only scientific and objective methodology that allows neurologists to accurately assess the extent of both gray and white matter pathology in the course of MS. The bookend methodology is a novel neuroimaging procedure that is based on dynamic susceptibility contrast MRI. The bookend technique, which utilizes a paramagnetic contrast agent, enables researchers to determine absolute quantification of flow and precisely quantifies cerebral perfusion by assessing the pre- and postgadolinium images.[5-7]

During this prospective study, the authors used the bookend technique to assess the frontal lobe gray matter perfusion in patients with secondary progressive MS who were also cognitively impaired. The cognitive status of the study subjects was also assessed with the standard cognitive battery called the *Minimal Assessment of Cognitive Function in MS*. The study subjects who showed decline in 2 individual tests were classified as "cognitively impaired." This study also included an arm of healthy control subjects who were evaluated with MRI to validate bookend assumptions. The obtained clinical and neuro-radiologic features were compared between the 2 groups. The investigators detected a global decrease in quantitative cerebral blood volume of gray and white matter of cognitively impaired MS patients. After adjusting for potential confounders while assessing sublobar level perfusion, only gray matter quantitative cerebral blood volume showed significant difference between cognitive groups. The detected hypoperfusion was localized to the bilateral medial superior frontal regions and left inferior, middle, and superior frontal regions of impaired MS patients compared with nonimpaired MS patients. The authors concluded that utilizing bookend methodology enabled them to detect a significant reduction in the gray matter quantitative cerebral blood volume in functionally relevant areas on the brain in patients with secondary progressive MS who suffered from cognitive decline.

A. Minagar, MD

References

1. Huijbregts SCJ, Kalkers NF, de Sonneville LMJ, de Groot V, Reuling IE, Polman CH. Differences in cognitive impairment of relapsing remitting, secondary, and primary progressive MS. *Neurology.* 2004;63:335-339.

2. Rao SM, Leo GJ, Ellington L, Nauertz T, Bernardin L, Unverzagt F. Cognitive dysfunction in multiple sclerosis. II. Impact on employment and social functioning. *Neurology.* 1991;41:692-696.
3. Adams RA, Passino M, Sachs BD, Nuriel T, Akassoglou K. Fibrin mechanisms and functions in nervous system pathology. *Mol Interv.* 2004;4:163-176.
4. Aviv RI, Francis PL, Tenenbein R, et al. Decreased frontal lobe gray matter perfusion in cognitively impaired patients with secondary-progressive multiple sclerosis detected by the bookend technique. *AJNR Am J Neuroradiol.* 2012;33:1779-1785.
5. Carroll TJ, Horowitz S, Shin W, et al. Quantification of cerebral perfusion using the "bookend technique": an evaluation in CNS tumors. *Magn Reson Imaging.* 2008;26:1352-1359.
6. Shin W, Cashen TA, Horowitz SW, Sawlani R, Carroll TJ. Quantitative CBV measurement from static T1 changes in tissue and correction for intravascular water exchange. *Magn Reson Med.* 2006;56:138-145.
7. Shin W, Horowitz S, Ragin A, Chen Y, Walker M, Carroll TJ. Quantitative cerebral perfusion using dynamic susceptibility contrast MRI: evaluation of reproducibility and age-and gender-dependence with fully automatic image postprocessing algorithm. *Magn Reson Med.* 2007;58:1232-1241.

Effect of Aquatic Exercise Training on Fatigue and Health-Related Quality of Life in Patients With Multiple Sclerosis

Kargarfard M, Etemadifar M, Baker P, et al (Univ of Isfahan, Iran; Isfahan Univ of Med Sciences, Iran; Univ of Queensland, Herston, Australia)
Arch Phys Med Rehabil 93:1701-1708, 2012

Objective.—To examine the effectiveness of aquatic exercise training on fatigue and health-related quality of life (HRQOL) in women with multiple sclerosis (MS).

Design.—Randomized controlled trial, 4-week and 8-week follow-up.

Setting.—Referral center of a multiple sclerosis society.

Participants.—Women (N = 32) diagnosed with relapsing-remitting MS (mean age ± SD, 32.6 ± 8.0 y) were recruited into this study. After undergoing baseline testing by a neurologist, participants were randomly assigned to either an intervention (aquatic exercise) or a control group.

Interventions.—The intervention consisted of 8 weeks supervised aquatic exercise in a swimming pool (3 times a week, each session lasting 60 min).

Main Outcome Measures.—At baseline, 4 weeks, and 8 weeks, fatigue and HRQOL were assessed by a blind assessor using the Modified Fatigue Impact Scale and the Multiple Sclerosis Quality of Life-54 questionnaire, respectively. A mixed-model approach to repeated-measures analysis of variance was used to detect within- and between-subject effects.

Results.—Findings are based on 21 patients (10 from the exercise group and 11 from the control group) who had data available on outcomes. There was no significant difference between the 2 groups at the baseline. Patients in the aquatic exercise group showed significant improvements in fatigue and subscores of HRQOL after 4 and 8 weeks compared with the control group. Results obtained from the intention-to-treat analysis were consistent with those of per-protocol analysis.

Conclusions.—The findings suggest that aquatic exercise training can effectively improve fatigue and HRQOL of patients with MS and should be considered in the management of this relatively common public health problem.

► Multiple sclerosis (MS) is a progressive, disabling neurological disease of the human central nervous system that affects young individuals. MS causes fatigue, loss of mental and physical productivity, and significantly compromises quality of life. Most MS patients with relapsing-remitting MS are young women, and their most common complaint is fatigue. The fatigue in MS has a number of etiologies, which include the underlying disease process, depression, and side effects of some of the disease-modifying drugs. Because the detailed pathogenesis of fatigue in MS remains largely unknown and unexplored, the existing medications and treatments for fatigue are only symptomatic and do not target the root of the problem. During this single-center, randomized, controlled trial, which involved 32 female patients with relapsing-remitting MS, Kargarfard et al assessed the efficacy of aquatic exercise training on fatigue and other health-related quality of life in patients. The study consisted of 4 weeks of randomized trial and 8 weeks of follow-up. The study participants were initially examined by a neurologist and were then randomly assigned to either aquatic exercise, which consisted of 8 weeks of supervised aquatic exercise in a swimming pool (3 times a week, each session lasting 60 minutes), or a control group. The investigators assessed fatigue and health-related quality of life at the onset of the study and then at 4 and 8 weeks. They utilized the Modified Fatigue Impact Scale and the Multiple Sclerosis Quality of Life-54 questionnaire, respectively, and used mixed-model approach to repeated-measures analysis of variance to identify within- and between-subject effects. The 2 arms of the study did not differ significantly at baseline. However, according to the results of this interesting trial, patients in the aquatic exercise group showed significant improvements in fatigue and subscores of health-related quality of life after 4 and 8 weeks compared with the control group. The obtained results from the intention-to-treat analysis were consistent with those of per-protocol analysis. The authors concluded that aquatic exercise training can effectively reduce fatigue and improve health-related quality of life of MS patients. Their findings once again emphasize the important positive role of continuous exercise in the life of MS patients and highlight the role of treating neurologists in instructing and educating MS patients about the issue of regular exercise and physical activity in their disease management.

A. Minagar, MD

Heterogeneity of cortical lesions in multiple sclerosis: Clinical and pathologic implications

Kooi E-J, Strijbis EMM, van der Valk P, et al (VU Univ Med Ctr, Amsterdam, the Netherlands)

Neurology 79:1369-1376, 2012

Objective.—Autopsy cases show that cortical lesions (CLs) in multiple sclerosis (MS) lack lymphocyte/macrophage influx, blood-brain barrier breakdown, and complement activation. However, some CLs were demonstrated to harbor activated microglia. Here, we assessed the clinical significance of microglia activation in CLs in a large autopsy sample, and we investigated possible interrelationships with other pathologic characteristics.

Methods.—We cross-sectionally investigated the clinicopathologic characteristics of 22 patients with MS with extensive subpial demyelination (CL group) and 19 patients with MS with only little demyelination of the cerebral cortex (non-CL group).

Results.—A subset of the patients in the CL group (12 patients) showed rims of activated microglia (RAM) at the border of the CLs (RAM-CL group), whereas the other 10 patients in this group did not show microglia activation (non–RAM-CL group). A subsequent comparison between groups showed that patients with MS harboring RAM-CLs were significantly younger at the time of their death (53.5 years) than patients harboring mainly non-RAM-CLs (68.7 years; $p < 0.05$) or patients without extensive numbers of CLs (66.9 years; $p < 0.01$). In addition, a significantly shorter disease duration was found for the RAM-CL group (mean 20.9 years) than for the non-CL group (mean 34.5 years; $p < 0.05$). We also found that the presence of RAM-CLs is associated with a higher number of chronic active white matter (WM) lesions (Spearman $p = 0.74$; $p < 0.0001$).

Conclusions.—RAM-CLs were found in a subset of patients with MS who also have more active WM inflammation and a less favorable disease course.

▶ A number of recent neuroimaging studies have further elucidated the role of gray matter involvement in pathogenesis of multiple sclerosis (MS) and the significant role of cortical gray matter lesions in cognitive decline, progressive disability, and disease progression. However, despite the wealth of neuroimaging studies on such a significant subject, neuropathologic studies with focus on the nature of these lesions are few and far between. This neuropathologic study is an autopsy-based evaluation of the cortical lesions in MS patients that sheds light into their underlying nature. Neuropathologic features of cortical gray matter lesions are dissimilar to those of white matter and include absence of lymphocyte/macrophage influx, lack of blood-brain barrier disruption, and complement activation. However, some of these cortical lesions contain activated microglia. The authors of this interesting study aimed to evaluate the clinical importance of microglia activation in cortical lesions and assessed the possible interrelationships with other pathologic features. During the course of this cross-sectional study, the investigators assess clinical and pathologic features of 22 MS patients with widespread subpial demyelination and 19 MS patients with minimal cerebral cortex demyelination. The investigators detected that of the 22 MS patients with cortical lesions, 12 had rims of activated microglia at the border of the lesions, whereas 10 patients did not show such a feature. Interestingly, MS patients whose cortical lesions contained rims of activated macrophages had passed away at a younger age than those MS patients without the rims of activated microglia at their cortical lesions or MS patients without high numbers of cortical lesions. In addition, MS patients with cortical lesions that carried rims of activated microglia had significantly shorter disease duration than those MS patients who had cortical lesions without rims of activated microglia. Lastly, the presence of MS cortical lesions with rims of activated microglia was accompanied by the presence of larger numbers of chronic active white matter lesions. The authors concluded that the cortical gray matter lesions with rims of activated microglia were associated with more active white matter inflammatory lesions and a worse outcome. This solid scientific study adds much to our understanding of the pathologic nature of cortical gray matter lesions in MS patients.

A. Minagar, MD

Gray Matter Pathology in MS: A 3-Year Longitudinal Study in a Pediatric Population

Calabrese M, Seppi D, Romualdi C, et al (Univ Hosp of Padua, Italy; Univ of Padua, Italy)

AJNR Am J Neuroradiol 33:1507-1511, 2012

Background and Purpose.—GM pathology is considered a major determinant of disability in MS, but the comprehension of its origin and progression rate is limited by the uncertainty of dating the biologic disease onset. Thus, we planned a longitudinal study aimed at analyzing and comparing cortical pathology in pediatric and adult MS patients at clinical onset.

Materials and Methods.—Within 12 months from clinical onset, 35 patients with cMS and 57 with aMS were included in a longitudinal study. At T0, GMf and CL number and volume were analyzed. Percentages of Δ-GMf and number of new CLs were assessed every year for 3 years (T1-T3). Twenty-eight age- and sex-matched NCs constituted the reference population.

Results.—At T0, GMf did not differ between cMS and NC ($P = .18$), while it was lower in patients with aMS compared with both NCs ($P < .001$) and patients with cMS ($P < .001$). The number of patients with CLs, as well as CL number and volume, were higher in patients with aMS than in those with cMS ($P < .001$). At T3, Δ-GMf was higher in both patients with cMS (1.6% ± 0.5%; range 0.7%-3.4%; $P < .001$) and aMS (1.6% ± 0.6%; range 0.6%−3.4%; $P < .001$) compared with NCs (0.7% ± 0.2%; range 0.4%−1.1%), whereas no difference was observed between patients with cMS and aMS ($P = .93$). Δ-GMf significantly correlated with increased CL volume (cMS: $r = 0.46$; aMS: $r = 0.48$) and with the appearance of new CLs (cMS: $r = 0.51$; aMS: $r = 0.49$).

Conclusions.—Our findings suggest that focal (CLs) and diffuse (atrophy) GM damage are strictly associated with the biologic onset of MS, and proceed linearly and partly independently of WM pathology.

▶ With new knowledge about the underlying pathogenesis of multiple sclerosis (MS), it is no longer considered and researched as a white matter disease of the human central nervous system. Based on the current knowledge, which stems from both very in-depth neuroimaging and neuropathologic studies, MS is a whole brain disease that affects both gray and white matters. The pathogenesis of MS has 2 arms of neuroinflammation and neurodegeneration, which often run in parallel and eventually lead to inflammatory demyelination, resulting in both neuronal and axonal loss. In the long run it is the neurodegenerative arm of MS pathogenesis that becomes the dominant event and causes progressive and irreversible disability. Exactly what factors play a significant role and how these factors trigger the neurodegenerative arm of MS remain unknown.

The authors designed and executed a longitudinal study to assess and evaluate cortical neuropathology in 2 cohorts of patients, those with childhood-onset MS vs those with adulthood-onset MS. The investigators included 35 patients with childhood-onset MS and 57 patients with adult-onset MS within 1 year from clinical onset. At the beginning of the longitudinal study, they analyzed the gray matter fraction and the number of cortical lesions in both arms of the study. Then, they analyzed the changes of gray matter fraction and new cortical lesions once a year for 3 years. The control group consisted of 28 age- and sex-matched healthy individuals who were used as reference. Based on the results of this study, at study onset the gray matter fraction did not significantly differ between patients with childhood MS and normal controls; however, it was less in adult patients with MS compared with the normal controls and study subjects with childhood-onset MS. Patients with adult-onset MS had more cortical lesions and higher volume of cortical lesions compared with the patients with childhood-onset MS. During the third year of the study, both patient groups showed more change in gray matter fraction compared with healthy controls, whereas no differences were detected between the 2 patient groups. Changes in gray matter fraction demonstrated significant correlation with increased cortical lesion volume and with the development of new cortical lesions. The authors concluded that both focal cortical lesions and diffuse atrophy of gray matter occur as components of biological initiation of MS and are at least partially independent of white matter neuropathology. This study once more highlights the significance of further studies of the gray matter pathology in MS patients.

A. Minagar, MD

Placebo-Controlled Phase 3 Study of Oral BG-12 for Relapsing Multiple Sclerosis

Gold R, for the DEFINE Study Investigators (St Josef-Hosp/Ruhr-Univ Bochum, Germany; et al)
N Engl J Med 367:1098-1107, 2012

Background.—BG-12 (dimethyl fumarate) was shown to have antiinflammatory and cytoprotective properties in preclinical experiments and to result in significant reductions in disease activity on magnetic resonance imaging (MRI) in a phase 2, placebo-controlled study involving patients with relapsing–remitting multiple sclerosis.

Methods.—We conducted a randomized, double-blind, placebo-controlled phase 3 study involving patients with relapsing–remitting multiple sclerosis. Patients were randomly assigned to receive oral BG-12 at a dose of 240 mg twice daily, BG-12 at a dose of 240 mg three times daily, or placebo. The primary end point was the proportion of patients who had a relapse by 2 years. Other end points included the annualized relapse rate, the time to confirmed progression of disability, and findings on MRI.

Results.—The estimated proportion of patients who had a relapse was significantly lower in the two BG-12 groups than in the placebo group (27% with BG-12 twice daily and 26% with BG-12 thrice daily vs. 46% with placebo, $P < 0.001$ for both comparisons). The annualized relapse rate at 2 years was 0.17 in the twice-daily BG-12 group and 0.19 in the thrice-daily BG-12 group, as compared with 0.36 in the placebo group, representing relative reductions of 53% and 48% with the two BG-12 regimens, respectively ($P < 0.001$ for the comparison of each BG-12 regimen with placebo). The estimated proportion of patients with confirmed progression of disability was 16% in the twice daily BG-12 group, 18% in the thrice-daily BG-12 group, and 27% in the placebo group, with significant relative risk reductions of 38% with BG-12 twice daily ($P = 0.005$) and 34% with BG-12 thrice daily ($P = 0.01$). BG-12 also significantly reduced the number of gadolinium-enhancing lesions and of new or enlarging T2-weighted hyperintense lesions ($P < 0.001$ for the comparison of each BG-12 regimen with placebo). Adverse events associated with BG-12 included flushing and gastrointestinal events, such as diarrhea, nausea, and upper abdominal pain, as well as decreased lymphocyte counts and elevated liver aminotransferase levels.

Conclusions.—In patients with relapsing-remitting multiple sclerosis, both BG-12 regimens, as compared with placebo, significantly reduced the proportion of patients who had a relapse, the annualized relapse rate, the rate of disability progression, and the number of lesions on MRI.

▶ BG-12 (dimethyl fumarate) is an oral medication with anti-inflammatory and cytoprotective features that is currently under investigation for approval in the treatment of patients with relapsing-remitting multiple sclerosis (MS). Based on the results of a phase-2, placebo-controlled trial, treatment of patients with relapsing-remitting MS with BG-12 led to significant reductions in disease activity on magnetic resonance imaging (MRI). Based on such positive results, Gold et al designed and conducted a 2-year randomized, double-blind, placebo-controlled phase 3 study to assess the efficacy of oral BG-12 in treatment of patients with relapsing-remitting MS. During this clinical trial, MS patients were randomly assigned to oral BG-12 at a dose of 240 mg twice daily, BG-12 at a dose of 240 mg 3 times daily, or placebo. The primary aim of the trial was to determine the proportion of MS patients who experienced a relapse by 2 years. Other goals of the trial consisted of determination of the annualized relapse rate, the time to confirmed progression of disability, and MRI outcomes. Based on the results of this significant trial, the estimated proportion of patients who experienced one relapse was significantly lower in the 2 BG-12 groups than in the placebo group (27% with BG-12 twice daily and 26% with BG-12 thrice daily vs 46% with placebo, $P < .001$ for both comparisons). In addition, the annualized relapse rate at 2 years was 0.17 in the twice-daily BG-12 group and 0.19 in the thrice-daily BG-12 group compared with 0.36 in the placebo group, which indicated relative decreases of 53% and 48% with the 2 BG-12 treatment groups, respectively ($P < .001$ for the comparison of each BG-12 regimen with placebo). The estimated proportion of patients with confirmed progression of disability was 16% in the twice-daily BG-12 group, 18% in the thrice-daily BG-12 group, and 27% in the placebo group, representing significant relative risk reductions of 38% ($P = .005$) and 34% ($P = .01$), respectively, in the BG-12 dosing groups. Treatment with BG-12 was associated with significant reduction of the number of gadolinium-enhancing lesions and reduction of new or enlarging T2-weighted hyperintense lesions. Adverse events associated with treatment of MS patients with BG-12 consisted of flushing and gastrointestinal events, such as diarrhea, nausea, and upper abdominal pain, as well as decreased lymphocyte counts and elevated liver aminotransferase levels. Treatment of MS patients with BG-12 reduces relapse rate, decreases the rate of disability progression, and improves MRI outcomes. Once approved by the US Food and Drug Administration, BG-12 will be the third oral treatment for relapsing-remitting MS. The fact that this medication is oral and does not have certain side effects that occur after the use of injectable treatments for MS indicates that it may improve the compliance rate among this population.

A. Minagar, MD

Cortical lesion load associates with progression of disability in multiple sclerosis

Calabrese M, Poretto V, Favaretto A, et al (Univ Hosp of Padova, Italy)

Brain 135:2952-2961, 2012

Cortical inflammatory lesions have been correlated with disability and cortical atrophy in multiple sclerosis. The extent to which cortical lesion load is associated with longer-term physical and cognitive disability in different multiple sclerosis phenotypes has not yet been investigated. Thus, a 5-year prospective longitudinal study was carried on in a large group of patients with multiple sclerosis. Three hundred and twelve consecutive patients suffering from multiple sclerosis (157 relapsing remitting, 35 paediatric, 45 benign, 44 primary progressive and 31 secondary progressive) were enrolled in a 5-year prospective clinical and neuroimaging study. Several magnetic resonance parameters (including cortical lesion number and volume, contrast-enhancing cortical lesions and grey matter atrophy) were analysed to find associations with clinical and cognitive outcomes. Patients with high cortical lesion load had higher Expanded Disability Status Scale increase (median = 1.5; range = 0–3) during the study than both patients with low cortical lesion load (median = 1.0; range = 1–3, $P < 0.001$) and without cortical lesions (median = 0.5; range = −1 to 2, $P < 0.001$). Compared with clinically stable patients, 101 (32.4) patients showing clinical progression at 5 years had the highest rate of cortical lesion accumulation ($P < 0.001$). Stepwise regression analysis revealed significant and independent contributions from age ($\beta = 0.55$), cortical lesion volume

($\beta = 0.58$), T_2 white matter lesion volume ($\beta = 0.34$) and grey matter fraction ($\beta = 0.42$) as predictors (final model with $r^2 = 0.657$, $P < 0.001$) of Expanded Disability Status Scale change. Disease duration ($\beta = 0.52$, $P < 0.001$), cortical lesion volume ($\beta = 0.67$, $P < 0.001$), grey matter fraction ($\beta = 0.56$, $P < 0.001$) and T_2 white matter lesion volume ($\beta = 0.31$, $P = 0.040$) at baseline were found to be independent predictors of cognitive status at the end of the study. While confirming the relevance of cortical pathology in all multiple sclerosis phenotypes, but benign, our study suggests that grey matter and white matter changes in multiple sclerosis occur, at least, partly independently, and that grey matter, more than white matter, damage is associated with physical and cognitive disability progression. Thus, the combination of grey and white matter parameters gives a more comprehensive view of multiple sclerosis pathology and allows a better understanding of the progressive phase of the disease, which, however, seems more related to cortical damage than to subcortical white matter changes.

▶ Recent advances in neuroimaging of multiple sclerosis (MS) have advanced our knowledge of MS as a whole brain disease with pathological involvement of both gray and white matters. Now we realize that cortical inflammatory lesions in MS are damaging and are associated with cortical atrophy and neurological disability. This original research paper is an attempt to determine the extent these lesions lead to cognitive decline and disability in MS patients with various disease phenotypes. This 5-year prospective study included a large cohort of MS patients with these courses: relapsing-remitting, secondary progressive, primary progressive, benign, and pediatric MS. The authors analyzed a number of neuroimaging outcomes, including cortical lesion number and volume, contrast-enhancing cortical lesions, and gray matter atrophy, and attempted to identify correlations and clinical and cognitive parameters. The investigators detected that study subjects with more cortical lesions experienced more disability as evidenced by higher Expanded Disability Status Scale (EDSS) progression compared with those without cortical lesions. Furthermore, those patients with clinical deterioration at 5 years had developed the highest number of cortical lesion load. The authors also assessed the patients for contributions from age, cortical lesion volume, T2-weighted white matter lesion volume, and gray matter fraction as predicting factors for alteration of the EDSS and found these variables to be independent predictors of cognitive status at the termination of the study. The important finding of this study was that (except for the patients with benign MS) gray matter pathology, at least partially, occurs independent of the white matter pathology. It is the gray matter neuropathology that leads to deterioration of physical and cognitive status of the MS patients. This interesting article once again pinpoints the significance of gray matter pathology and lesion load in the long-term prognosis of MS patients.

A. Minagar, MD

Impact of Fingolimod Therapy on Magnetic Resonance Imaging Outcomes in Patients With Multiple Sclerosis

Radue E-W, for the FTY720 Research Evaluating Effects of Daily Oral Therapy in Multiple Sclerosis (FREEDOMS) Study Group (Univ Hosp, Basel, Switzerland; et al)

Arch Neurol 69:1259-1269, 2012

Objective.—To assess the impact of fingolimod (FTY720) therapy on magnetic resonance imaging measures of inflammatory activity and tissue damage in patients participating in a 2-year, placebo-controlled, phase 3 study.

Design.—Patients with active relapsing-remitting multiple sclerosis were randomized to receive fingolimod, 0.5 mg; fingolimod, 1.25 mg; or placebo for 2 years. Standardized magnetic resonance imaging scans were obtained at months 0, 6, 12, and 24 and centrally evaluated for number and volume of T1 gadolinium-enhancing, T2 hyperintense, and T1 hypointense lesions and for percentage of brain volume change. Findings were compared across subgroups by treatment and baseline characteristics.

Setting.—Worldwide, multicenter clinical trial.

Patients.—Patients were part of the fingolimod FTY720 Research Evaluating Effects of Daily Oral Therapy in Multiple Sclerosis (FREEDOMS) clinical trial for relapsing-remitting multiple sclerosis (N = 1272).

Main Outcome Measures.—We measured the effect of therapy on acute inflammatory activity, burden of disease, and irreversible loss of brain volume.

Results.—Fingolimod therapy resulted in rapid and sustained reductions in inflammatory lesion activity as assessed by gadolinium-enhancing and new/newly enlarged T2 lesions after 6, 12, and 24 months of therapy ($P < .001$, all comparisons vs placebo). Changes in T2 hyperintense and T1 hypointense lesion volume also significantly favored fingolimod ($P < .05$, all comparisons). Fingolimod, 0.5 mg (licensed dose), significantly reduced brain volume loss during months 0 to 6, 0 to 12, 12 to 24, and 0 to 24 ($P < .05$, all comparisons) vs placebo, and subgroup analyses confirmed these effects over 2 years irrespective of the presence/absence of gadolinium-enhancing lesions, T2 lesion load, previous treatment status, or level of disability.

Conclusion.—These results, coupled with the significant reductions in relapse rates and disability progression reported previously, support the positive impact on long-term disease evolution.

Trial Registration.—clinicaltrials.gov Identifier: NCT00289978.

▶ Fingolimod (Gilenya, Novartis) is the first immunomodulating drug approved by US Food and Drug Administration for treatment of patients with relapsing-remitting multiple sclerosis (MS). The mechanism of action of fingolimod is unique and very interesting. It acts as a modulator of sphingosine 1-phosphate receptor and, by sequestering lymphocytes within the lymph nodes, reduces their number in the peripheral circulation and circumvents their participation in the autoimmune reaction against putative central nervous system antigens. The authors present results from the FREEDOMS randomized, placebo-controlled, intent-to-treat clinical trial evaluating the effects of fingolimod (FTY720) therapy on acute inflammatory activity, burden of disease, and loss of brain volume in a group of 1272 patients with MS as evidenced by magnetic resonance imaging (MRI). The study evaluated the effects of 2 different doses of FTY720 (0.5 mg and 1.25 mg) compared with placebo in MRI changes at 6 months, 12 months, and 24 months.

The study found that both doses of fingolimod were effective in reducing inflammatory lesions at each assessment interval as well as lesion volume and brain volume loss. Patients randomly assigned to the placebo group also experienced improvements in these areas, although the changes from baseline were not statistically significant, and the effects in the placebo group dissipated after 12 months. The authors illustrated the benefits of fingolimod over time in included figures; however, the time range for the number of patients free from new or inflammatory lesions were expressed in time intervals of months 0 to 12, months 12 to 24, and months 0 to 24, and no graphic display was used to show the main effects at 6 months. Because the most significant findings were at 6 months for both groups, the inclusion of this time interval would be beneficial.

The authors did an excellent job describing the results of the study and the potential benefits of fingolimod in patients with MS.

A. Minagar, MD

Ginkgo biloba does not improve cognitive function in MS: A randomized placebo-controlled trial

Lovera JF, Kim E, Heriza E, et al (Louisiana State Univ Health Sciences Ctr—New Orleans; Portland VA Med Ctr, OR; et al)

Neurology 79:1278-1284, 2012

Objective.—To determine whether *Ginkgo biloba* extract (ginkgo) improves cognitive function in persons with multiple sclerosis (MS).

Methods.—Persons with MS from the Seattle and Portland VA clinics and adjacent communities who scored 1 SD or more below the mean on one of 4 neuropsychological tests (Stroop Test, California Verbal Learning Test II [CVLT-II], Controlled Oral Word Association Test [COWAT], and Paced Auditory Serial Addition Task [PASAT]) were randomly assigned to receive either one 120-mg tablet of ginkgo (EGb-761; Willmar Schwabe GmbH and Co, Germany) or one placebo tablet twice a day for 12 weeks. As the primary outcome, we compared the performance of the 2 groups on the 4 tests at exit after adjusting for baseline performance.

Results.—Fifty-nine subjects received placebo and 61 received ginkgo; 1 participant receiving placebo and 3 receiving ginkgo were lost to follow-up. Two serious adverse events (AEs) (myocardial infarction and severe depression) believed to be unrelated to the treatment occurred in the ginkgo group; otherwise, there were no significant differences in AEs. The differences (ginkgo − placebo) at exit in the z scores for the cognitive tests were as follows: PASAT −0.2 (95% confidence interval [CI]-0.5 to 0.1); Stroop Test −0.5 (95% CI −0.9 to −0.1); COWAT 0.0 (95% CI −0.2 to 0.3); and CVLT-II 0.0 (95% CI −0.3 to 0.3); none was statistically significant.

Conclusions.—Treatment with ginkgo 120 mg twice a day did not improve cognitive performance in persons with MS.

▶ The authors present the results of a randomized, placebo-controlled, intent-to-treat study comparing the effects of ginkgo biloba on cognitive impairment in a cohort of patients with multiple sclerosis (MS). A total of 121 patients with MS were randomly assigned to receive either 120 mg ginkgo (EGb-761) twice per day or placebo twice per day for 12 weeks. Primary outcome measures included the patients' scores on a series of neuropsychological assessments, designed to measure cognitive functioning in the areas of working memory, memory, sustained attention, selective attention, speed, response inhibition, and verbal fluency. Final data analysis indicated no statistically significant differences between groups in changes from baseline to the end of the study on any of the measures of cognitive function. However, some minor improvements were noted, which could be clinically relevant.

The authors report study limitations to include underrepresented minorities, short duration of ginkgo biloba intake (12 weeks), and minimal impairments in subjects at baseline. Study findings may have been strengthened by providing rationale for excluding those patients (n = 7) whose Beck Depression Inventory scores were higher than 28, indicating severe depression, as severe depression has been reported to be significantly correlated with cognitive impairments, and many patients with MS are severely depressed. Including stratifying results may have provided insight into possible cognitive benefits of ginkgo biloba in this select group of patients. Further, the mean age of the subjects in this study was 51.3 (ginkgo group) and 53.0 (placebo group). However, the average age of initial MS diagnosis is reported to be around age 30, making the subjects in this study substantially older, which can be attributed to the environment from which the subjects were recruited (Veterans Administration Hospital). Replicating this study with a more diverse age group may yield different findings.

Overall, the study was well designed and provided insight into considerations of herbal supplements for cognitive impairments in patients with MS. However, because ginkgo biloba has been reported to cause liver problems, its use should be cautionary, at best, in patients with MS who are being treated with disease-modifying therapies processed through the liver, which are also known to potentially cause liver issues.

A. Minagar, MD

6 Neoplastic Disease

Refractory temporal lobe epilepsy caused by angiocentric glioma complicated with focal cortical dysplasia: a surgical case series

Liu CQ, Zhou J, Qi X, et al (Capital Med Univ, Beijing, People's Republic of China)
J Neurooncol 110:375-380, 2012

Angiocentric glioma (AG) is a rare, epilepsy-associated, low-grade neoplasm with a characteristic perivascular growth pattern. Here, we review the histological types, surgical interventions, and postoperative seizure in our three cases of AG with drug-resistant epilepsy. Some patients with AG present focal cortical dysplasia. For these patients, extended lesionectomy including the adjacent cortical dysplasia is necessary to achieve a seizure-free outcome. Surgical planning based on comprehensive evaluation of epilepsy and cortical dysplasia is therefore an important step for all patients.

▶ The authors of this interesting study present 3 cases of angiocentric glioma, a rare epilepsy-associated low-grade neoplasm. To date, only around 50 such cases have been reported in the literature. The authors discuss each of the 3 cases in terms of their presenting symptomology and management. These 3 cases not only represent rare lesions but also present 3 patients who are resistant to medical treatment of epilepsy. This case series constitutes a significant addition to the scientific literature in that it highlights the importance of completing a thorough preoperative evaluation, which includes video electroencephalogram as well as magnetoencephalography. This comprehensive approach to preoperative evaluation results in more favorable tumor resection, thus reducing the likelihood of recurring seizures or tumor relapse. The reported cases provide further information on a relatively new area of neuro-oncology with limited case examples. It also provides an in-depth discussion about management of all patients who have brain tumors with epilepsy.

A. Minagar, MD

An experimental study on acute brain radiation injury: Dynamic changes in proton magnetic resonance spectroscopy and the correlation with histopathology

Li H, Li J-P, Lin C-G, et al (State Key Laboratory of Oncology in Southern China, Guangzhou, People's Republic of China; Dongguan People's Hosp, People's Republic of China)

Eur J Radiol 81:3496-3503, 2012

Purpose.—To investigate the correlation between the alterations of single-voxel ^{1}H MRS and the histopathological characteristics of radiation brain injury following radiation.

Materials and Methods.—Twenty-seven rabbits were randomized into nine groups to receive radiation with a single dose of 25 Gy. The observation time points included a pre-radiation and 1, 2, 3, 4, 5, 6, 7, and 8 wk following radiation. Each treatment group underwent conventional MRI and single-voxel ^{1}H MRS, N-acetyl aspartate (NAA), choline (Cho), and creatine (Cr) were observed over the region of interest, and the presence or absence of lactate (Lac) and lipid (Lip) was detected. Histological specimens of each group were obtained after image acquisition.

Results.—The values of Cho were significantly increased in the first 3 wk, and decreased over the following 5 wk after radiation. Levels of NAA showed a trend toward a decrease 5 wk after radiation. The levels of Cr were not changed between before and after radiation. The Cho/NAA metabolic ratio was significantly increased in weeks 6, 7, and 8 following irradiation, compared to pre-radiation values. Vascular and glial injury appeared on 2 wk after RT in the histology samples, until 4 wk after RT, necrosis of the oligodendrocytes, neuronal degeneration and demyelination could be observed.

Conclusions.—MRS is sensitive to detect metabolic changes following radiation, and can be used in the early diagnosis of radiation brain injury.

▶ Radiation therapy (RT) is commonly used for treatment of tumors of head and neck and is one of the major treatment procedures for these patients. During RT, both cancerous and normal brain tissues are exposed to the radiation, and this, in turn, leads to both short-term and long-term brain injuries. Development of such neurologic deficits is a major restricting factor for application of RT in this cohort of patients. Patients who have undergone RT are imaged again, and routinely the question is raised as to whether the postradiation changes are indicative of radiation-induced necrosis of tumoral tissue or recurrence of the original tumor. One particular magnetic resonance imaging modality that is commonly used to differentiate these 2 scenarios is magnetic resonance spectroscopy (MRS). The authors of this valuable article have taken another step ahead and attempted to determine if the use of MRS can establish radiation-induced brain injury at an early stage. The authors devised an innovative rabbit model to assess acute radiation-induced brain injury using both MRS and histopathologic examination and sought any correlations between these 2 tests. Using both procedures, they determined that MRS was sensitive in detecting metabolic alterations after brain radiation and should be utilized for early diagnosis of radiation-induced brain injury. This study is valuable and unique because it brings neuroimaging and neuropathology together and provides treating physicians with a practical and noninvasive test for assessment of such a significant neurologic issue.

A. Minagar, MD

Differentiation of glioblastoma and primary CNS lymphomas using susceptibility weighted imaging

Radbruch A, Wiestler B, Kramp L, et al (Univ of Heidelberg Med Ctr, Germany; et al)

Eur J Radiol 82:552-556, 2013

Introduction.—Reliable differentiation between glioblastoma and primary CNS lymphoma (PCNSL) using conventional MR imaging is challenging, since both entities may show similar appearance on structural MR imaging. Here we analyzed if the appearance of intratumoural susceptibility signals (ITSS) on susceptibility weighted imaging (SWI) may differentiate between both entities.

Methods and Materials.—SWI and contrast enhanced T1-weighted images were acquired from 15 patients with newly diagnosed PCNSL (14 B-cell PCNSL, 1 T-cell PCNSL) and 117 patients with newly diagnosed glioblastoma with a 3 Tesla MR. Additional phase images were available in 8 patients with PCNSL and 88 patients with glioblastoma. Appearance of ITSS was assessed by two readers on SWI and the size of the enhancing lesions on contrast enhanced T1-weighted images were measured. Furthermore it was assessed if ITSS displayed more clearly on SWI or on phase images.

Results.—ITSS were detected in 106 (reader 1) and 109 (reader 2) glioblastoma, respectively. Both readers identified ITSS within the T-cell PCNSL while both readers did not identify any ITSS within the 14 Bcell PCNSL. Interrarter variability as determined by Cohen κ was excellent for glioblastoma ($\kappa = 0.938$) and for PCNSL ($\kappa = 1$). The medium size of the enhancing lesion of the glioblastoma that did not harbour ITSS was significantly smaller than the size of the glioblastoma exhibiting ITSS ($p < 0.008$). All identified ITSS displayed more clearly on SWI than on phase images.

Conclusion.—Presence of ITSS differentiates reliably between glioblastoma and B-cell PCNSL and provides a fast bases for the clinical decision without causing any postprocessing work.

▶ Clinicians who treat patients who have brain tumors occasionally encounter patients who present a significant diagnostic challenge, as neither the treating neuro-oncologist nor the neuroradiologist can say conclusively whether the brain lesion on magnetic resonance imaging is glioblastoma or central nervous system (CNS) lymphoma. Both of these lesions imitate each other, and because their treatments and prognoses are different, it is important to differentiate them as accurately as possible. The authors of this informative study have addressed this challenging situation by analyzing the appearance of intratumoral susceptibility signals (ITSS) on susceptibility weighted imaging (SWI) to set them apart. Two different readers assessed SWI and contrast-enhanced T2-weighted images of 15 patients with newly diagnosed primary CNS lymphoma (PCNSL) and 88 patients with glioblastoma. The investigators detected ITSS in patients with glioblastoma and also in patients with T-cell PCNSL. However, ITSS were not detected in patients with B-cell PCNSL. The authors concluded that ITSS enables clinicians to set glioblastoma apart from patients with B-cell PCNSL. This particular study enhances our knowledge about the fundamental differences between these 2 dissimilar tumors and presents a practical approach to solving this problem.

A. Minagar, MD

Long-term follow-up of vanishing tumors in the brain: How should a lesion mimicking primary CNS lymphoma be managed?

Okita Y, Narita Y, Miyakita Y, et al (Natl Cancer Ctr Hosp, Tokyo, Japan)

Clin Neurol Neurosurg 114:1217-1221, 2012

Objectives.—The spontaneous disappearance of a tumor is referred to as a vanishing tumor. Most vanishing tumors in the brain are eventually diagnosed as malignant tumors or multiple sclerosis. However, their long-term clinical course remains unclear. This study aims to elucidate the management of vanishing tumors in the brain.

Patients and Methods.—We defined a vanishing tumor as a case in which the tumor spontaneously disappeared or decreased to less than 70% of the initial tumor volume before definitive diagnosis and treatment (other than steroid treatment). Ten cases of vanishing tumors are reviewed.

Results.—Nine patients underwent biopsy at least once. Five patients, all of whom had malignant tumors (primary central nervous system lymphoma: 4, germinoma: 1) that recurred in 4–45 months (median: 7 months), underwent a second biopsy after the reappearance of the tumors. Five patients (tumefactive demyelinating lesion: 1, undiagnosed: 4) who had no relapse are alive, and their median follow-up time is 44 months. No cases have yet been reported of malignant brain tumors that recurred more than 5 years after spontaneous regression.

Conclusions.—Patients with vanishing tumors should be followed up carefully by magnetic resonance imaging for at least 5 years, even after the disappearance of an enhancing lesion.

▶ Neurologists and neurosurgeons around the globe often see patients with brain lesions that cannot be easily characterized by utilizing conventional neuroimaging techniques and spinal tap. In addition, many of these lesions decrease in size significantly or disappear either spontaneously or with systemic administration of corticosteroids. Diagnosis of these lesions is a formidable challenge for the clinicians, and doctors frequently end up doing brain biopsy for neuropathologic examination. Interestingly, most of these lesions turn out to be demyelinating lesions or malignant brain tumors. This report by Okita et al addresses such challenges and proposes a practical approach to treatment of these patients. This informative report defined a vanishing tumor as a case in which the tumor spontaneously disappeared or decreased to less than 70% of the initial tumor volume before definitive diagnosis and treatment. The authors reviewed 10 patients with vanishing tumors and followed them up for a median of 44 months with regular brain magnetic resonance imaging, even after the initial lesion had resolved. The authors conclude with the important practical recommendation that long-term follow-up of these patients with serial imaging is strongly recommended.

A. Minagar, MD

Diffusion Tensor Imaging Provides an Insight Into the Microstructure of Meningiomas, High-Grade Gliomas, and Peritumoral Edema

De Belder FE, Oot AR, Van Hecke W, et al (Antwerp Univ Hosp and Univ of Antwerp, Belgium; et al)

J Comput Assist Tomogr 36:577-582, 2012

Objective.—Fractional anisotropy (FA) is a measure for the degree of microstructural organization. Several studies have used FA values to assess microstructural organization of brain tumors and peritumoral edema. The purpose of our study was to validate FA and apparent diffusion constant (ADC) values in the diagnosis of meningiomas versus high-grade glial tumors, with the focus on the ability of diffusion tensor imaging (DTI) to reveal tumor ultrastructure. Our hypothesis was that FA and ADC values significantly differ between high-grade gliomas and meningiomas, and in the peritumoral edema.

Methods.—Diffusion tensor imaging values were obtained from 20 patients with meningiomas (21 tumors) and 15 patients with high-grade gliomas. Regions of interest were outlined in FA and ADC maps for solid-enhancing tumor tissue and peritumoral edema. Fractional anisotropy and ADC values were normalized by comparison to normal-appearing white matter (NAWM) in the contralateral hemisphere. Differences between meningiomas and high-grade gliomas were statistically analyzed.

Results.—Meningiomas showed a significantly higher FA tumor/FA NAWM ratio ($P = 0.0001$) and lower ADC tumor/ADC NAWM ratio ($P = 0.0008$) compared to high-grade gliomas. On average, meningiomas also showed higher FA values in peritumoral edema than high-grade gliomas ($P = 0.016$). Apparent diffusion constant values of peritumoral edema for the 2 tumor groups did not differ significantly ($P = 0.5$).

Conclusions.—Diffusion tensor imaging can be used to reveal microstructural differences between meningiomas and high-grade gliomas and may contribute toward predicting the histopathology of intracranial tumors.

We advocate that diffusion tensor imaging should be included in the standard imaging protocol for patients with intracranial tumors.

▶ Introduction of magnetic resonance imaging (MRI) and its various sequences has fundamentally altered our understanding and management of brain tumors. Now more than ever before in history we can noninvasively visualize brain tumors and, based on the neuroimaging findings, meticulously plan the next step in management of these lesions. The authors of this interesting neuroimaging and neuro-oncology article have used fractional anisotropy (FA), an index of the degree of microstructural organization of tissues, and apparent diffusion constant (ADC) to neuroradiologically differentiate meningiomas from high-grade gliomas, with the focus on the ability of diffusion tensor imaging (DTI) to reveal tumor ultrastructure. The investigators' null hypothesis was that FA and ADC values significantly differentiate these tumors from each other. The authors looked at FA and ADC maps of 20 patients with meningiomas and 15 patients with high-grade gliomas. They reported that application of FA, ADC map, and DTI could separate these lesions meaningfully and may be able to predict the underlying neuropathology of the intracranial tumor. The authors' comment about adding DTI to the standard MRI protocols for visualizing brain tumor is excellent with great practical use. This informative article paves the path toward better use of MRI for diagnosis and differentiation of central nervous system tumors and has significant clinical application for neuro-oncologists and neurosurgeons.

A. Minagar, MD

A randomized trial on the efficacy of methylphenidate and modafinil for improving cognitive functioning and symptoms in patients with a primary brain tumor

Gehring K, Patwardhan SY, Collins R, et al (Tilburg Univ, The Netherlands; Univ of Houston, TX; The Michael E. DeBakey VA Med Ctr, Houston, TX; et al)
J Neurooncol 107:165-174, 2012

Limited research is available regarding the efficacy of psychostimulants in treating cognitive function in primary brain tumor patients. An open-label, randomized, pilot trial examined both the general and differential efficacy of 4 weeks of methylphenidate (MPH) and modafinil (MOD) in 24 brain tumor patients. Participants completed cognitive tests and self-report measures of fatigue, sleep disturbance, mood and quality of life at baseline and after 4 weeks.

Following stimulant treatment, there was evidence of a beneficial effect on test performance in speed of processing and executive function requiring divided attention. Patients with the greatest deficit in executive function at baseline appeared to derive the greatest benefit following stimulant therapy. Inconsistent, differential effects were found on a measure of attention in favor of MPH and on a measure of processing speed in favor of MOD. There was also evidence of a general beneficial effect on patient-reported measures of fatigue, mood, and quality of life, with no statistically significant differences between treatment arms in these measures over time. The results from this small pilot study should be interpreted with caution, but appear to warrant additional research, in larger study samples, targeting fatigue, processing speed and executive function, and exploring different doses of stimulants. Future studies may also wish to explore the specific patient factors that may be associated with responsiveness to psychostimulant treatment.

▶ Primary brain tumors and their treatment modalities are commonly associated with significant cognitive decline, which leaves patients encountering major restrictions imposed on their daily living activities. These patients usually suffer from attention deficit and slowness of their capabilities to process data. Physicians who treat patients with primary brain tumors and cognitive decline have limited therapeutic options because this is an underresearched field and a significantly unknown area.

This article highlights the efforts of a group of investigators who, in the context of an open-labeled clinical trial, have assessed the impact of the psychostimulants, methylphenidate, and modafinil in treatment of cognitive deficits in these patients. During this pilot trial, the investigators determined both the general and differential impacts of 4 weeks' treatment with methylphenidate and modafinil in 24 patients with primary brain tumor. They found that treatment of these patients with these medications was associated with improvement on certain test performance in speed of processing and executive function. This study is very interesting and has great practical use because it addresses a frequently observed and often inadequately addressed problem in patients with primary brain tumor. The shortcomings of this study were the small number of participants and being open labeled, which may cause certain bias in interpretation of the test results. Despite these issues, it certainly is a great start for larger double-blind, placebo-controlled clinical trials to follow this preliminary study.

A. Minagar, MD

Valproic acid sensitizes human glioma cells for temozolomide and γ-radiation

Van Nifterik KA, Van den Berg J, Slotman BJ, et al (VU Univ Med Ctr, Amsterdam, The Netherlands; et al)

J Neurooncol 107:61-67, 2012

Temozolomide (TMZ) is given in addition to radiotherapy in glioma patients, but its interaction with the commonly prescribed antiepileptic drug valproic acid (VPA) is largely unknown. Induction of DNA demethylation by VPA could potentially induce expression of the O^6-methylguanine-DNA-methyltransferase (MGMT) protein, causing resistance to TMZ and thereby antagonizing its effect. Therefore, this study investigates the interaction between VPA, TMZ, and γ-radiation. Two glioma cell lines were used that differ in TMZ sensitivity caused by the absence (D384) or presence (T98) of the MGMT protein. VPA was administered before

(24/48 h) or after (24 h) single doses of γ-radiation; or, after 24 h, VPA treatment was accompanied by a single dose of TMZ for another 24 h. For trimodal treatment the combination of VPA and TMZ was followed by single doses of γ-radiation. In both cell lines VPA caused enhancement of the radiation response after preincubation ($DMF_{0.2}$ 1.4 and 1.5) but not after postirradiation ($DMF_{0.2}$ 1.1 and 1.0). The combination of VPA and TMZ caused enhanced cytotoxicity ($DMF_{0.2}$ 1.7) in both the TMZ-sensitive cell line (D384) and the TMZ-resistant cell line (T98). The combination of VPA and TMZ caused a significant radiation enhancement ($DMF_{0.2}$ 1.9 and 1.6) that was slightly more effective than that of VPA alone. VPA does not antagonize the cytotoxic effects of TMZ. Preincubation with VPA enhances the effect of both γ-radiation and TMZ, in both a TMZ-sensitive and a TMZ-resistant human glioma cell line. VPA combined with TMZ may lead to further enhancement of the radiation response.

▶ Patients with glioma who present with seizures are often treated with a potent antiepileptic—valproic acid (VPA). VPA induces demethylation of DNA, which, in turn, can induce expression of O-6-methylguanine-DNA-methyltransferase protein (MGMT). Such upregulation and expression of MGMT can theoretically cause resistance to therapeutic effects of temozolomide (TMZ). This by itself can pose a significant challenge to neuro-oncologists.

The authors of this original research article addressed this issue and explored the validity of such a concept. They used an in vitro model to assess the interactions among TMZ, VPA, and γ-radiation. This significant study reveals an opposite finding that VPA does not antagonize the cytotoxic effect of TMZ, and preincubation with VPA enhances the effect of both γ-radiation and TMZ in both a TMZ-sensitive and a TMZ-resistant human glioma cell line. This laboratory finding has a huge clinical application for treatment of patients with glioma and adds more to our present knowledge about treatment of gliomas. Another article by Ryu et al[1] supports such findings and introduces VPA as an anticancer drug that may have synergistic effects with TMZ against gliomas.

A. Minagar, MD

Reference

1. Ryu CH, Yoon WS, Park KY, et al. Valproic acid downregulates the expression of MGMT and sensitizes temozolomide-resistant glioma cells. *J Biomed Biotechnol.* 2012:987495.

Risk of ischemia in glioma surgery: comparison of first and repeat procedures

Dützmann S, Geßler F, Bink A, et al (Johann Wolfgang Goethe-Univ, Frankfurt/Main, Germany)

J Neurooncol 107:599-607, 2012

The role of repeat resection in the multimodal treatment of gliomas is unclear. Repeat surgery theoretically carries a higher risk of inducing neurological deficits, which might even out any advantage of cytoreduction. We sought to determine whether the occurrence of perioperative infarction is higher for repeat surgery than for first surgery, and sought to identify factors associated with the occurrence of postoperative infarction. Therefore, we searched our database to identify patients who were operated for primary or recurrent glial tumors between October 2007 and October 2010. We analyzed 177 procedures, of which 130 (73.4%) were first surgeries and 47 (26.5%) were repeat. Initial WHO grades, KPS scores, and age were evenly distributed between the groups. Forty-six (26.0%) patients had new DWI lesions on their postoperative MRI scan. Eighteen (10.2%) patients had new lesions greater than 4 cm^3. Among these were 11 (6.2%) patients, for whom the new lesion caused neurologic deficit. There was no difference between first and repeat surgery with regard to the occurrence of new DWI lesions (27.7 vs. 21.3%, $P = 0.77$) or neurological deficits (10.0 vs. 10.6%, $P = 1.0$). Tumor location in the insula, operculum, and temporal lobe was found to be significantly associated with the occurrence of new DWI lesions. We conclude that repeat surgery should not be withheld as a treatment option for patients with recurrent gliomas for fear of a higher risk of postoperative infarction or new neurologic deficit than the first surgery.

▶ Existing treatment modalities for malignant gliomas include chemotherapy, surgical resection, and radiation therapy. Many research papers have addressed various aspects of these procedures and have focused on their benefits vs disadvantages and adverse effects. However, the role of repeat surgical resection of the recurring tumor, if and whenever possible, has not received much attention. In this informative article, the authors have addressed the risk of ischemic infarct during the initial glioma respective surgery vs repeat resection. The methodology of study was solely based on retrospective data collection and analysis to find new ischemic lesions on diffusion-weighted brain magnetic resonance imaging. They could not find any significant differences in occurrence of ischemic strokes during the first surgical procedure vs the repeat resection procedure. They concluded that in patients with recurrent gliomas, surgical treatment should not be withheld because the risk of perisurgical ischemic stroke is not increased. This valuable study addresses a practical question that arises every day and provides clinicians with useful pragmatic points as to how to approach this problem.

A. Minagar, MD

Differentiation between Brain Glioblastoma Multiforme and Solitary Metastasis: Qualitative and Quantitative Analysis Based on Routine MR Imaging

Chen XZ, Yin XM, Ai L, et al (Capital Med Univ, Beijing, P.R. China; China Coal General Hosp, Beijing, P.R. China)

AJNR Am J Neuroradiol 33:1907-1912, 2012

Background and Purpose.—The differentiation between cerebral GBM and solitary MET is clinically important and may be radiologically challenging. Our hypothesis is that routine MR imaging with qualitative and quantitative analysis is helpful for this differentiation.

Materials and Methods.—Forty-five GBM and 21 solitary metastases were retrospectively identified, with their preoperative routine MR imaging analyzed. According to the comparison of the area of peritumoral T2 prolongation with that of the lesion, the tumors were classified into grade I (prolongation area ≤ tumor area) and grade II (prolongation area > tumor area). The signal intensities of peritumoral T2 prolongation were measured on T2WI and normalized to the values of the contralateral normal regions by calculating the ratios. The ratio (nSI) of both types of tumors was compared in grade I, grade II, and in tumors without grading. The best cutoff values to optimize the sensitivity and specificity were determined for optimal differentiation.

Results.—The nSI of GBM was significantly higher than that of MET without T2 prolongation grading ($P < .001$), resulting in AUC = 0.725. The difference was significant ($P = .014$) in grade I tumors (GBM, 38; MET, 9), with AUC = 0.741, and in grade II tumors (GBM, 7; MET, 12), with AUC = 0.869 ($P = .017$). Both types of tumors showed a different propensity in T2 prolongation grading ($\chi^2 = 12.079$, $P = .001$).

Conclusions.—Combined with qualitative and quantitative analysis of peritumoral T2 prolongation, routine MR imaging can help in the differentiation between brain GBM and solitary MET.

▶ Differentiating the brain glioblastoma multiforme (GBM) from solitary brain metastasis is a difficult but necessary task that needs to be done accurately to plan further treatment of these lesions. These cancerous lesions on routine brain MRI appear similar and present with the presence of mass that contains necrosis, postcontrast enhancement, and peritumoral segments with T2-weighted prolongation.

The authors of this interesting and practically useful article hypothesized that routine MRI of brain with qualitative and quantitative analyses should enable clinicians to differentiate these lesions. The authors examined 45 GBMs and 21 solitary brain metastases and found that MRI analysis of the peritumoral area, based on prolongation of T2-weighted signal intensities, was able to differentiate these 2 lesions. They concluded that use of routine brain MRI with both qualitative and quantitative analyses of the peritumoral T2 prolongation characteristic can assist clinicians in differentiating these 2 lesions. Although the number of analyzed specimens in this study is small, it still provides practical methods to address such a diagnostic challenge.

A. Minagar, MD

Detection of *IDH1* mutation in the plasma of patients with glioma

Boisselier B, Gállego Pérez-Larraya J, Rossetto M, et al (Université Pierre et Marie Curie-Paris 6, France; Groupe Hospitalier Pitié-Salpêtrière, Paris, France; et al)

Neurology 79:1693-1698, 2012

Objective.—The $IDH1^{R132H}$ mutation is both a strong prognostic predictor and a diagnostic hallmark of gliomas and therefore has major clinical relevance. Here, we developed a new technique to detect the $IDH1^{R132H}$ mutation in the plasma of patients with glioma.

Methods.—Small-size DNA (150-250 base pairs) was extracted from the plasma of 31 controls and 80 patients with glioma with known $IDH1^{R132H}$ status and correlated with MRI data. The $\mathrm{IDH1}^{\mathrm{R132H}}$ mutation was detected by a combination of coamplification at lower denaturation temperature and digital PCR.

Results.—The small size DNA concentration was 1.2 ng/mL (range 0.1-6.6) in controls vs 1.2 ng/mL (range 0.1-50.3) in patients with glioma (p = not significant) and 0.9 ng/mL (0.0-3.0) in low-grade gliomas vs 1.5 ng/mL in high-grade gliomas ($p < 0.01$). The small size DNA concentration correlated with enhancing tumor volume (1.6 ng/mL [0.4-24.9] when <10 cm^3 and 14.0 ng/mL [0.6-50.3] when ≥10 cm^3). The $IDH1^{R132H}$ mutation was detected in 15 out of 25 plasma DNA mixtures (60%) from patients with mutated tumors and in none of the 14 patients with a nonmutated tumor. The sensitivity increased with enhancing tumor volume (3/9 in nonenhancing tumors, 6/10 for enhancing volume < 10 cm^3, and 6/6 for enhancing volume < 10 cm^3).

Conclusion.—With a specificity of 100% and a sensitivity related to the tumor volume and contrast enhancement, $IDH1^{R132H}$ identification has a valuable diagnostic accuracy in patients not amenable to biopsy.

▶ In this interesting article, the authors present findings from a study conducted to assess the diagnostic accuracy of $IDH1^{R132H}$ mutation in patients with glioma. Study findings reveal that extracting small size DNA from patients diagnosed with glioma provided significantly accurate clinical information, with $IDH1^{R132H}$ mutations detected in 60% of patients with mutated tumors and none detected in patients with nonmutated tumor. Furthermore, the small size DNA was significantly correlated with enhancing tumor volume and showed significant specificity in detecting low-grade versus high-grade gliomas. The findings of this study offer valuable insight to diagnostic options in patients with glioma. Obtaining small size DNA for the diagnosis of glioma is a less invasive procedure than biopsy and could be a feasible and preferred alternative in patient diagnosis. Further, obtaining such relevant clinical information could alter the course of treatment and patient management in patients with glioma. The extraction of small size DNA to identify $IDH1^{R132H}$ mutation could become the mainstay for clinical decision making in treating patients with glioma, particularly in those patients with gliomas nonamenable to biopsy.

A. Minagar, MD

Correlation between language function and the left arcuate fasciculus detected by diffusion tensor imaging tractography after brain tumor surgery

Hayashi Y, Kinoshita M, Nakada M, et al (Kanazawa Univ, Japan)

J Neurosurg 117:839-843, 2012

Object.—Disturbance of the arcuate fasciculus in the dominant hemisphere is thought to be associated with language-processing disorders, including conduction aphasia. Although the arcuate fasciculus can be visualized in vivo with diffusion tensor imaging (DTI) tractography, its involvement in functional processes associated with language has not been shown dynamically using DTI tractography. In the present study, to clarify the participation of the arcuate fasciculus in language functions, postoperative changes in the arcuate fasciculus detected by DTI tractography were evaluated chronologically in relation to postoperative changes in language function after brain tumor surgery.

Methods.—Preoperative and postoperative arcuate fasciculus area and language function were examined in 7 right-handed patients with a brain tumor in the left hemisphere located in proximity to part of the arcuate fasciculus. The arcuate fasciculus was depicted, and its area was calculated using DTI tractography. Language functions were measured using the Western Aphasia Battery (WAB).

Results.—After tumor resection, visualization of the arcuate fasciculus was increased in 5 of the 7 patients, and the total WAB score improved in 6 of the 7 patients. The relative ratio of postoperative visualized area of the arcuate fasciculus to preoperative visualized area of the arcuate fasciculus was increased in association with an improvement in postoperative language function ($p = 0.0039$).

Conclusions.—The role of the left arcuate fasciculus in language functions can be evaluated chronologically in vivo by DTI tractography after brain tumor surgery. Because increased postoperative visualization of the fasciculus was significantly associated with postoperative improvement in language functions, the arcuate fasciculus may play an important role in language function, as previously thought. In addition, postoperative changes in the arcuate fasciculus detected by DTI tractography could represent a predicting factor for postoperative language-dependent functional outcomes in patients with brain tumor.

▶ Arcuate fasciculus of the dominant hemisphere is perceived to be involved in language functions, and its disturbances in the dominant hemisphere are associated with language-processing disorders such as conduction aphasia. Neuroanatomically, arcuate fasciculus can be visualized using diffusion tensor imaging. However, its actual function associated with language using diffusion tensor imaging tractography has not yet been visualized.

In this interesting neuroimaging study, the authors assessed its role in language activities by studying post–brain tumor surgery changes using diffusion tensor imaging tractography. The authors examined arcuate fasciculus in 7 right-handed patients with brain tumors. The brain tumors were located in the left hemisphere in the area near the arcuate fasciculus. The authors assessed the language functions using the Western Aphasia Battery. The results of this study demonstrated improvement of language function in 6 of 7 patients, and this was associated with an increase in visualization of arcuate fasciculus. This study is among the first neuroimaging studies to assess the role of arcuate fasciculus objectively and chronologically. The knowledge gained from this study can not only be used in our practice toward predicting postoperative language changes in patients with brain tumor who will undergo surgery, but it also enhances behavioral neurology and the neuroanatomy of the language and its functions.

A. Minagar, MD

Cognitive functioning early after surgery of gliomas in eloquent areas

Satoer D, Vork J, Visch-Brink E, et al (Univ Med Ctr, Rotterdam, The Netherlands)
J Neurosurg 117:831-838, 2012

Object.—Patients with gliomas frequently have cognitive deficits, and surgery can exacerbate these deficits. Preoperative assessment is therefore crucial in patients undergoing surgery for glioma in eloquent areas, because the proximity of functional areas increases the risk of permanent postoperative cognitive disturbances. Although pre- and postoperative language and motor function in patients with glioma have been investigated frequently, data on good cognition studies are scarce. Most studies have focused on clinical neurological functioning or have only used brief neurological instruments. The authors investigated whether surgery for glioma in eloquent areas influences cognition early after surgery, by using an elaborate test protocol.

Methods.—Twenty-eight patients with gliomas of the left hemisphere in language and nonlanguage areas were assessed before and 3 months after surgery with a comprehensive neuropsychological test protocol. The authors performed a correlation analysis between change in cognitive performance and tumor characteristics (that is, location, volume, pathological features, and histological grade) and between cognitive change and treatment-related factors (the extent of the resection and postoperative treatment with chemo- and radiotherapy).

Results.—Both pre- and postoperatively, the mean performance of the patients was worse than the performance of the normal population in the language domain, the memory domain, and the executive functions ($p < 0.05$). Postoperatively, a decline was found in the language domain ($t = 2.34$, $p = 0.027$) and in the executive functions ($t = 2.45$, $p = 0.022$). However, cognitive change postsurgery was influenced by the location of the tumor; the decrease of cognitive score in the language domain was only observed in patients with tumors in or close to language areas ($t = 2.33$, $p = 0.029$). No effect on cognitive change was found for the other tumor characteristics and treatment-related factors.

Conclusions.—This study underlines the importance of the use of a neuropsychological test protocol before and after surgery in patients with glioma, because several tasks in the domains of language, memory, and executive functions appeared to deteriorate after surgery. Tumor resection in language areas increases the risk of cognitive deficits in the language domain postoperatively.

▶ These authors discuss the use of a comprehensive neuropsychological test protocol to assess cognitive and executive functioning in patients presenting with glioma. Findings revealed that using the neuropsychological test protocol before and after surgical resection of glioma in the reported study sample enabled investigators to see a distinction between the patients and the normal population before surgery in the domains of language, memory, and executive functions. Additionally, postsurgical differences were noted in the same areas but were significantly correlated with tumor location. This study is important because it provides insight into the effects of glioma on cognitive functioning, both before and after surgery. Because tumor resection in the language areas of the brain increases the risk of language deficits, neuropsychological tests should be conducted prior to considering surgery to determine the patient's current level of cognition. If the glioma is located in a language area of the brain and the patient presents with significant language deficiency preoperatively, other treatment options may need to be explored to prevent further cognitive decline. This interesting article also enhances our knowledge in the behavioral neurology aspects of patients with glioma prior and after the performance of a neurosurgical procedure.

A. Minagar, MD

Diagnostic performance of whole brain volume perfusion CT in intra-axial brain tumors: Preoperative classification accuracy and histopathologic correlation

Xyda A, Haberland U, Klotz E, et al (Georg-August Univ, Goettingen, Germany; Siemens AG Healthcare Sector, Forchheim, Germany; et al)

Eur J Radiol 81:4105-4111, 2012

Background.—To evaluate the preoperative diagnostic power and classification accuracy of perfusion parameters derived from whole brain volume perfusion CT (VPCT) in patients with cerebral tumors.

Methods.—Sixty-three patients (31 male, 32 female; mean age 55.6 ± 13.9 years), with MRI findings suspected of cerebral lesions, underwent VPCT. Two readers independently evaluated VPCT data. Volumes of interest (VOIs) were marked circumscript around the tumor according to maximum intensity projection volumes, and then mapped automatically onto the cerebral blood volume (CBV), flow (CBF) and permeability Ktrans perfusion datasets. A second VOI was placed in the contra lateral cortex, as control. Correlations among perfusion values, tumor grade, cerebral hemisphere and VOIs were evaluated. Moreover, the diagnostic power of VPCT parameters, by means of positive and negative predictive value, was analyzed.

Results.—Our cohort included 32 high-grade gliomas WHO III/IV, 18 low-grade I/II, 6 primary cerebral lymphomas, 4 metastases and 3 tumor-like lesions. Ktrans demonstrated the highest sensitivity, specificity and positive predictive value, with a cut-off point of 2.21 mL/100 mL/min, for both the comparisons between high-grade versus low-grade and low-grade versus primary cerebral lymphomas. However, for the differentiation between high-grade and primary cerebral lymphomas, CBF and CBV proved to have 100% specificity and 100% positive predictive value, identifying preoperatively all the histopathologically proven high-grade gliomas.

Conclusion.—Volumetric perfusion data enable the hemodynamic assessment of the entire tumor extent and provide a method of preoperative differentiation among intra-axial cerebral tumors with promising diagnostic accuracy.

▶ These authors present findings of a study aimed at determining the preoperative diagnostic and classification accuracy of perfusion parameters from whole brain volume perfusion computed tomography (VPCT) in patients with cerebral tumors. This well-designed study found that the use of cerebral blood flow and cerebral blood volume provided 100% specificity and 100% positive predictive values in identifying high-grade gliomas. Because this information can be obtained preoperatively, its use in the diagnosis and management of patients with cerebral tumors is a remarkable revelation, which could alter treatment approaches. Such diagnostic abilities further expand the applicability of imaging in the diagnostic workup of patients. This large, prospective study provides a significant contribution to the scientific literature because it is the first of its kind to prospectively study the use of VPCT in patients with various tumor lesions. Using VPCT in the differential diagnosis of patients with cerebral tumors should be considered in standard preoperative clinical decision making. The findings of this excellent original article enable treating physicians of patients with cerebral tumors to identify better treatment approaches.

A. Minagar, MD

Diffuse brainstem glioma: prognostic factors

Dellaretti M, Reyns N, Touzet G, et al (CHRU Hôpital Roger Salengro, Lille, France; et al)

J Neurosurg 117:810-814, 2012

Object.—Brainstem gliomas were regarded as a single entity prior to the advent of MRI; however, several studies investigating MRI have recognized that these lesions are a heterogeneous group, and certain subgroups have a better prognosis for long-term survival. The aim of this study was to conduct a retrospective analysis of prognostic factors of patients with brainstem gliomas confirmed by histopathological diagnosis, particularly regarding assessment of whether histological grade, age, and MRI findings are prognostic factors for patient survival.

Methods.—The study evaluated 100 patients diagnosed with brainstem glioma. There were 63 adults (40 men and 23 women; age range 18–75 years, mean 41 years) and 37 children (19 boys and 18 girls; age range 2–12 years, mean 6.9 years).

Results.—The mean overall survival of this population, measured from the date of biopsy, was 57 months for diffuse low-grade glioma and 13.8 months for diffuse high-grade glioma ($p < 0.001$). The mean survival among patients with nonenhancing contrast lesions on MRI was 54.2 months, whereas for patients with enhancing lesions, it was 21.7 months ($p < 0.001$). Comparisons between the Kaplan-Meier survival curves of adults and children revealed similar median survival periods of 25 and 16 months, respectively ($p > 0.05$). The multivariate analysis (Cox proportional hazards regression) revealed that only histological grade was a significant prognostic factor ($p < 0.001$).

Conclusions.—The study revealed that histological grade and MRI features were significant prognostic factors for survival in these patients, but in multivariate analysis, only histological grade remained a significant factor.

▶ The authors present findings from a retrospective review of diffuse brainstem glioma in 100 patients (63 adults and 37 children) to assess for potential prognostic factors. Because patients with brainstem glioma and their family members always question their treating physicians about the long-term prognosis of this tumor, it is very important to provide them with some meaningful answers. Historically, the treatment of brainstem gliomas has been primarily based on magnetic resonance imaging (MRI) findings with no consideration given to histopathologic diagnosis. The current retrospective study makes a significant contribution to the published literature as it highlights the importance of histologic grade as a factor in survival. Based on the findings of the current study, both findings on MRI and histologic grade should be considered in the treatment and management of patients suffering from diffuse brainstem glioma. In addition, the authors emphasize the role of histologic grade as a significant prognostic factor in these patients. Having a more in-depth understanding of the role of histologic grade may allow treating physicians to pursue alternative modes of treatment, such as long-term therapies, which may have been previously avoided because of presumed time allowances. Although this study is a retrospective review of data and comes with its potential limitations because of the lack of sufficient knowledge about diffuse brainstem gliomas, it is still a great effort to improve our understanding of the prognosis of these tumors.

A. Minagar, MD

Cranial Irradiation Increases Risk of Stroke in Pediatric Brain Tumor Survivors

Campon CJ, Kranick SM, Kasner SE, et al (The Perelman School of Medicine at the Univ of Pennsylvania, Philadelphia; et al)

Stroke 43:3035-3040, 2012

Background and Purpose.—The purposes of this study were to determine the incidence of neurovascular events as late complications in pediatric patients with brain tumor and to evaluate radiation as a risk factor.

Methods.—Patients were ascertained using the tumor database of a pediatric tertiary care center. Included patients had a primary brain tumor, age birth to 21 years, initial treatment January 1, 1993, to December 31, 2002, and at least 2 visits with neuro-oncology. Radiation exposure included: whole brain, whole brain plus a focal boost, or focal brain. The primary outcome was stroke or transient ischemic attack.

Results.—Of 431 subjects, 14 had 19 events of stroke or transient ischemic attack over a median follow-up of 6.3 years. The incidence rate was 548/100 000 person-years. Overall, 61.5% of subjects received radiation, including 13 of 14 subjects with events. Median time from first radiation to first event was 4.9 years. The stroke/transient ischemic attack hazard ratio for any brain irradiation was 8.0 (95% CI, 1.05–62; $P = 0.045$); for the circle of Willis, radiation was 9.0 (95% CI, 1.2–70; $P = 0.035$); and for focal noncircle of Willis, radiation was 3.4 (95% CI, 0.21–55; $P = 0.38$).

Conclusions.—The incidence of neurovascular events in this population is 100-fold higher than in the general pediatric population and cranial irradiation is an important risk factor. By defining the incidence of this late effect, physicians are better able to counsel parents regarding treatment, monitor patients at risk, and target a population for primary stroke prevention in future studies.

► Although radiation therapy provides clinicians with a great tool for treatment of pediatric patients with brain tumors, it also has its own morbidities and complications. These complications may be even more prominent in children than adults since their brains are not fully developed and they are still evolving and growing.[1-3] Some of the better recognized complications of cranial radiation include neuroendocrine abnormalities,[4] cognitive decline,[1,2] cavernous malformations,[5] and vasculopathy, including stroke.[1,6-11] In addition, because of improvements in the survival rate of the children with brain tumors and the fact they are still growing, further research about the late complications of radiation therapy is necessary.

The authors of this informative article reviewed the data collected at a pediatric tertiary care center about children with brain tumors who were treated with 3 modes of radiation therapy for development of stroke or transient ischemic attack. The results of this study revealed an increased risk of stroke, up to 100-fold higher, in this population compared with the general population. Although this study was a retrospective analysis of data with its inherent limitations, it alerts clinicians to the risk of stroke in this group of patients and further emphasizes the fact that we should always follow this particular group of patients for the danger of upcoming stroke. It also emphasizes that we need to do larger prospective studies for primary stroke prevention in these patients.

A. Minagar, MD

References

1. Crossen JR, Garwood D, Glatstein E, Neuwelt EA. Neurobehavioral sequelae of cranial irradiation in adults: a review of radiation-induced encephalopathy. *J Clin Oncol.* 1994;12:627-642.
2. Fouladi M, Gilger E, Kocak M, et al. Intellectual and functional outcome of children 3 years old or younger who have CNS malignancies. *J Clin Oncol.* 2005;23: 7152-7160.
3. Monje ML, Vogel H, Masek M, Ligon KL, Fisher PG, Palmer TD. Impaired human hippocampal neurogenesis after treatment for central nervous system malignancies. *Ann Neurol.* 2007;62:515-520.
4. Gurney JG, Kadan-Lottick NS, Packer RJ, et al. Endocrine and cardiovascular late effects among adult survivors of childhood brain tumors: Childhood Cancer Survivor Study. *Cancer.* 2003;97:663-673.
5. Burn S, Gunny R, Phipps K, Gaze M, Hayward R. Incidence of cavernoma development in children after radiotherapy for brain tumors. *J Neurosurg.* 2007;106: 379-383.
6. Fouladi M, Langston J, Mulhern R, et al. Silent lacunar lesions detected by magnetic resonance imaging of children with brain tumors: a late sequela of therapy. *J Clin Oncol.* 2000;18:824-831.
7. Belka C, Budach W, Kortmann RD, Bamberg M. Radiation induced CNS toxicity—molecular and cellular mechanisms. *Br J Cancer.* 2001;85:1233-1239.
8. Giglio P, Gilbert MR. Cerebral radiation necrosis. *Neurologist.* 2003;9:180-188.
9. Bitzer M, Topka H. Progressive cerebral occlusive disease after radiation therapy. *Stroke.* 1995;26:131-136.
10. Grenier Y, Tomita T, Marymont MH, Byrd S, Burrowes DM. Late postirradiation occlusive vasculopathy in childhood medulloblastoma. Report of two cases. *J Neurosurg.* 1998;89:460-464.
11. Rogers LR. Cerebrovascular complications in cancer patients. *Neurol Clin.* 2003; 21:167-192.

Comparison of a Strategy Favoring Early Surgical Resection vs a Strategy Favoring Watchful Waiting in Low-Grade Gliomas

Jakola AS, Myrmel KS, Kloster R, et al (St Olavs Univ Hosp, Trondheim; Univ Hosp of Northern Norway, Tromsø)
JAMA 308:1881-1888, 2012

Context.—There are no controlled studies on surgical treatment of diffuse low-grade gliomas (LGGs), and management is controversial.

Objective.—To examine survival in population-based parallel cohorts of LGGs from 2 Norwegian university hospitals with different surgical treatment strategies.

Design, Setting, and Patients.—Both neurosurgical departments are exclusive providers in adjacent geographical regions with regional referral practices. In hospital A diagnostic biopsies followed by a "wait and scan" approach has been favored (biopsy and watchful waiting), while early resections have been advocated in hospital B (early resection). Thus, the treatment strategy in individual patients has been highly dependent on the patient's residential address. Histopathology specimens from all adult patients diagnosed with LGG from 1998 through 2009 underwent a blinded histopathological review to ensure uniform classification and inclusion. Follow-up ended April 11, 2011. There were 153 patients (66 from the center favoring biopsy and watchful waiting and 87 from the center favoring early resection) with diffuse LGGs included.

Main Outcome Measure.—The prespecified primary end point was overall survival based on regional comparisons without adjusting for administered treatment.

Results.—Initial biopsy alone was carried out in 47 (71%) patients served by the center favoring biopsy and watchful waiting and in 12 (14%) patients served by the center favoring early resection ($P < .001$). Median follow-up was 7.0 years (interquartile range, 4.5-10.9) at the center favoring biopsy and watchful waiting and 7.1 years (interquartile range, 4.2-9.9) at the center favoring early resection ($P = .95$). The 2 groups were comparable with respect to baseline parameters. Overall survival was significantly better with early surgical resection ($P = .01$). Median survival was 5.9 years (95% CI, 4.5-7.3) with the approach favoring biopsy only while median survival was not reached with the approach favoring early resection. Estimated 5-year survival was 60% (95% CI, 48%-72%) and 74% (95% CI, 64%-84%) for biopsy and watchful waiting and early resection, respectively. In an adjusted multivariable analysis the relative hazard ratio was 1.8 (95% CI, 1.1-2.9, $P = .03$) when treated at the center favoring biopsy and watchful waiting.

Conclusions.—For patients in Norway with LGG, treatment at a center that favored early surgical resection was associated with better overall survival than treatment at a center that favored biopsy and watchful waiting. This survival benefit remained after adjusting for validated prognostic factors.

▶ Surgical management of patients with diffuse low-grade gliomas remains a controversial subject because of the lack of any controlled therapeutic studies in this group of patients. During this retrospective study, the Norwegian investigators reviewed and compared the results from 2 different Norwegian hospitals with 2 dissimilar therapeutic approaches of early resection of the tumor versus diagnostic biopsy followed by "watchful wait and scan" approach. The main outcome of this study was the overall survival based on regional comparisons without adjusting for the type of employed therapy. Based on the results of this study, after a median follow-up period of 7 years, the overall survival rate for patients who underwent early resection was significantly superior to the conservative approach of "watchful wait and scan." Although the results of this study clearly support the early resection, it is based on retrospective analysis of data and lacks class I evidence. Despite the existence of such a pitfall, this study still is interesting because of the lack of other studies that address such an important health issue and because the main target of this particular study, "the survival of the patients," remains unaffected by the retrospective gathering of the data. This study will be even more robust and useful if the authors follow the same cohorts of patients for longer periods and assess them for neurological complications of the underlying tumor, the survival rate beyond 7 years, and chance of malignant transformation and recurrence of the original tumor.

A. Minagar, MD

7 Neuromuscular Disease

Comprehensive analysis of the *TRPV4* gene in a large series of inherited neuropathies and controls

Fawcett KA, Murphy SM, Polke JM, et al (UCL Inst of Neurology and Natl Hosp for Neurology and Neurosurgery, UK)

J Neurol Neurosurg Psychiatry 83:1204-1209, 2012

Background.—*TRPV4* mutations have been identified in Charcot–Marie–Tooth type 2 (CMT2), scapuloperoneal spinal muscular atrophy and distal hereditary motor neuropathy (dHMN).

Objective.—We aimed to screen the *TRPV4* gene in 422 British patients with inherited neuropathy for potentially pathogenic mutations.

Methods.—We sequenced *TRPV4* coding regions and splice junctions in 271 patients with CMT2 and 151 patients with dHMN. Mutations were clinically and genetically characterised and screened in ≥345 matched controls.

Results.—13 missense and nonsense variants were identified, of which five were novel and absent from controls (G20R, E218K, N302Y, Y567X and T701I). N302Y and T701I mutations were present in typical CMT2 cases and are potentially pathogenic based on in silico analyses. G20R was detected in a patient with dHMN and her asymptomatic father and is possibly pathogenic with variable expressivity. The Y567X variant segregated with disease in a family with severe CMT2 but also with a *MFN2* mutation reported to cause a mild CMT2 phenotype. Although Y567X caused nonsense mediated mRNA decay, the amount of TRPV4 protein on western blotting of patient lymphoblasts was no different to control. Y567X is therefore unlikely to be pathogenic. E218K is unlikely to be pathogenic based on segregation.

Conclusions.—In this comprehensive analysis of the *TRPV4* gene, we identified mutations in <1% of patients with CMT2/dHMN. We found that *TRPV4* likely harbours many missense and nonsense non-pathogenic variants that should be analysed in detail to prove pathogenicity before results are given to patients.

▶ Genetic testing is often nonrevealing in patients with axonal Charcot-Marie-Tooth (CMT) type 2 disease. Mutation in vanilloid transient receptor potential cation channel 4 (*TRPV4*) gene is an uncommon cause of CMT 2, distal hereditary motor neuropathy (dHMN), scapuloperoneal muscular atrophy, and a variety of autosomal dominant skeletal dysplasias.[1-3] *TRPV4* is a nonselective ionic channel, and pathogenic mutations probably cause disease through gain of function.

This study involved screening for *TRPV4* mutations in a large cohort of subjects with CMT 2 and dHMN who had tested negative for available genetic testing. The use of this test in routine assessment of patients with axonal neuropathy should be limited because less than 1% of the subjects had a *TRPV4* mutation and many nonpathologic genetic variations were also detected. On the other hand, testing for *TRPV4* mutations has a higher yield in patients with CMT 2 or dHMN who also have skeletal dysplasia or vocal cord or diaphragmatic paresis. This study is important because it demonstrates the low diagnostic yield of *TRPV4* genetic testing in patients with distal neuropathy.

K. Rezania, MD

References

1. Landouré G, Zdebik AA, Martinez TL, et al. Mutations in TRPV4 cause Charcot-Marie-Tooth disease type 2C. *Nat Genet.* 2010;42:170-174.
2. Cho TJ, Matsumoto K, Fano V, et al. TRPV4-pathy manifesting both skeletal dysplasia and peripheral neuropathy: a report of three patients. *Am J Med Genet A.* 2012;158A:795-802.
3. Deng HX, Klein CJ, Yan J, et al. Scapuloperoneal spinal muscular atrophy and CMT2C are allelic disorders caused by alterations in TRPV4. *Nat Genet.* 2010; 42:165-169.

Curcumin derivatives promote Schwann cell differentiation and improve neuropathy in R98C CMT1B mice

Patzkó A, Bai Y, Saporta MA, et al (Wayne State Univ, Detroit, MI; et al)

Brain 135:3551-3566, 2012

Charcot–Marie–Tooth disease type 1B is caused by mutations in myelin protein zero. R98C mice, an authentic model of early onset Charcot–Marie–Tooth disease type 1B, develop neuropathy in part because the misfolded mutant myelin protein zero is retained in the endoplasmic reticulum where it activates the unfolded protein response. Because oral curcumin, a component of the spice turmeric, has been shown to relieve endoplasmic reticulum stress and decrease the activation of the unfolded protein response, we treated R98C mutant mice with daily gastric lavage of curcumin or curcumin derivatives starting at 4 days of age and analysed them for clinical disability, electrophysiological parameters and peripheral nerve morphology. Heterozygous R98C mice treated with curcumin dissolved in sesame oil or phosphatidylcholine curcumin performed as well as wild-type littermates on a rotarod test and had increased numbers of large-diameter axons in their sciatic nerves. Treatment with the latter two compounds also increased compound muscle action potential amplitudes and the innervation of neuromuscular junctions in both heterozygous and homozygous R98C animals, but it did not improve nerve conduction velocity, myelin thickness, G-ratios or myelin period. The expression of c-Jun and suppressed cAMP-inducible POU (SCIP)—transcription factors that inhibit myelination when overexpressed—was also decreased by treatment. Consistent with its role in reducing endoplasmic reticulum stress, treatment with curcumin dissolved in sesame oil or phosphatidylcholine curcumin was associated with decreased X-box binding protein (XBP1) splicing. Taken together, these data demonstrate that treatment with curcumin dissolved in sesame oil or phosphatidylcholine curcumin improves the peripheral neuropathy of R98C mice by alleviating endoplasmic reticulum stress, by reducing the activation of unfolded protein response and by promoting Schwann cell differentiation.

▶ This study is important because it may result in identification of molecular targets for future pharmacologic interventions in patients with Charcot-Marie-Tooth (CMT) disease. In this study, curcumin, when given in the form of phosphatidylcholine curcumin or when dissolved in sesame oil, improved the phenotype in a mouse model of CMT type 1B. Different myelin protein zero (MPZ) mutations cause neuropathy thorough different pathogenic pathways; as a result, the phenotype of MPZ mutation is a spectrum from severe peripheral nerve demyelination to a primarily axonal neuropathy.[1] The study drug likely worked through suppressing the toxic gain of function of mutated MPZ, resulting in endoplasmic reticulum (ER) stress (although it is also possible that the drug worked on other pathways such as nuclear factor-kappa B). One of the challenges of conducting clinical trials using curcumin or similar compounds in human clinical trials is to identify CMT 1B patients with MPZ mutations that result in ER stress. On the other hand, curcumin can also be tried in other types of CMT in which ER stress could have a significant pathogenic role. Should patients with CMT 1B use curcumin (which is available as an over-the-counter product) based on the results of this study? I would be hesitant to make this recommendation at this time: An adult human would have to take 10 to 12 g of curcumin a day to achieve tissue levels reached in the mouse, which causes a bad aftertaste[2]; furthermore, curcumin will theoretically only work on a subgroup of CMT 1B patients.

K. Rezania, MD

References

1. Shy ME, Jáni A, Krajewski K, et al. Phenotypic clustering in MPZ mutations. *Brain.* 2004;127:371-384.
2. Singh S. Indian pharma enters the global arena. *Cell.* 2007;128:811-814.

Novel mutation in *VCP* gene causes atypical amyotrophic lateral sclerosis

González-Pérez P, Cirulli ET, Drory VE, et al (Univ of Massachusetts Med School, Worcester; Duke Univ School of Medicine, Durham, NC; Tel-Aviv Sourasky Med Ctr, Israel; et al)

Neurology 79:2201-2208, 2012

Objective.—To identify the genetic variant that causes autosomal dominantly inherited motor neuron disease in a 4-generation Israeli-Arab family using genetic linkage and whole exome sequencing.

Methods.—Genetic linkage analysis was performed in this family using Illumina single nucleotide polymorphism chips. Whole exome sequencing was then undertaken on DNA samples from 2 affected family members using an Illumina 2000 HiSeq platform in pursuit of potentially pathogenic genetic variants that comigrate with the disease in this pedigree. Variants meeting these criteria were then screened in all affected individuals.

Results.—A novel mutation (p.R191G) in the valosin-containing protein (*VCP*) gene was identified in the index family. Direct sequencing of the *VCP* gene in a panel of DNA from 274 unrelated individuals with familial amyotrophic lateral sclerosis (FALS) revealed 5 additional mutations. Among them, 2 were previously identified in pedigrees with a constellation of inclusion body myopathy with Paget disease of the bone and frontotemporal dementia (IBMPFD) and in FALS, and 2 other mutations (p.R159C and p.R155C) in IBMPFD alone. We did not detect *VCP* gene mutations in DNA from 178 cases of sporadic amyotrophic lateral sclerosis.

Conclusions.—We report a novel *VCP* mutation identified in an amyotrophic lateral sclerosis family (p.R191G) with atypical clinical features. In our experience, *VCP* mutations arise in approximately 1.5% of FALS cases. Our study supports the view that motor neuron disease is part of the clinical spectrum of *VCP*-associated disease.

▶ Mutations in valosin-containing protein (VCP) have been associated with inclusion body myopathy, Paget disease of the bone, and frontotemporal dementia.[1] More recently, VCP mutations have been associated with familial amyotrophic lateral sclerosis (FALS).[2]

In this study, a family with autosomal dominant FALS was assessed with genetic linkage analysis and whole genome sequencing. After a disease-associated novel VCP mutation was found in the index family, *VCP* gene was sequenced in 275 unrelated patients with FALS, and 5 more patients with different VCP mutations were then identified. Consistent with a previous study,[2] this study showed that VCP mutations account for about 2% of cases with FALS. Furthermore, it confirmed the belief that VCP mutations may present with a spectrum of neuromuscular phenotypes, including inclusion body myopathy and ALS. Paget disease of bone and frontal lobe dementia are among the other manifestations of VCP mutations. The presence of severe bone pain and frontotemporal dementia in patients with neuromuscular disease should raise the suspicion for VCP mutations. Other more common causes of FALS and frontotemporal dementia include mutations in TDP-43 and hexanucleotide expansion in C9ORF72.

K. Rezania, MD

References

1. Weihl CC, Pestronk A, Kimonis VE. Valosin-containing protein disease: inclusion body myopathy with Paget's disease of the bone and fronto-temporal dementia. *Neuromuscul Disord.* 2009;19:308-315.
2. Johnson JO, Mandrioli J, Benatar M, et al. Exome sequencing reveals VCP mutations as a cause of familial ALS. *Neuron.* 2010;68:857-864.

GSK3β mediates muscle pathology in myotonic dystrophy

Jones K, Wei C, Iakova P, et al (Baylor College of Medicine, Houston, TX; et al)
J Clin Invest 122:4461-4472, 2012

Myotonic dystrophy type 1 (DM1) is a complex neuromuscular disease characterized by skeletal muscle wasting, weakness, and myotonia. DM1 is caused by the accumulation of CUG repeats, which alter the biological activities of RNA-binding proteins, including CUG-binding protein 1 (CUGBP1). CUGBP1 is an important skeletal muscle translational regulator that is activated by cyclin D3–dependent kinase 4 (CDK4). Here we show that mutant CUG repeats suppress Cdk4 signaling by increasing the stability and activity of glycogen synthase kinase 3β (GSK3β). Using a mouse model of DM1 (HSA^{LR}), we found that CUG repeats in the 3′ untranslated region (UTR) of human skeletal actin increase active GSK3β in skeletal muscle of mice, prior to the development of skeletal muscle weakness. Inhibition of GSK3β in both DM1 cell culture and mouse models corrected cyclin D3 levels and reduced muscle weakness and myotonia in DM1 mice. Our data predict that compounds normalizing GSK3β activity might be beneficial for improvement of muscle function in patients with DM1.

▶ Myotonic dystrophy type 1 (DM1) is a complex multisystem disease, with muscle weakness and myotonia its most important manifestations. DM1 is caused by the expansion of noncoding CTG repeats in the 3 untranslated regions of the dystrophia myotonica-protein kinase (*DMPK*) gene.[1] Expanded CTG repeats are pathogenic as they result in genesis of RNA CUG repeats that misregulate several CUG RNA-binding proteins, including CUG-binding protein 1 (CUGBP1).[2] The number of repeat size is associated with the severity of the disease (ie, congenital DM1 cases have higher repeat size). The expression of CUGBP1 is increased in congenital DM1 and has also been associated with delay of myogenesis in the CUGBP1 transgenic mouse model.[3] Using human muscle biopsy samples and a mouse model of DM1 (HSA^{LR} mice), this study investigates the abnormalities in upstream enzymes that regulate CUGBP1 and concludes that an increased level of active glycogen synthase kinase 3β (GSK3β) has an essential role in high CUGBP1 levels in DM1. It was also shown that inhibition of GSK3β by lithium and TDZD-8 (4-benzyl-2-methyl-1,2,4-thiadiazolidine-3,5-dione) improves weakness and myotonia in HSA^{LR} mice. Importantly, findings of this study suggest that GSK3β is a viable therapeutic target in DM1 and may result in future potential treatments for this currently incurable disease.

K. Rezania, MD

References

1. Brook JD, McCurrach ME, Harley HG, et al. Molecular basis of myotonic dystrophy: expansion of a trinucleotide (CTG) repeat at the 3′ end of a transcript encoding a protein kinase family member. *Cell.* 1992;4:799-808.
2. Timchenko LT, Timchenko NA, Caskey CT, Roberts R. Novel proteins with binding specificity for DNA CTG repeats and RNA CUG repeats: implications for myotonic dystrophy. *Hum Mol Genet.* 1996;5:115-121.
3. Timchenko NA, Patel R, Iakova P, Cai ZJ, Quan L, Timchenko LT. Overexpression of CUG triplet repeat-binding protein, CUGBP1, in mice inhibits myogenesis. *J Biol Chem.* 2004;279:13129-13139.

Dysfunction of the neuromuscular junction in spinal muscular atrophy types 2 and 3

Wadman RI, Vrancken AFJE, van den Berg LH, et al (Univ Med Ctr Utrecht, the Netherlands)

Neurology 79:2050-2055, 2012

Objective.—Spinal muscular atrophy (SMA) is pathologically characterized by degeneration of anterior horn cells. Recent observations in animal models of SMA and muscle tissue from patients with SMA suggest additional abnormalities in the development and maturation of the neuromuscular junction. We therefore evaluated neuromuscular junction function in SMA with repetitive nerve stimulation.

Methods.—In this case-control study, repetitive nerve stimulation was performed in 35 patients with SMA types 2, 3, and 4, 20 healthy controls, and 5 controls with motor neuron disease.

Results.—Pathologic decremental responses (>10%) during 3-Hz repetitive nerve stimulation were observed in 17 of 35 patients (49%) with SMA types 2 and 3, but not in healthy controls or controls with motor neuron disease. None of the patients or controls had an abnormal incremental response of >60%. The presence of an abnormal decremental response was not specific for the type of SMA, nor was it associated with compound muscle action potential amplitude, clinical scores, or disease duration. Two of 4 patients with SMA type 3 who tried pyridostigmine reported increased stamina.

Conclusions.—These data suggest dysfunction of the neuromuscular junction in patients with SMA types 2 and 3. Therefore, drugs that facilitate neuromuscular transmission are candidate drugs for evaluation in carefully designed, placebo-controlled, clinical trials (Fig 1).

▶ Abnormalities of the neuromuscular junction (NMJ) are shown to precede motor neuron death in animal models with spinal muscular atrophy (SMA).[1] This study found abnormal NMJ function in patients with SMA types 2, 3, and

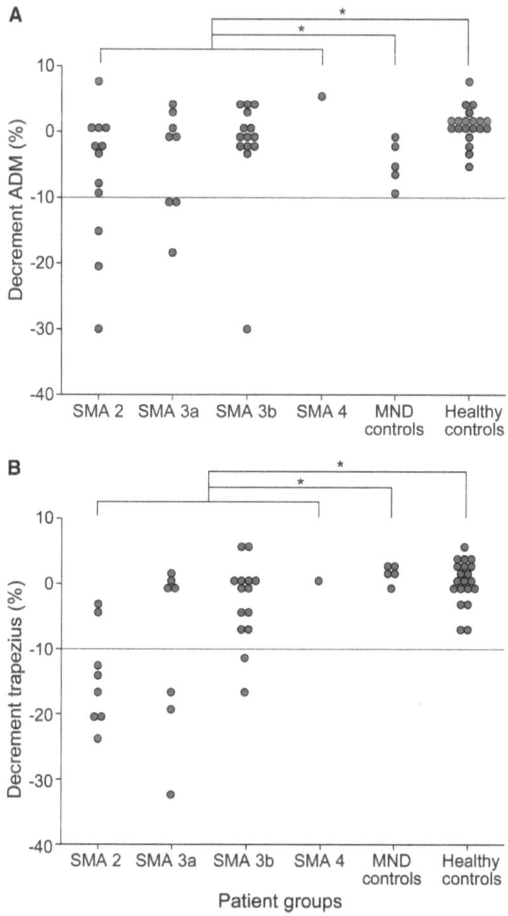

FIGURE 1.—Levels of decrement in the musculus abductor digiti minimi (ADM) (A) and m. trapezius (B). Decrement observed during 3-Hz stimulation in (A) m. abductor digiti minimi and (B) m. trapezius. Levels of decrement in patients with spinal muscular atrophy (SMA) are more pronounced than in healthy controls or controls with motor neuron disease (MND) ($p < 0.05$). Decrement in the m. trapezius in early-onset patients (SMA type 2 and 3a) is more pronounced than in late-onset SMA ($p < 0.01$). (Reprinted from Wadman RI, Vrancken AFJE, van den Berg LH, et al. Dysfunction of the neuromuscular junction in spinal muscular atrophy types 2 and 3. *Neurology.* 2012;79:2050-2055, with permission from American Academy of Neurology.)

4, but not in patients with other motor neuron diseases and normal controls (Fig 1). This study has some limitations. It would have been useful to confirm the abnormal NMJ with single-fiber electromyography in cases that had a borderline abnormal repetitive stimulation. Also, a lack of abnormalities in repetitive nerve stimulation in patients with other motor neuron diseases could be related to the small number of subjects in that group. It would have been interesting to see if the abnormal decrement in compound muscle action potential amplitude in repetitive stimulation ameliorated or normalized after injection of a short-acting acetylcholine esterase blocker (such as edrophonium) before a clinical trial using a longer-acting medication (such as pyridostigmine) is considered in SMA patients. However, given its favorable side effect profile, pyridostigmine can be tried as an off-label use in patients with SMA.

K. Rezania, MD

Reference

1. Martinez TL, Kong L, Wang X, et al. Survival motor neuron protein in motor neurons determines synaptic integrity in spinal muscular atrophy. *J Neurosci.* 2012;32:8703-8715.

Characterization of a Family With c9FTD/ALS Associated With the GGGGCC Repeat Expansion in *C9ORF72*

Savica R, Adeli A, Vemuri P, et al (Mayo Clinic, Rochester, MN)
Arch Neurol 69:1164-1169, 2012

Background.—The hexanucleotide repeat in the chromosome 9 open reading frame 72 (*C9ORF72*) gene was recently discovered as the underlying genetic cause of many families with frontotemporal dementia (FTD) and/or amyotrophic lateral sclerosis (ALS) linked to chromosome 9 (c9FTD/ALS). We report the clinical, neuropsychologic, and neuroimaging findings of a family with the *C9ORF72* mutation and clinical diagnoses bridging the FTD, parkinsonism, and ALS spectrum.

Objective.—To characterize the antemortem characteristics of a family with c9FTD/ALS associated with the GGGGCC repeat expansion in *C9ORF72*.

Design.—Clinical series.

Setting.—Tertiary care academic medical center.

Patients.—The members of a family affected by the mutation with features of FTD and/or ALS.

Main Outcome Measures.—Clinical, neuropsychologic, and neuroimaging assessments.

Results.—All 3 examined subjects had the hexanucleotide expansion detected in *C9ORF72*. All had personality/behavioral changes early in the course of the disease. One case had levodopa-unresponsive parkinsonism, and 1 had ALS. Magnetic resonance imaging showed symmetric bilateral frontal, temporal, insular, and cingulate atrophy.

Conclusions.—This report highlights the clinical and neuroimaging characteristics of a family with c9FTD/ALS. Further studies are needed to better understand the phenotypical variability and the cliniconeuroimaging-neuropathologic correlations.

► A hexanucleotide GGGGCC repeat expansion in the chromosome 9 open reading frame 72 (*C9ORF72*) gene is the most common cause of familial amyotrophic lateral sclerosis (ALS).[1,2] This mutation is also a common cause of frontotemporal dementia (FTD) and ALS and FTD and overall. The presence of cognitive and behavioral impairment on neuropsychological testing and abnormal nonmotor cortex on 3 T MRI predicts the carrier state for *C9ORF72* hexanucleotide expansion.[3] The pattern of magnetic resonance imaging (MRI) abnormalities can be useful in differentiating *C9ORF72* mutation from FTD caused by other mutations because atrophy of parietal, occipital, and cerebellar cortex is more often present in the former.[4]

This article reports on a family with *C9ORF72* mutation, 3 members of which underwent detailed neuropsychological testing, MRI, and positron emission tomography studies. Interestingly, 1 of the 3 cases had levodopa nonresponsive parkinsonism and cerebellar atrophy was noted in another case (see Fig 3 in the original article). This article adds to the accumulating evidence that neurodegenerative diseases, such as parkinsonism, cerebellar degeneration, and dementia with Alzheimer phenotype, could be associated with *C9ORF72* mutation.

K. Rezania, MD

References

1. Renton AE, Majounie E, Waite A, et al. A hexanucleotide repeat expansion in C9ORF72 is the cause of chromosome 9p21-linked ALS-FTD. *Neuron.* 2011;2: 257-268.
2. DeJesus-Hernandez M, Mackenzie IR, Boeve BF, et al. Expanded GGGGCC hexanucleotide repeat in noncoding region of C9ORF72 causes chromosome 9p-linked FTD and ALS. *Neuron.* 2011;72:245-256.
3. Byrne S, Elamin M, Bede P, et al. Cognitive and clinical characteristics of patients with amyotrophic lateral sclerosis carrying a C9orf72 repeat expansion: a population-based cohort study. *Lancet Neurol.* 2012;11:232-240.
4. Whitwell JL, Weigand SD, Boeve BF, et al. Neuroimaging signatures of frontotemporal dementia genetics: C9ORF72, tau, progranulin and sporadics. *Brain.* 2012; 135:794-806.

Myasthenia gravis in the elderly

Hellmann MA, Mosberg-Galili R, Steiner I (Tel Aviv Univ, Israel)
J Neurol Sci 325:1-5, 2013

Objective.—The objective of the study is to examine clinical, therapeutic and prognostic factors of myasthenia gravis (MG) in the elderly.

Patients and Methods.—We reviewed all MG files of patients who attended the neuro-immunology clinic at Rabin Medical Center, Petah Tikva, Israel from January 1995 until September 2011 for demographic data, MG presentation, and course and response to treatment. Patients were classified as elderly if disease onset was above 69 years.

Results.—Out of 137 patients with MG, 29 developed MG after age 69. The 108 young onset patients had a male:female ratio of 0.9:1 whereas the eighth and ninth decade onset had a significant male predominance with ratios of 2.6:1 and 4.5:1 respectively. There was no difference in the presenting symptomatology and the rate of sero-negativity in the elderly patients when compared to the early onset patients was similar. The older patients had much less thymic pathology and their acetylcholine

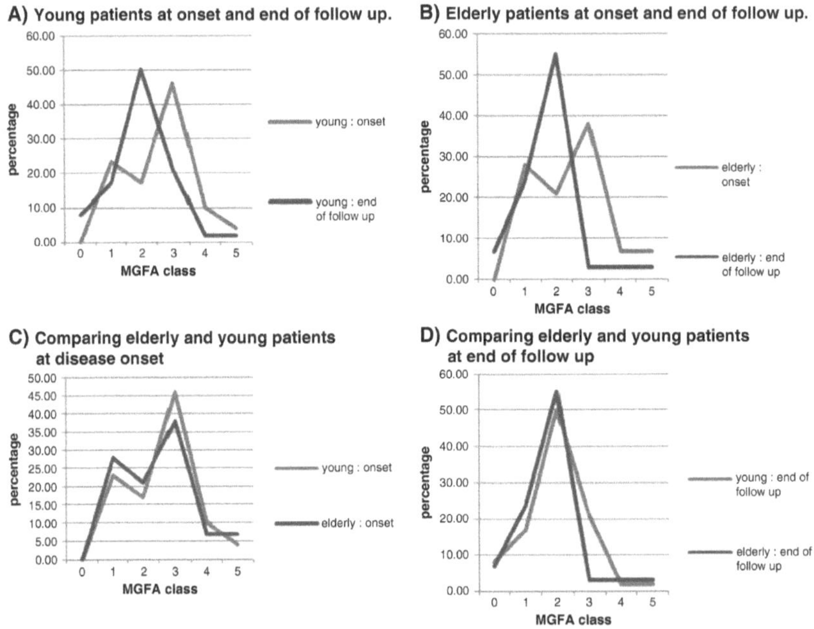

FIGURE 1.—MGFA class at onset and end of follow up. A. Young patients at onset and end of follow up. B. Elderly patients at onset and end of follow up. C. Comparing elderly and young patients at disease onset. D. Comparing elderly and young patients at end of follow up. (Reprinted from Journal of the Neurological Sciences. Hellmann MA, Mosberg-Galili R, Steiner I. Myasthenia gravis in the elderly. *J Neurol Sci.* 2013;325:1-5, Copyright 2013, with permission from Elsevier.)

receptor (AChR) antibody titer was lower. This was associated with better response to therapy and a good prognosis.

Conclusion.—MG onset in the elderly is not uncommon, is more prevalent in males, is associated with lower titer of AChR antibodies, is readily responsive to therapy and carries a good prognosis (Fig 1).

▶ Myasthenia gravis (MG) is rather common in the elderly population.[1] MG may, however, be an underdiagnosed disease in the elderly, because its manifestations may be mistaken for other comorbidities that are common in that age group, ie, fatigue and ptosis are rather common and other manifestations could be attributed to cerebrovascular accidents and cardiovascular disease. Previous studies have suggested that MG in patients older than 50 years of age could have higher rates of severe morbidity and mortality, partly as a result of increased prevalence of medical comorbidities.[2,3] However, more recent studies have questioned that notion. This retrospective study assessed the characteristics of MG in patients older than 70 years of age. Similar to another recent study,[2] this study showed that MG is generally not more severe than it is in younger individuals. Furthermore, this study showed that similar to some other autoimmune diseases, men are predominantly affected in the older age group. Because the diagnosis and appropriate treatment of MG may dramatically improve the quality of life of the patient, physicians should have a high level of suspicion when seeing older patients with symptoms suggestive of MG.

K. Rezania, MD

References

1. Zivković SA, Clemens PR, Lacomis D. Characteristics of late-onset myasthenia gravis. *J Neurol.* 2012;259:2167-2171.
2. Thomas CE, Mayer SA, Gungor Y, et al. Myasthenic crisis: clinical features, mortality, complications, and risk factors for prolonged intubation. *Neurology.* 1997;5:1253-1260.
3. Donaldson DH, Ansher M, Horan S, Rutherford RB, Ringel SP. The relationship of age to outcome in myasthenia gravis. *Neurology.* 1990;5:786-790.

Extensive genetics of ALS: A population-based study in Italy

Chiò A, On behalf of PARALS (Univ of Torino and AOU San Giovanni Battista of Torino, Italy; et al)

Neurology 79:1983-1989, 2012

Objective.—To assess the frequency and clinical characteristics of patients with mutations of major amyotrophic lateral sclerosis (ALS) genes in a prospectively ascertained, population-based epidemiologic series of cases.

Methods.—The study population includes all ALS cases diagnosed in Piemonte, Italy, from January 2007 to June 2011. Mutations of *SOD1*, *TARDBP*, *ANG*, *FUS*, *OPTN*, and *C9ORF72* have been assessed.

Results.—Out of the 475 patients included in the study, 51 (10.7%) carried a mutation of an ALS-related gene (*C9ORF72*, 32; *SOD1*, 10; *TARDBP*, 7; *FUS*, 1; *OPTN*, 1; *ANG*, none). A positive family history for ALS or frontotemporal dementia (FTD) was found in 46 (9.7%) patients. Thirty-one (67.4%) of the 46 familial cases and 20 (4.7%) of the 429 sporadic cases had a genetic mutation. According to logistic regression modeling, besides a positive family history for ALS or FTD, the chance to carry a genetic mutation was related to the presence of comorbid FTD (odds ratio 3.5; $p = 0.001$), and age at onset ≤54 years (odds ratio 1.79; $p = 0.012$).

Conclusions.—We have found that ~11% of patients with ALS carry a genetic mutation, with *C9ORF72* being the commonest genetic alteration. Comorbid FTD or a young age at onset are strong indicators of a possible genetic origin of the disease (Table 2).

▶ Familial amyotrophic lateral sclerosis (fALS) accounts for 5% to 23% of the cases of ALS, whereas the rest of the cases are sporadic.[1] Mutations in an increasing number of genes are recognized to be associated with fALS. Genetic testing can expedite the correct diagnosis in some ALS patients, but it should be offered only in selected cases after genetic counseling.[1]

TABLE 2.—Main Clinical Characteristics of Patients With Different Mutations and Without Known Mutations

	No. of Cases	% of Cases[a]	Gender (Female), n (%)	Median Age at Onset, y (IQR)	Site at Onset (Bulbar), n (%)	FTD, n (%)
C9ORF72	32	6.7	10 (31.3)	62.6 (55.7–67.3)	14 (43.8)	17 (53.1)
SOD1	10	2.1	8 (80.0)	57.0 (46.7–70.7)	1 (10.0)	0
TARDBP	7	1.5	3 (42.9)	66.8 (60.0–68.2)	3 (42.9)	2 (28.6)
Wild type, fALS	15	3.2	7 (46.7)	61.3 (55.1–68.0)	5 (33.3)	2 (13.3)
Wild type, sALS	409	86.1	187 (45.7)	66.6 (59.5–73.3)	126 (30.8)	66 (16.1)
Overall	475[b]	—	216 (45.7)	66.3 (59.1–73.0)	149 (31.4)	87 (18.3)
p			NS	0.0001	0.31	0.0001

Abbreviations: fALS = familial amyotrophic lateral sclerosis; FTD = frontotemporal dementia; IQR = interquartile range; NS = not significant; sALS = sporadic amyotrophic lateral sclerosis.

[a]Calculated on 475 cases.

[b]The 2 cases with *FUS* and *OPTN* missense mutations are not indicated in the table; both patients had a spinal phenotype and were cognitively normal.

This is a large population study of the prevalence of different mutations in patients with fALS and sporadic disease. This study is therefore free of referral bias. Consistent with some of the previous reports, hexanucleotide expansion in chromosome 9 open reading frame 72 (C9ORF72) followed by mutations in superoxide dismutase 1 (*SOD1*) and TAR DNA binding protein (TARDBP) were the most common causes of fALS.[1,2] A pathologic mutation was found in 11% of the cases and interestingly in about 5% of the sporadic cases. The authors recommended genetic testing in patients with concomitant frontotemporal dementia (FTD), family history of ALS or FTD, and age of onset younger than 55 years old, because the odds of finding abnormalities in the genetic testing were significantly higher in these patients. These guidelines, however, must be confirmed in future large studies. This study also redemonstrated that other available genes associated with ALS (besides those mentioned above) account for only a small percentage of fALS cases.

K. Rezania, MD

References

1. Andersen PM, Abrahams S, Borasio GD, et al. EFNS guidelines on the clinical management of amyotrophic lateral sclerosis (MALS)—revised report of an EFNS task force. *Eur J Neurol.* 2012;19:360-375.
2. Renton AE, Majounie E, Waite A, et al. A hexanucleotide repeat expansion in C9ORF72 is the cause of chromosome 9p21-linked ALS-FTD. *Neuron.* 2011; 72:257-268.

Reliability and accuracy of skeletal muscle imaging in limb-girdle muscular dystrophies

ten Dam L, van der Kooi AJ, van Wattingen M, et al (Univ of Amsterdam, the Netherlands)

Neurology 79:1716-1723, 2012

Objective.—To evaluate the reliability and accuracy of skeletal muscle CT to correctly identify different muscular dystrophies manifesting with limb-girdle weakness.

Methods.—Four evaluators assessed scans from 118 patients with limb-girdle muscular dystrophy (LGMD) caused by mutations in 7 different genes and from 32 controls. The conditions studied were scans of genetically confirmed cases of Becker muscular dystrophy (BMD) (n = 28), LGMD2C–F (sarcoglycanopathies) (n = 11), LGMD2I (n = 4), LGMD1B (n = 26), LGMD2A (n = 24), Bethlem myopathy (n = 14), and LGMD2L (n = 11). The control group (n = 32) consisted of patients with neuromuscular disorders manifesting with limb-girdle weakness in which the aforementioned muscular dystrophies were excluded. The scans were compared with the characteristic patterns described in literature.

Results.—The overall interobserver agreement was poor ($\kappa = 0.27$), with markedly higher scores for BMD ($\kappa = 0.51$) and Bethlem myopathy ($\kappa = 0.59$). The sensitivity to detect selective patterns in relation to the genetic diagnosis was 40% if all LGMDs were taken together. The specificity was 58%, positive predictive value (PPV) 77%, and 1 − negative predictive value (NPV) 79%. Markedly better scores were observed for BMD (sensitivity 91%, PPV 66%, 1 − NPV 3%) and Bethlem myopathy (sensitivity 90%, PPV 69%, 1 − NPV 1%).

Conclusions.—Our findings suggest that muscle CT might be an adjunct to the clinical diagnosis of BMD and Bethlem myopathy. However, pattern recognition was cumbersome in the other LGMDs (Fig 1, Tables 1 and 2).

▶ Imaging (CT scan or MRI) of skeletal muscle is commonly used to find an appropriate muscle for biopsy in myopathies. The pattern of skeletal involvement in muscle CT or MRI, such as atrophy, hypertrophy, and fatty replacement, is proposed in differentiating different forms of muscular dystrophies (Fig 1, Table 1).[1,2]

This study used CT scan and assessors who were blinded to the diagnosis in predicting the correct type of muscular dystrophies. Except for Becker muscular dystrophy and Bethlem myopathy, where the sensitivity was around 90%, this study found low sensitivity and interobserver agreement in the diagnosis of other muscular dystrophies (Table 2). The authors therefore recommended the use of muscle CT scan if Becker dystrophy and Bethlem myopathy are suspected clinically. Given the low interobserver agreement and because additional testing, such as genetic testing or muscle biopsy, is generally needed to confirm the correct diagnosis, the routine use of muscle CT scan in the diagnosis of limb girdle muscular dystrophies should be limited.

K. Rezania, MD

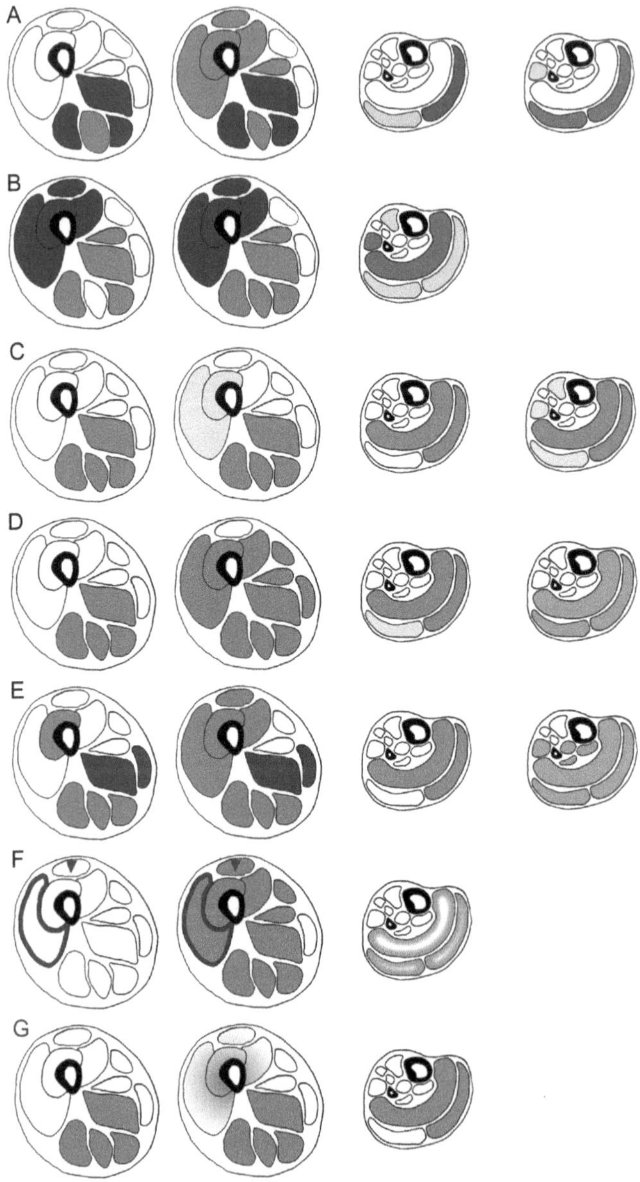

FIGURE 1.—Overview of the patterns of muscle involvement in the muscular dystrophies under examination. Patterns of muscle involvement in Becker muscular dystrophy (A), LGMD2C–F (B), LGMD2I (C), LGMD1B (D), LGMD2A (E), Bethlem myopathy (F), and LGMD2L (G) based on the literature search. The replacement of muscle tissue by fat is reflected by the gray color of (part of) the muscle. The first column shows a cross-section at the level of the thigh in an early stage of the disease, the second shows the disease in a more advanced stage. The third and fourth columns show cross-sections through the lower leg, at an early and more advanced stage, respectively. LGMD = limb-girdle muscular dystrophy. (Reprinted from ten Dam L, van der Kooi AJ, van Wattingen M, et al. Reliability and accuracy of skeletal muscle imaging in limb-girdle muscular dystrophies. *Neurology*. 2012;79:1716-1723, with permission from AAN Enterprises, Inc.)

TABLE 1.—Summary of Most Common Patterns of Muscle Involvement Derived from Literature Search[5-8,10,14,16-27]

	Thigh	Calf	Hypertrophy
BMD	Involvement of the biceps femoris, semimembranosus, and adductor magnus muscles; in an advanced stage more generalized involvement	Less changes as compared to the thigh, when affected usually both heads of the gastrocnemius muscle	Frequent; gracilis, sartorius, adductor longus, semitendinosus, and both heads of the gastrocnemius muscle
LGMD2C–F	Predominant anterior involvement, especially the vastus intermedius muscle	Predominant affliction of the soleus and peroneal muscles	Frequent; gracilis and sartorius muscles
LGMD2I	Predominant posterior involvement; vastus muscles also involved in an advanced stage of the disease	Generalized involvement of both the posterior and anterior compartments	Frequent; gracilis muscles
LGMD1B	Predominant involvement of posterior muscles or generalized in advanced stage of the disease	Medial or both heads of the gastrocnemius and the soleus muscle	Rare
LGMD2A	Selective involvement of the posterior muscles, especially the adductor magnus, and often the vastus intermedius muscle	Medial head of the gastrocnemius and the soleus muscles	Rare
LGMD2L	Predominant posterior affliction, with patchy involvement of the quadriceps muscles	Confined to the medial head of the gastrocnemius and the soleus muscles	Not mentioned (3/7 show hypertrophy of the gracilis and sartorius muscles)
Bethlem myopathy	Striking involvement of the central part of the rectus femoris and the peripheral part of the vastus muscles	Rim between gastrocnemius and soleus muscle visible	Rare

Abbreviations: BMD = Becker muscular dystrophy; LGMD = limb-girdle muscular dystrophy.
Editor's Note: Please refer to original journal article for full references.

TABLE 2.—Test Characteristics of Muscle CT After the Consensus Meeting[a]

	Prevalence	Sensitivity	Specificity	PPV	1 − NPV
Overall	86/110 (78)	34/86 (40)	14/24 (58)	34/44 (77)	52/66 (78)
BMD	23/110 (21)	21/23 (91)	76/87 (87)	21/32 (66)	2/78 (3)
LGMD2C–F	9/110 (8)	2/9 (22)	93/101 (92)	2/10 (20)	7/100 (7)
LGMD2I	3/110 (3)	0/3 (0)	96/107 (90)	0/11 (0)	3/99 (3)
LGDM1B	18/110 (16)	1/18 (6)	88/92 (96)	1/5 (20)	17/105 (16)
LGMD2A	15/110 (14)	1/15 (7)	92/95 (97)	1/4 (25)	14/106 (13)
Bethlem myopathy	10/110 (9)	9/10 (90)	96/100 (96)	9/13 (69)	1/97 (1)
LGMD2L	8/110 (7)	0/8 (0)	99/102 (97)	0/3 (0)	8/107 (7)

Abbreviations: BMD = Becker muscular dystrophy; LGMD = limb-girdle muscular dystrophy; NPV = negative predictive value; PPV = positive predictive value.
[a]Values are n (%). The prevalence indicates the proportion of patients with the target disorder in this study/total number of scans in this study. Sensitivity indicates the proportion of patients with the target disorder who have positive test/scan results, whereas specificity indicates the proportion of patients without the target disorder who have negative test/scan results. PPV indicates the proportion of patients with positive test/scan results who have the target disorder, whereas 1 − NPV refers to the proportion of patients with negative test/scan results who have the target disorder.

References

1. Lamminen AE. Magnetic resonance imaging of primary skeletal muscle diseases: patterns of distribution and severity of involvement. *Br J Radiol.* 1990;63:946-950.
2. Mercuri E, Clements E, Offiah A, et al. Muscle magnetic resonance imaging involvement in muscular dystrophies with rigidity of the spine. *Ann Neurol.* 2010;67: 201-208.

Awaji Criteria for the Diagnosis of Amyotrophic Lateral Sclerosis: A Systematic Review

Costa J, Swash M, de Carvalho M (Univ of Lisbon, Portugal)
Arch Neurol 69:1410-1416, 2012

Objective.—To estimate the potential diagnostic added value of the Awaji criteria for diagnosis of amyotrophic lateral sclerosis (ALS), which have been compared with the previously accepted gold standard the revised El Escorial criteria in several studies.

Data Sources.—MEDLINE and Web of Science (until October 2011).

Study Selection.—We searched for studies testing the diagnostic accuracy of the Awaji criteria vs the revised El Escorial criteria in patients referred with suspected ALS.

Data Extraction.—Evaluation and data extraction of identified studies were done independently. The Quality Assessment of Diagnostic Accuracy Studies list was used to assess study quality. We determined the proportion of patients classified as having probable/definite ALS and derived indices of diagnostic performance (sensitivity, specificity, and diagnostic odds ratio). Quantitative data synthesis was accomplished through random-effects meta-analysis, and heterogeneity was assessed with the I^2 test.

Data Synthesis.—Eight studies were included (3 prospective and 5 retrospective) enrolling 1187 patients. Application of Awaji criteria led to a 23% (95% CI, 12% to 33%; $I^2 = 84\%$) increase in the proportion of patients classified as having probable/definite ALS. Diagnostic performance of the Awaji criteria was higher than the revised El Escorial criteria (pooled sensitivity: 81.1% [95% CI, 72.2% to 90.0%; $I^2 = 91\%$] vs 62.2% [95% CI, 49.4% to 75.1%; $I^2 = 93\%$]; pooled diagnostic odds ratio, 35.8 [95% CI, 15.2 to 84.7; $I^2 = 3\%$] vs 8.7 [95% CI, 2.2 to 35.6; $I^2 = 50\%$]). Diagnostic accuracy of Awaji criteria was higher in bulbar- than in limb-onset cases.

Conclusion.—The Awaji criteria have a significant clinical impact allowing earlier diagnosis and clinical trial entry in ALS.

▶ Amyotrophic lateral sclerosis (ALS) is a progressive, universally fatal, paralyzing disease that is characterized by degeneration of the upper and lower motor neurons. The extent of lower motor neuron involvement based on the revised El Escorial criteria is commonly used to support the diagnosis of ALS. Revised El Escorial criteria have a very high specificity but a rather low sensitivity when used in early stages of the disease.[1] This could result in delay of diagnosis in patients with early ALS and those with bulbar-onset disease, and it may result in unnecessary diagnostic workup and inappropriate use of potentially toxic treatments.

Awaji recommendations were proposed by a consensus of experts to increase the sensitivity of electromyogram in the diagnosis of ALS.[2] The presence of fasciculations, especially those with a complex morphology, is considered equivalent to positive waves and fibrillations in cases with clinical suspicion for ALS in Awaji but not in El Escorial criteria.[2]

This article is a meta-analysis of previous literature that includes 8 studies involving 1187 patients who were referred to a tertiary center for clinical suspicion for ALS or motor neuron disease. Comparing the diagnostic odds ratio (DOR) of each study as well as the pooled DOR using either criteria (see Fig 2 in the original article), the study showed higher sensitivity of Awaji (81%) vs El Escorial criteria (62%), whereas the specificity of the 2 sets of criteria was the same (98%). For bulbar-onset ALS, the sensitivity was 83% and 46% for Awaji and El Escorial criteria, respectively. It is estimated that when using the El Escorial criteria, about 22% of patients with ALS die without reaching a level of diagnosis more certain than possible ALS.[3] It is hoped that earlier diagnosis of ALS using Awaji criteria will result in participation of a larger proportion of patients with early disease in ALS clinical trials.

K. Rezania, MD

References

1. Makki AA, Benatar M. The electromyographic diagnosis of amyotrophic lateral sclerosis: does the evidence support the El Escorial criteria? *Muscle Nerve.* 2007;35:614-619.
2. de Carvalho M, Dengler R, Eisen A, et al. Electrodiagnostic criteria for diagnosis of ALS. *Clin Neurophysiol.* 2008;119:497-503.
3. Traynor BJ, Codd MB, Corr B, Forde C, Frost E, Hardiman OM. Clinical features of amyotrophic lateral sclerosis according to the El Escorial and Airlie House diagnostic criteria: a population-based study. *Arch Neurol.* 2000;57:1171-1176.

8 Neuro-otology

Recent advances in central acute vestibular syndrome of a vascular cause
Kim H-A, Lee H (Keimyung Univ School of Medicine, Daegu, South Korea)
J Neurol Sci 321:17-22, 2012

Acute vestibular syndrome (AVS) is characterized by acute onset of spontaneous prolonged vertigo (lasting days), spontaneous nystagmus, postural instability, and autonomic symptoms. Peripheral AVS commonly presents as vestibular neuritis, but may also include other disorders such as Meniere's disease. Vertigo in central AVS due to vertebrobasilar ischemic stroke is usually accompanied by other neurological dysfunction. However it can occur in isolation and mimicking peripheral AVS, particularly with cerebellar strokes. Recent large prospective studies have demonstrated that approximately 11% of patients with isolated cerebellar infarction presented with isolated vertigo mimicking peripheral AVS, and the bedside head impulse test is the most useful tool for differentiating central from peripheral AVS. Herein we review the keys to the diagnosis of central AVS of a vascular cause presenting with isolated vertigo or audiovestibular loss.

▶ Acute vestibular syndrome (AVS) is recognized by the presence of acute onset spontaneous prolonged vertigo that may last up to several days, spontaneous nystagmus, postural instability, and autonomic manifestations.[1,2] Patients with AVS also experience head-motion intolerance and lack of gait stability. AVS originates from peripheral or central causes. Peripheral AVS frequently stems from vestibular neuritis or Ménière's disease, whereas central etiologies for AVS include more serious conditions such as vertebrobasilar ischemic stroke. The AVS of central nervous system origin is usually accompanied by other neurological deficits of brainstem or cerebellar origin. Vestibular neuritis may clinically imitate AVS of central origin and may be misdiagnosed as such. Interestingly, up to 11% of patients who suffer from isolated cerebellar ischemic infarcts may manifest with isolated vertigo resembling peripheral AVS. The bedside head impulse test is the most useful tool for differentiating central forms of AVS from peripheral ones. The authors of this comprehensive review present a detailed discussion on the keys to the diagnosis of central AVS of a vascular origin manifesting with isolated vertigo or audiovestibular loss. This article has high practical value for all clinicians, particularly those who visit patients with AVS in the emergency department.

A. Minagar, MD

References

1. Hotson JR, Baloh RW. Acute vestibular syndrome. *N Engl J Med.* 1998;339: 680-685.
2. Guntinas-Lichius O. Acute vestibular syndrome. *N Engl J Med.* 1999;340:151-152.

Gamma Knife Treatment of Growing Vestibular Schwannoma in Norway: A Prospective Study

Varughese JK, Wentzel-Larsen T, Pedersen P-H, et al (Univ of Bergen, Norway; Haukeland Univ Hosp, Bergen, Norway)

Int J Radiat Oncol Biol Phys 84:e161-e166, 2012

Purpose.—Gamma Knife radiosurgery (GKRS) has been increasingly used in the treatment of vestibular schwannoma (VS). Very few studies relate tumor control and post-treatment growth rates to pretreatment growth rates.

Methods and Materials.—We prospectively included 45 consecutive VS patients who were initially treated conservatively and then received GKRS between 2000 and 2007 because of demonstrated tumor growth. Pretreatment and post-treatment tumor volumes were estimated. Patients underwent audiograms, reported their symptoms, and responded to the Short Form General Health Survey (SF-36) questionnaire on each visit.

Results.—Volume doubling times before and after treatment were 1.36 years (95% confidence intervals, 1.14–1.68) and −13.1 years (95% confidence intervals, −111.0 to −6.94), respectively. Tumor control, defined as a post-GKRS growth rate ≤0, was achieved in 71.1% of patients, with highest odds for tumor control among older patients and those with larger tumors. The 5-year retreatment-free survival rate was 93.9% (95% confidence intervals, 76.5–98.5). None of the clinical endpoints investigated showed statistically significant changes after GKRS, but improvement was seen in a few SF-36 parameters.

Conclusions.—GKRS alters the natural course of the tumor by reducing growth. Mathematic models yield poorer tumor control rates than those found by clinical assessment. Symptoms were unaffected by treatment, but quality of life was improved.

▶ Gamma knife radiosurgery (GKRS) is a noninvasive medical procedure that is increasingly being used for treatment of both benign and malignant brain tumors. Although GKRS is currently used for the treatment of vestibular schwannoma (VS), few studies compare and relate tumor control and posttreatment growth rates with pretreatment growth rates. This prospective study by Varughese et al assessed and determined the efficacy of GKRS for treatment of VS, determining and comparing posttreatment growth rates with pretreatment growth rates. The study included 45 consecutive VS patients who were initially treated conservatively and then were treated with GKRS between 2000 and 2007 because of demonstrated tumor growth. Pre- and posttreatment tumor volumes were estimated. In addition, all patients underwent audiograms, reported their symptoms, and responded to the

Short Form General Health Survey (SF-36) questionnaire during each visit. The results of this study showed that the volume doubling times before and after treatment were 1.36 years (95% confidence intervals, 1.14–1.68) and −13.1 years (95% confidence intervals, −111.0 to −6.94), respectively. Tumor control, which was defined as a post-GKRS growth rate ≤ 0, was achieved in most (71.1%) patients, with highest odds for tumor control among older patients and those who had larger tumors. The 5-year retreatment-free survival rate was 93.9% (95% confidence intervals, 76.5–98.5). In addition, improvement was seen in a few SF-36 parameters. This interesting study clearly showed that GKRS was capable of altering the natural course of VS by reducing the tumor growth and that GKRS is safe and effective, having low complication rates and improving the quality of life of the patients.

A. Minagar, MD

Current epidemiology and management trends in acoustic neuroma

Gal TJ, Shinn J, Huang B (Univ of Kentucky, Lexington; Kentucky Cancer Registry, Lexington)

Otolaryngol–Head Neck Surg 142:677-681, 2010

Objective.—The objective of this study was to assess the epidemiology of acoustic neuroma and determine current trends in therapy using tumor registry techniques.

Study Design.—Analysis of a national database.

Subjects and Methods.—The Surveillance Epidemiology and End Results (SEER) database is a national tumor registry that began to identify and abstract benign and borderline tumors of the brain and central nervous system in the year 2004. Coding for International Classification of Diseases for Oncology (ICD-O-3) codes for schwannoma (9560/0) with collaborative staging (CS) coding for acoustic nerve (72.4) was used to identify acoustic neuromas. Demographic data, tumor size, and treatment data were analyzed.

Results.—A total of 1621 patients with acoustic neuroma were identified, for an incidence rate of 1.1/100,000. Mean age was 53.1 years. Tumors were equally distributed across gender and tumor laterality, with the majority (84%) occurring in Caucasians. Nine hundred sixty-four patients (59.5%) were treated with surgery, whereas 341 (21.0%) were treated with radiation. A total of 1.6 percent received combined therapy over the study period, with the remaining patients receiving either no treatment or unknown therapy. Of tumors less than 2 cm, 27.2 percent were treated with radiotherapy. Statistically significant associations were observed with the increased use of radiotherapy for small (< 2 cm) tumors ($P = 0.0001$).

Conclusion.—Unlike data from single series, which usually represent individual treatment preferences and techniques, use of SEER data allows for the assessment of demographics and treatment trends at the national level. The results and potential applications are discussed.

▶ Acoustic neuroma, which is also recognized as vestibular schwannoma, is a benign intracranial tumor of the myelin-forming cells of the 8th cranial nerve. Clinically, acoustic neuroma manifests with sensorineural hearing loss, deafness, impairment of balance and gait, vertigo with nausea and vomiting, and feeling of pressure in the ear. Acoustic neuroma is the most common tumor of the cerebellopontine angle. The authors of this epidemiological study aimed to evaluate and determine the epidemiology of acoustic neuroma and show the present trends in its treatment by using tumor registry techniques. They employed the Surveillance Epidemiology and End Results (SEER) database. SEER is a national tumor registry that was initiated to identify and abstract benign and borderline tumors of the brain and central nervous system in 2004. They used the diagnostic codes for acoustic neuroma to extract the cases. In addition, they analyzed demographic data, tumor size, and treatment modalities. The investigators identified 1621 patients with acoustic neuroma with an incidence rate of 1.1/100 000. Mean patient age was 53.1 years and tumors were equally distributed across gender and tumor laterality. Based on their obtained results, the majority (84%) occurred in Caucasian individuals. A total of 964 (59.5%) were treated with surgery, whereas 341 (21.0%) received radiation. A total of 1.6% of patients were treated with combined therapy over the study period, with the remaining patients receiving either no treatment or unknown therapy. Of tumors smaller than 2 cm, 27.2% were treated with radiotherapy. The investigators detected statistically significant associations between the increased use of radiotherapy for small (< 2 cm) tumors ($P = .0001$). This interesting and comprehensive study using SEER presents our readers with an excellent view of demographics and treatment trends at the national level.

A. Minagar, MD

Neuroanatomical correlates of tinnitus revealed by cortical thickness analysis and diffusion tensor imaging

Aldhafeeri FM, MacKenzie I, Kay T, et al (The Univ of Liverpool, UK; Aintree Univ Hosps NHS Foundation Trust, Liverpool, UK)

Neuroradiology 54:883-892, 2012

Introduction.—Tinnitus is a poorly understood auditory perception of sound in the absence of external stimuli. Convergent evidence proposes that tinnitus perception involves brain structural alterations as part of its pathophysiology. The aim of this study is to investigate the structural brain changes that might be associated with tinnitus-related stress and negative emotions.

Methods.—Using high-resolution magnetic resonance imaging and diffusion tensor imaging, we investigated grey matter and white matter (WM) alterations by estimating cortical thickness measures, fractional anisotropy and mean diffusivity in 14 tinnitus subjects and 14 age- and sex-matched non-tinnitus subjects.

Results.—Significant cortical thickness reductions were found in the prefrontal cortex (PFC), temporal lobe and limbic system in tinnitus subjects compared to non-tinnitus subjects. Tinnitus sufferers were found to have disrupted WM integrity in tracts involving connectivity of the PFC, temporal lobe, thalamus and limbic system.

Conclusion.—Our results suggest that such neural changes may represent neural origins for tinnitus or consequences of tinnitus and its associations.

▶ Tinnitus is defined as an unknown auditory phenomenon that is recognized by the perception of the noise in the human ear while there is no external objective source for such stimulus. The pathophysiology of tinnitus is largely unrecognized and currently there is no cure for it. To find a cure for this unpleasant and bothersome condition, we have to learn more about the neurophysiology behind the tinnitus. Functional neuroimaging studies have demonstrated abnormal activity of the auditory areas,[1] the limbic system,[2] amygdala,[3] and prefrontal cortex.[4] The authors of this neuroimaging study aimed to investigate the structural brain alterations that might be associated with tinnitus-related stress and negative emotions. The investigators used high-resolution magnetic resonance imaging and diffusion tensor imaging to assess gray matter and white matter (WM) changes by estimating cortical thickness measures, fractional anisotropy, and mean diffusivity in 14 patients with tinnitus and 14 age- and sex-matched non-tinnitus subjects. The results of this interesting research article indicate that significant cortical thickness reductions were detected in the prefrontal cortex (PFC), temporal lobe, and limbic system in patients with tinnitus compared with those without tinnitus. Patients with tinnitus had disrupted WM integrity in tracts involving connectivity of the PFC, temporal lobe, thalamus, and limbic system. This informative, original research article provides objective evidence for abnormal alteration of certain areas of the human brain that may be the neuro-anatomic basis for tinnitus. Indeed, this type of study enables scientists to proceed toward finding a cure for tinnitus.

A. Minagar, MD

References

1. Mühlnickel W, Elbert T, Taub E, Flor H. Reorganization of auditory cortex in tinnitus. *Proc Natl Acad Sci U S A*. 1998;95:10340-10343.
2. Lockwood AH, Salvi RJ, Coad ML, Towsley ML, Wack DS, Murphy BW. The functional neuroanatomy of tinnitus: evidence for limbic system links and neural plasticity. *Neurology*. 1998;50:114-120.
3. Mirz F, Gjedde A, Sødkilde-Jrgensen H, Pedersen CB. Functional brain imaging of tinnitus-like perception induced by aversive auditory stimuli. *Neuroreport*. 2000; 11:633-637.
4. Mirz F, Pedersen B, Ishizu K, et al. Positron emission tomography of cortical centers of tinnitus. *Hear Res*. 1999;134:133-144.

Endolymphatic Space Imaging in Idiopathic Sudden Sensorineural Hearing Loss With Vertigo

Chen X, Zhang X-D, Gu X, et al (First Clinical Med College of Fujian Med Univ, Fuzhou, Fujian Province, P.R. China; First Affiliated Hosp of Fujian Med Univ, Fuzhou, Fujian Province, P.R. China)
Laryngoscope 122:2265-2268, 2012

Objectives/Hypothesis.—To investigate endolymphatic space images in patients with idiopathic sudden sensorineural hearing loss (ISNHL) and vertigo using three-dimensional fluid-attenuated inversion recovery magnetic resonance imaging (3D-FLAIR MRI).

Study Design.—This is a prospective study of an analysis using the imaging technology of 3D-FLAIR MRI for patients with ISNHL and vertigo.

Methods.—3D-FLAIR MRI was performed 24 hours after intratympanic injection of gadolinium–diethylenetriamine penta-acetic acid.

Results.—In four of seven cases of ISNHL with vertigo, endolymphatic hydrops were confirmed in the cochlea and/or the vestibule of the affected ears.

Conclusions.—The results of the study imply that there may be some relationship between endolymphatic hydrops and ISNHL with vertigo.

▶ Patients with idiopathic sudden sensorineural hearing loss (ISNHL) present with unexplained sensorineural hearing loss for less than 72 hours with or without tinnitus or vertigo. Although the cause of ISNHL remains unrecognized, a number of etiologies, such as viral infection, disruption of the cochlear membrane, circulatory abnormalities, immunologic causes, and disintegration of the cochlear membranes, have been proposed.[1] Using 3-dimensional fluid-attenuated inversion recovery magnetic resonance imaging (3D-FLAIR MRI), the authors of this study aimed to investigate endolymphatic space images in patients with ISNHL and vertigo. During this prospective study, 3D-FLAIR MRI was performed in 7 study subjects with ISNHL and vertigo. The investigators detected endolymphatic hydrops, which was located in the cochlea or the vestibule of the affected ears in 4 of the 7 study patients. Although this interesting study does not establish a straightforward causal relationship between the endolymphatic hydrops and development of ISNHL, it clearly sheds more light into the pathogenesis of this unknown condition and assists us in better outlining the underlying pathology of ISNHL. It also suggests a need for further research into the role of endolymphatic space in ISNHL.

A. Minagar, MD

Reference

1. Eisenman D, Arts HA. Effectiveness of treatment for sudden sensorineural hearing loss. *Arch Otolaryngol Head Neck Surg*. 2000;126:1161-1164.

Short-term audiologic effect of intratympanic gadolinium contrast agent application in patients with Ménière's disease

Louza JPR, Flatz W, Krause E, et al (Univ of Munich, Germany)

Am J Otolaryngol 33:533-537, 2012

Objectives.—The aim of this study was to assess whether gadolinium-based contrast agent influences short-term hearing function in patients with Ménière's disease undergoing intratympanically enhanced inner-ear magnetic resonance imaging.

Design.—This is a prospective cohort study.

Setting.—This study was conducted a tertiary referral university hospital, ENT department.

Participants.—In this study, 21 adult patients with definite, unilateral Ménière's disease were included. According to the criteria of the Committee on Hearing and Equilibrium, all patients were in stage 1 or 2 of the disease, with largely preserved hearing function.

Outcomes.—All patients underwent clinical and audiologic testing before and 24 hours after intratympanic application of gadolinium-based contrast agent. The effects of the contrast medium on the hearing function were assessed by analysis of frequency thresholds, pure-tone average from 500 Hz to 3 kHz, and speech audiometry.

Results.—Pure-tone average and single-frequency thresholds in audiometry showed no statistically significant difference after the application of intratympanic gadolinium-based contrast agent. Furthermore, speech audiometry scores remained stable after the application of the contrast agent.

Conclusions.—This study did not demonstrate clinically significant short-term effects of intratympanic application of gadolinium-based contrast agent on hearing function in patients with Ménière's disease in initial stages.

▶ For many years the diagnosis of Ménière's disease (MD) was made based on the constellation of clinical symptoms of hearing loss, tinnitus, vertigo and aural fullness. With the introduction of magnetic resonance imaging (MRI) of inner ear, which can demonstrate endolymphatic hydrops, the diagnosis of MD has taken a new course and has become more robust and based on objective evidence.[1] The MRI technique to visualize the endolymphatic hydrops utilizes gadolinium as contrast material. Nephrogenic systemic fibrosis is a rare, but well recognized, complication of the use of gadolinium contrast for MRI. Few studies have explored the effects of gadolinium contrast on the function of the inner ear.[2,3] The authors of this prospective study aimed to evaluate if gadolinium-based contrast agent affects short-term hearing function in patients suffering from MD who were undergoing intratympanically enhanced inner-ear MRI. The investigators recruited 21 adult patients with definite, unilateral MD and, based on the criteria of the Committee on Hearing and Equilibrium, all patients were in stage 1 or 2 of the disease, with largely preserved hearing function. All study subjects were examined using clinical and audiologic testing before and 24 hours after intratympanic application of gadolinium-based contrast agent. The investigators assessed the effects of the contrast medium on hearing function by analyzing of frequency thresholds, pure-tone average from 500 Hz to 3 kHz, and speech audiometry. They found that pure-tone average and single-frequency thresholds in audiometry showed no statistically significant difference after the utilization of intratympanic gadolinium-based contrast agent. In addition, speech audiometry scores remained stable after the application of the contrast agent. The authors of this interesting research paper concluded that the use of intratympanic application of gadolinium-based contrast agent did not have any short-term negative effects on hearing function in patients with MD in initial stages.

A. Minagar, MD

References

1. Nakashima T, Naganawa S, Sugiura M, et al. Visualization of endolymphatic hydrops in patients with Ménière's disease. *Laryngoscope*. 2007;117:415-420.
2. Kakigi A, Nishimura M, Takeda T, et al. Effects of gadolinium injected into the middle ear on the stria vascularis. *Acta Oto-Laryngol*. 2008;128:841-845.
3. Tanaka H, Tanigawa T, Suzuki M, et al. Effects of MR contrast agents (Omniscan™) on vestibular end organs. *Acta Oto-Laryngol*. 2010;130:17-24.

Audiovestibular Dysfunction Associated with Adoptive Cell Immunotherapy for Melanoma

Seaman BJ, Guardiani EA, Brewer CC, et al (Georgetown Univ Med Ctr, Washington, DC; Natl Insts of Health, Bethesda, MD)
Otolaryngol Head Neck Surg 147:744-749, 2012

Objective.—To understand the audiologic and vestibular toxicities associated with adoptive cell immunotherapy (ACI) targeting pigment-pathway antigens on melanoma and to investigate the use of intratympanic steroid injections in the treatment of these toxicities.

Study Design.—Prospective nonrandomized study.

Setting.—Tertiary clinical research center.

Methods.—Thirty-two patients with progressive metastatic melanoma who failed conventional therapy underwent ACI with T cells genetically modified to target MART-1 (n = 18) or gp100 (n = 14). All patients received serial audiometric testing. Vestibular testing was performed on patients with vestibular complaints. Patients with significant deficits received intratympanic steroid injections.

Results.—Of 32 patients, 15 had no hearing change, 9 had mild hearing loss, and 8 had moderate hearing loss following treatment. Ten patients received intratympanic steroid injections for mild (n = 2) or moderate (n = 7) hearing loss or for significant imbalance (n = 1). Of those with mild hearing loss (n = 9), all but 1 recovered to pretreatment hearing levels. Four of 8 patients with moderate hearing loss recovered to baseline hearing levels, and 4 had partial recovery. All 7 patients with posttreatment vestibular complaints had demonstrable vestibular dysfunction. Three of these patients demonstrated recovery to normal vestibular function. The number of modified T cells infused for therapy correlated with the degree of audiovestibular deficit.

Conclusion.—Adoptive cell immunotherapy targeting pigment-pathway cell proteins, a novel therapy for melanoma, can induce hearing loss and vestibular dysfunction. The presumed mechanism of autoimmune attack on normal melanocytes in the cochlear stria vascularis and in the vestibular organs demonstrates the importance of melanocytes in normal inner ear function.

▶ Treatment of progressive metastatic melanoma poses a formidable therapeutic challenge to the clinicians and demands novel therapies. Targeting tumor-associated antigens is a modern method for treatment of metastatic melanomas. One way to achieve this goal rests on adoptive cell immunotherapy (ACI). During ACI, T-lymphocytes specific for these tumor antigens are utilized, which are activated and expanded in vitro and then administered to the patient after lymphodepletion. Because tissue-specific antigens are also expressed by various normal cells throughout the human body, their targeting by ACI translates into unwanted toxicities. The authors of this interesting article aimed to explore and unravel the audiologic and vestibular toxicities associated with ACI, which targets pigment-pathway antigens on melanoma, and to assess the use of intratympanic steroid injections in the treatment of such toxicities. During the course of this prospective nonrandomized study, 32 patients with progressive metastatic melanoma who did not respond to conventional therapy were treated with ACI with T cells genetically modified to target (melanoma antigen recognized by T cells 1) MART-1 ($n = 18$) or gp100 ($n = 14$). All study subjects underwent serial audiometric testing. In addition, vestibular testing was performed on patients with vestibular complaints. Those study subjects who suffered from significant deficits were treated with intratympanic steroid injections. Of the 32 patients who participated in this study, 15 experienced no hearing change, 9 had mild hearing loss, and 8 had moderate hearing loss after treatment. Ten patients were treated with intratympanic corticosteroid injections for mild ($n = 2$) or moderate ($n = 7$) hearing loss or for significant imbalance ($n = 1$). Of those with mild hearing loss ($n = 9$), all except one improved to the pretreatment hearing levels. Four of 8 patients with moderate hearing loss improved to baseline hearing levels, and 4 had partial recovery. All 7 study participants with posttreatment vestibular complaints had demonstrable vestibular dysfunction. However, 3 of these patients recovered to normal vestibular function. The number of modified T-lymphocytes infused for treatment correlated with the degree of audiovestibular deficit. The authors concluded that ACI may cause hearing loss and vestibular dysfunction possibly via an autoimmune attack on normal melanocytes in the cochlear stria vascularis and in the vestibular organs. These findings further emphasize the significance of melanocytes in normal inner ear function.

A. Minagar, MD

Quality of Life of Patients With Bilateral Vestibulopathy

Guinand N, Boselie F, Guyot J-P, et al (Univ Hosp Maastricht, the Netherlands; Univ Hosps of Geneva, Switzerland)

Ann Otol Rhinol Laryngol 121:471-477, 2012

Objectives.—Currently, there is no evidence of an effective treatment for patients with bilateral vestibulopathy (BV). Their main complaints are oscillopsia and imbalance. Opinions about the impact of BV on their quality of life are controversial, and their handicap is not always recognized, even among otoneurologists. The aim of this study was to objectively assess the health status of BV patients in order to evaluate the need for pursuing efforts toward the development of new treatments.

Methods.—The Short-Form Health Survey (SF-36), the Dizziness Handicap Inventory (DHI), the Short Falls Efficacy Scale–International (Short FES-I), and an oscillopsia severity questionnaire were submitted to 39 BV patients. The SF-36 scores were compared to the scores of a general Dutch population. The DHI scores were correlated to the oscillopsia severity scores. The Short FES-I scores were compared to scores in an elderly population. Residual otolithic function was correlated to all scores, and hearing to SF-36 scores.

Results.—Compared to the general Dutch population, the BV patients scored significantly worse on the "physical functioning," "role physical," "general health," "vitality," and "social functioning" SF-36 variables ($p < 0.05$). The DHI scores were strongly correlated with the oscillopsia severity scores ($r = 0.75$; $p < 0.000001$). The Short FES-I scores indicated a slight to moderate increase in the patients' fear of falling. No significant score differences were found between BV patients with residual otolithic function and patients with complete BV. There was no correlation between hearing status and SF-36 scores.

Conclusions.—The results correlate with our clinical impression that BV has a strong negative impact on physical and social functioning, leading to a quality-of-life deterioration. There is a clear need for a therapeutic solution. Efforts toward the development of a vestibular implant are justified.

▶ The vestibular system functions include regulation of balance control, spatial orientation, and image stabilization during head movements. Bilateral vestibulopathy (BV), which stems from injuries to the inner ears, manifests with abnormalities of balance, motor coordination, and hearing. Patients commonly complain of oscillopsia and imbalance. Presently, there is no effective therapy for BV, and the quality of life of patients with BV is significantly compromised. The authors of this novel study aimed to objectively evaluate the health status of patients with BV to further demonstrate the need for innovative therapies. The investigators used the short-form health survey (SF-36), the dizziness handicap inventory (DHI), the short falls efficacy scale-international (short FES-I), and an oscillopsia severity questionnaire to assess 39 patients with BV. The obtained SF-36 scores were compared with the scores of a general Dutch population that served as controls. The DHI scores were correlated with the oscillopsia severity scores, and the short

FES-I scores were compared with scores in an elderly population. Residual otolithic function was correlated to all scores, and hearing was correlated to SF-36 scores. The results of this study demonstrated that when compared with the general Dutch population, patients with BV scored significantly worse on the "physical functioning," "role physical," "general health," "vitality," and "social functioning" SF-36 variables ($P < .05$). In addition, the DHI scores revealed a strong correlation with the oscillopsia severity scores ($r = 0.75$; $P < .000001$). The short FES-I scores indicated a slight-to-moderate increase in BV patients' fear of falling. The investigators of this significant epidemiological study concluded that their obtained results correlated with the clinical impression that BV negatively impacts the physical and social functioning of these patients. It leads to a significant decline of their quality of life. Such a significant deterioration of the quality of life again places more emphasis on the need to develop more effective treatments with these patients, including new procedures to develop vestibular implants.

A. Minagar, MD

Traumatic Tympanic Membrane Perforations: Clinical and Audiometric Findings in 198 Patients

Hempel JM, Becker A, Müller J, et al (Ludwig Maximilian Univ, Munich, Germany)

Otol Neurotol 33:1357-1362, 2012

Objective.—To obtain clinical and audiometric findings in traumatic tympanic membrane perforations from a typical patient collective in a Western industrial nation because the appropriate data have an important relevance in medicolegal questions.

Study Design.—Retrospective data collection.

Setting.—Germany's largest university clinic for otorhinolaryngology, head and neck surgery.

Subject and Methods.—From the medical records of 198 patients with traumatic tympanic membrane perforations, the following data were collected: demographic data, date and mechanism of the trauma, otoscopic findings and collateral injuries, kind of therapy and its results, pure tone audiometry, and statement of tinnitus or vertigo in the course.

Results.—Most patients were young (mean age, 29.2 yr) and male (62%). Men and women are equally represented in perforations resulting from a physical blow to the ear (44.7% vs 46.7%); a collision was more often the cause in men (23.6% vs 14.7%), whereas an accidental perforation by insertion of a cotton bud was approximately 2 times more common on women (13.8% vs 25.3%). The left ear was more often affected than the right ear (58.5% vs 41.5%). Collateral damage was found in only 1% of the cases. In blows, collisions, barotraumas, and the insertion of sharp objects, the inferior parts of the tympanic membrane were most often affected; the most severe (subtotal) perforations were caused by explosions, weld beads, and insertion of cotton buds. For therapy, myringoplasty had an overall success rate of 88.9%; splinting with silicon foils, 51.6%; and "no therapy," 53.3%. Bone conduction thresholds for the affected ear were higher in low, middle, and high frequencies compared with the contralateral ear by trend, but a statistical difference was only found in the high frequencies. In follow-up examinations, the hearing thresholds in the high frequencies were no longer significantly different. A "c^5 dip" or "fis^5 dip" was found in 18.0% and 9.2%. Tinnitus and vertigo were reported in 30.8 and 8.1%, respectively, but only in 2.0% and 0% during follow-up.

Conclusion.—High-frequency hearing loss, tinnitus, and vertigo in traumatic tympanic membrane perforations have a good prognosis.

▶ Physicians frequently visit and treat patients with perforations of the tympanic membrane that may result from direct or indirect trauma to the ear. Aside from hearing loss, patients also complain of vertigo and tinnitus. Traumatic perforation of the tympanic membrane is associated with conductive and sensorineural hearing loss.[1-4] The authors of this original research article aimed to collect and analyze clinical and audiologic data of patients with traumatic tympanic membrane perforation in a Western industrial nation to further assess this condition because the obtained information carries important relevance in medicolegal questions. During this retrospective study, the investigators evaluated the medical records of 198 patients with tympanic membrane perforation and gathered data about demographic location, date, and mechanism of the trauma; otoscopic findings and collateral injuries; type of treatment and its results; pure tone audiometry; and statement of tinnitus or vertigo in the course. According to the results of this study, most of the patients were young, with a mean age of 29 years, and male (62% male vs 38% female). However, males and females were equally represented in perforations resulting from a physical blow to the ear (44.7% vs 46.7%), whereas collision was more frequently the cause in males (23.6% vs 14.7%). The accidental perforation by insertion of a cotton bud was approximately 2 times more common in females. The right ear was less affected than the left ear, and collateral damage was detected in a minority of patients. In blows, collisions, barotraumas, and the insertion of sharp objects, the inferior sections of the tympanic membrane were most often affected, whereas the most severe (subtotal) perforations were caused by explosions, weld beads, and insertion of cotton buds. In terms of treatment, myringoplasty had a general success rate of 88.9%; splinting with silicon foils, 51.6%; and "no therapy," 53.3%. Such treatments did have positive outcomes, and in follow-up assessments, there was sustained improvement of hearing. The authors concluded that high-frequency hearing loss, tinnitus, and vertigo in traumatic tympanic membrane perforations have a good prognosis and are responsive to available therapies.

A. Minagar, MD

References

1. Orji FT, Agu CC. Patterns of hearing loss in tympanic membrane perforation resulting from physical blow to the ear: a prospective controlled cohort study. *Clin Otolaryngol.* 2009;34:526-532.
2. Berger G, Finkelstein Y, Avraham S, Himmelfarb M. Patterns of hearing loss in non-explosive blast injury of the ear. *J Laryngol Otol.* 1997;111:1137-1141.

3. Dejgaard A. Pathophysiology and treatment of diabetic neuropathy. *Diabet Med.* 1998;15:97-112.
4. Koide Y, Tajima S, Yoshida M, Konno M. Biochemical changes in the inner ear induced by insulin, in relation to the cochlear microphonics. *Ann Otol Rhinol Laryngol.* 1960;69:1083-1097.

Benign paroxysmal positional vertigo in people with traumatic spinal cord injury: incidence, treatment efficacy and implications

Lee WK, Koh SW, Wee SK (Tan Tock Seng Rehabilitation Centre, Singapore)
Am J Otolaryngol 33:723-730, 2012

Purpose.—To determine the incidence of benign positional paroxysmal vertigo (BPPV) and its treatment efficacy as well as the safety of conventional and modified BPPV assessments and treatment techniques in traumatic spinal cord injury (SCI) population. Subsequently, arrive at implications for clinical practices and set foundation for future research.

Materials and Methods.—Consecutive traumatic SCI patients who were admitted to the rehabilitation centre during the period from August 2008 to December 2010 were screened for BPPV using the Dix-Hallpike test and roll test. The treatment efficacy was reflected by the number of treatment required for complete resolution of BPPV symptoms. Modified assessment and treatment techniques were employed for people with cervical SCI.

Results.—A total of 62 subjects were included and the overall incidence of BPPV was 14.5%. People with cervical SCI were 2.87 times more likely to have BPPV compared to people with thoracic/ lumbar SCI. The treatment efficacy for posterior and horizontal canal canalithiasis were 75% and 100% respectively with one manoeuvre. All BPPVs were resolved within three manoeuvres without any complication. All conventional and modified BPPV assessment and treatment techniques were found to be safe in people with traumatic SCI.

Conclusion.—This is the first study to look into the incidence and treatment efficacy of BPPV in people with traumatic SCI. The high incidence is worth clinicians' attentions. The treatments were also highly effective for immediate symptoms resolution. We recommend that assessments and treatments for BPPV could be incorporated into the standard care for people with traumatic SCI.

▶ Benign positional paroxysmal vertigo (BPPV) is a disorder of the inner ear that is characterized by bouts of positional vertigo caused by alterations of the head position.[1] Not much information is available regarding the frequency of BPPV in patients with traumatic spinal cord injury (SCI). The authors of this study aimed to assess the incidence of BPPV and the efficacy of its treatment in this unique patient population. The investigators included 62 consecutive patients with traumatic SCI who were treated at a rehabilitation center from August 2008 to December 2010. They examined the patients for the presence of BPPV utilizing the Dix-Hallpike test and roll test. The treatment efficacy was determined by the number of treatments required for complete symptomatic resolution of

BPPV. The investigators utilized modified assessment and treatment techniques for people with cervical SCI. Based on the results of this epidemiologic study, the overall incidence of BPPV was determined to be 14.5%. Interestingly, patients with cervical SCI were 2.87 times more likely to have BPPV compared with patients with thoracic/lumbar SCI. The treatment efficacies for posterior and horizontal canal canalithiasis were 75% and 100%, respectively, with one maneuver, and in all patients with BPPV the symptoms were resolved within 3 maneuvers without any complication. It was also determined that all conventional and modified BPPV assessment and treatment methods were safe in patients with traumatic SCI.

The authors concluded that this study, for the first time, addresses the BPPV in patients with traumatic SCI and provides clinicians with useful practical input regarding treatment of BPPV in this population of patients. The high frequency of BPPV in this patient population, as well as the high efficacy of immediate symptomatic resolution of BPPV, further stresses the necessity to look for this disorder in these patients. This interesting study also indicates that evaluation for and treatment of BPPV should be included in the standard management of patients with traumatic SCI.

A. Minagar, MD

Reference

1. Alvarenga GA, Barbosa MA, Porto CC. Benign paroxysmal positional vertigo without nystagmus: diagnosis and treatment. *Braz J Otorhinolaryngol.* 2011;77: 799-804.

A Randomized, Double-Blind, Placebo-Controlled Clinical Study to Assess Safety and Clinical Activity of OTO-104 Given as a Single Intratympanic Injection in Patients With Unilateral Ménière's Disease

Lambert PR, Nguyen S, Maxwell KS, et al (Med Univ of South Carolina, Charleston; Piedmont Ear Nose and Throat Associates, Winston-Salem, NC; et al)
Otol Neurotol 33:1257-1265, 2012

Objective.—To evaluate the safety, tolerability, and clinical activity of a single intratympanic injection of OTO-104, sustained-release dexamethasone formulation, in patients with unilateral Ménière's disease.

Study Design.—Prospective, double-blind, randomized, placebo-controlled, dose-escalation study of 16 weeks' (4—wk lead-in before dosing; 12—wk follow-up after dosing) duration for each patient.

Setting.—Fifteen centers (physician offices and academic or tertiary referral centers).

Patients.—Forty-four patients aged 22 to 75 years.

Intervention.—Single intratympanic injection of OTO-104 (3 or 12 mg) or placebo.

Main Outcome Measures.—Safety and tolerability were assessed via adverse event reports, otoscopy, audiometry, and tympanometry. Clinical activity was assessed primarily as changes in vertigo frequency.

Results.—OTO-104 was well tolerated, with no impact on hearing function. Plasma levels were observed in a few patients and were barely quantifiable. The most frequently reported adverse event considered related to investigational product was tympanic membrane perforation; no clinical sequelae were associated with these perforations and all were graded mild or moderate. At Month 3, the observed mean ± standard deviation (SD) change from baseline in vertigo frequency was −0.124 ± 0.153, −0.147 ± 0.166, and −0.211 ± 0.153 for the placebo, 3-mg OTO-104, and 12-mg OTO-104 groups, respectively; corresponding to 42%, 56% and 73% reductions in vertigo frequency, respectively. Similar results were observed for tinnitus, measured by the Tinnitus Handicap Inventory (THI−25).

Conclusion.—OTO-104 was safe and well tolerated. Although the sample size was small, the data suggest 12 mg of OTO-104 was associated with a clinically meaningful reduction in vertigo frequency compared to placebo 3 months after treatment.

▶ Ménière's disease (MD) is characterized by the presence of episodic vertigo, tinnitus, and hearing loss. This idiopathic chronic disease of the inner ear affects up to 0.2% of the population and currently remains incurable. It has been hypothesized that the imbalance between generation of endolymph and its absorption leads to endolymphatic hydrops. Existing medical and surgical treatments for MD only partially alleviate its symptoms and possess serious side effects. There is a strong need for development of more effective and safer treatments for MD. The authors of this clinical trial report aimed to assess the safety, tolerability, and clinical activity of a single intratympanic injection of OTO-104, sustained-release dexamethasone formulation, in patients with unilateral MD. This trial was designed as a prospective, double-blind, randomized, placebo-controlled, dose-escalation study of 16 weeks' (4-week lead-in before dosing; 12-week follow-up after dosing) duration for each study subject, and it was done in 15 medical centers. It included 44 patients from 22 to 75 years of age, and study outcome measures included assessment of the safety and tolerability of OTO-104 via adverse event reports, otoscopy, audiometry, and tympanometry. Clinical activity was evaluated by determining the alteration in vertigo frequency. Based on the results obtained from this trial, OTO-104 was well tolerated but had no effect on hearing function. The most commonly reported adverse event related to investigational product was tympanic membrane perforation with no clinical sequelae associated with these perforations. All cases of tympanic perforations were graded as mild or moderate. At month 3, the observed reduction in vertigo frequency for the placebo-treated group was only 42%, whereas the patients who were treated with the investigational medication—3 mg OTO-104 and 12 mg OTO-104 groups—showed 56% and 73% reductions, respectively. Similar results were obtained for tinnitus as measured by the Tinnitus Handicap Inventory. The authors concluded that OTO-104 was safe and well tolerated. Although the sample size was small, the data indicate that injection of 12 mg of OTO-104 was associated with a clinically meaningful reduction in vertigo frequency compared with the placebo 3 months after treatment.

A. Minagar, MD

Auditory and Vestibular Symptoms and Chronic Subjective Dizziness in Patients With Ménière's Disease, Vestibular Migraine, and Ménière's Disease With Concomitant Vestibular Migraine

Neff BA, Staab JP, Eggers SD, et al (Mayo Clinic School of Medicine, Rochester, MN)

Otol Neurotol 33:1235-1244, 2012

Objective.—To compare presentations of Ménière's disease (MD), vestibular migraine (VM), and Ménière's disease plus vestibular migraine (MDVM), with and without comorbid chronic subjective dizziness (CSD).

Study Design.—Retrospective review with diagnosis confirmed by consensus conference of investigators using published criteria for MD, VM, and CSD.

Setting.—Ambulatory, tertiary dizziness clinic.

Patients.—Approximately 147 consecutive patients with diagnoses of MD, VM, or MDVM, with/without comorbid CSD.

Interventions.—Diagnostic consultation.

Main Outcome Measures.—Similarities and differences between diagnostic groups in demographics; symptoms; and results of neurotologic, audiometric, and vestibular laboratory assessments.

Results.—Seventy-six patients had MD, 55 MD alone. Ninety-two patients had VM, 71 VM alone. Twenty-one patients had MDVM, representing about one-quarter of those diagnosed with MD or VM. Clinical features thought to differentiate VM from MD were found in all groups. Twenty-seven patients with VM (38%) had ear complaints (subjective hearing loss, aural pressure, and tinnitus) during episodes of vestibular symptoms and headache, including 10 (37%) with unilateral symptoms. Conversely, 27 patients with MD alone (49%) had headaches with migraine features that did not meet full IHS diagnostic criteria, migrainous symptoms (photophobia, headache with vomiting), or first-degree relative with migraine. Including MDVM patients, 59% (45/76) of all patients with MD had migrainous features. Thirty-two patients had CSD; most (29; 91%) were in the VM group.

Conclusion.—Comorbidity was common between MD and VM, and their symptoms overlapped. More specific diagnostic criteria are needed to differentiate these diseases and address their coexistence. CSD co-occurred with VM but was rarely seen with MD.

▶ Ménière's disease (MD) manifests with episodic vertigo, tinnitus, and hearing loss. Patients with unrelenting unsteadiness or dizziness between episodes of vertigo present diagnostic challenges to the clinicians. Two other diseases that may assist us to better understand the latter patients include vestibular migraine

(VM) and chronic subjective dizziness (CSD). VM is characterized by episodic vertigo associated with migraine headaches. CSD is recognized with persistent unsteadiness and nonvertiginous dizziness that is increasingly being diagnosed as a frequent residual of episodic vestibular conditions. MD, VM, and CSD share certain clinical features and imitate each other. It is also possible that patients with recurrent bouts of vertigo may suffer from more than one pathology and have concurrent MD and VM. The authors of this retrospective study aimed to compare the clinical manifestations of MS, VM, and MD plus vestibular migraine (MDVM), with and without comorbid CSD. During this study, the investigators reviewed the medical records of approximately 147 consecutive patients with diagnoses of MD, VM, or MDVM, with/without comorbid CSD. Study outcome measures included similarities and differences between diagnostic groups in demographics, symptoms, and results of neurotologic, audiometric, and vestibular laboratory assessments. Based on the results, 76 patients had MD with 55 having MD alone, whereas of the 92 patients with a diagnosis of VM, 71 had VM alone. Twenty-one patients had MDVM, representing about 25% of those who were diagnosed with MD or VM. Clinical features that set VM apart from MD were identified in all groups. Twenty-seven patients with VM (38%) had ear complaints such as subjective hearing loss, aural pressure, and tinnitus during episodes of vestibular symptoms and headache, including 10 (37%) with unilateral symptoms. On the other hand, 27 patients with MD alone (49%) had headaches with migraine features that did not meet full International Headache Society diagnostic criteria, migrainous symptoms (photophobia, headache with vomiting), or first-degree relative with migraine. In MDVM patients, 59% (45 of 76) of all patients who suffered from MD had migrainous features. Apart from this, 32 patients had CSD, most of whom (29; 91%) were in the VM group. The authors concluded that comorbidity was common between MD and VM, and their clinical manifestation overlapped. CSD was more common in patients with VM and rare among those with MD. Although this paper explores the clinical similarities and dissimilarities among these conditions, it also highlights the need for more robust diagnostic criteria to differentiate these diseases.

A. Minagar, MD

Irreversible Atorvastatin-Associated Hearing Loss

Liu M, Alafris A, Longo AJ, et al (Long Island Univ, Brooklyn, NY; UCB Pharma, Rochester, NY)

Pharmacotherapy 32:e27-e34, 2012

Drug-associated ototoxicity is a potentially irreversible adverse event. Among the several 3-hydroxy-3-methylglutaryl coenzyme A reductase inhibitors (statins) available in the United States, only atorvastatin is associated with tinnitus, but none are associated with any forms of hearing loss. A search of the published literature (1950—August 2011) revealed no published case reports of ototoxicity associated with statins. To our knowledge, we describe the first case of progressive, irreversible hearing loss in a 32-year-old man 18 months after starting atorvastatin therapy. He began taking atorvastatin 20 mg every evening for treatment of hypercholesterolemia. Six months later, he complained of occasional episodes of tinnitus, which resolved spontaneously. An audiogram was obtained and was normal. By 18 months, the tinnitus became continuous. Another audiogram revealed bilateral "cookie-bite" middle-frequency hearing loss. Atorvastatin was immediately discontinued, and the patient was fitted with hearing aids. Four years after drug discontinuation, his hearing loss had neither progressed nor regressed. Use of the Naranjo adverse drug reaction probability scale indicated a possible (score of 2) temporal and causal relationship between the patient's hearing loss and atorvastatin. Causes of "cookie-bite" hearing loss include chronic exposure to loud noises, presbycusis, genetic predisposition, and drugs. The manufacturer of atorvastatin has received three unpublished cases of deafness, but claims that causal relationships were not established. Despite these claims by the manufacturer, based on this case report, we recommend that clinicians and patients be aware of the risk of atorvastatin-associated tinnitus and permanent hearing loss. Further research is needed to better understand the mechanism and frequency of this adverse event.

▶ The introduction of 3-hydroxy-3-methylglutaryl coenzyme A reductase inhibitors (statins) to the medical world has fundamentally altered our approach and treatment of patients with hypercholesterolemia and hyperlipidemia. These medications were approved by the US Food and Drug Administration after comprehensive clinical trials demonstrated their efficacy in the treatment of patients with hypercholesterolemia and hyperlipidemia. However, statins, similar to many other medications, do have side effects. Some of these side effects are better known as myopathy, whereas the others are less common and less recognized. The authors of this interesting clinical article report a patient who developed irreversible hearing loss following the administration of atorvastatin. Of the statin medications available in the US market, only atorvastatin is associated with the development of tinnitus. This group of medications has not been reported to be ototoxic and do not cause hearing loss. This is the first case report about atorvastatin-associated hearing loss. In this particular case, the patient was followed for a number of years and the hearing loss associated with use of atorvastatin did not improve. Although this particular case does not establish a definite causal relationship between the use of atorvastatin and hearing loss and this observation should be interpreted with great caution, it also alerts clinicians to be aware of such potential adverse events. The chance of such association is minimal; however, treating physicians and patients should acknowledge a potential risk of hearing loss associated with use of atorvastatin and report any such events to the product manufacturer.

A. Minagar, MD

Tinnitus in Children: Association With Stress and Trait Anxiety

Kim YH, Jung HJ, Kang SI, et al (Seoul Natl Univ, South Korea; et al)

Laryngoscope 122:2279-2284, 2012

Objectives/Hypothesis.—The aim of this study was to investigate associations between tinnitus and stress factors including anxiety in elementary school students.

Study Design.—Cross-sectional study.

Methods.—We conducted a cross-sectional questionnaire survey in 940 students aged from 10 to 12 years. Data on 928 students were collected. The questionnaire comprised 96 questions that were classified into six categories: subjects' symptoms, stress factors, State Anxiety (transitory emotional condition characterized by feeling of tension and apprehension) Inventory for Children (SAIC), Trait Anxiety (general tendency to respond with anxiety to environmental threat) Inventory for Children (TAIC), visual analog scale of tinnitus, and Tinnitus Handicap Inventory (THI).

Results.—Four hundred thirty-five students (46.9%) had experienced tinnitus more than once, and 41 (4.4%) suffered from it continuously. Self-perception of hearing loss, dizziness, headache, and concerns about obesity had significant differences between tinnitus and nontinnitus groups, whereas other stress factors did not show any difference. TAIC scores showed statistically significant differences according to the frequency of tinnitus in children experiencing tinnitus, whereas SAIC scores did not. Annoyance, influence on daily life, disturbance of sleep, and study by tinnitus and THI scores showed significant differences according to the frequency of tinnitus.

Conclusions.—The present study confirms that many children are aware of tinnitus and that they may be susceptible to stressful environments. In particular, trait anxiety may be associated with tinnitus. Because both tinnitus and anxiety can affect the daily lives and health of children—as with adults—a detailed strategy for the management of tinnitus in children should be established.

▶ Tinnitus (ringing in the ear) is defined as a perception of sound within the human ear, although there is no corresponding external source. Tinnitus is not a disease but a symptom of a diverse group of underlying pathologies, such as multiple sclerosis, ear infections, or medication side effect. Tinnitus affects both adult and pediatric patients. However, our knowledge about children with tinnitus is limited. The aim of this study was to investigate associations between tinnitus and stress factors, including anxiety in elementary school students. The authors of this cross-sectional study aimed to explore this issue further and used a questionnaire survey in 940 students 10 to 12 years of age. They collected information on 928 students. The study questionnaire consisted of 96 questions that were categorized into 6 categories: subjects' symptoms, stress factors, State Anxiety (transitory emotional condition characterized by feeling of tension and apprehension) Inventory for Children (SAIC), Trait Anxiety (general tendency to respond with anxiety to environmental threat) Inventory for Children (TAIC), visual analog scale of tinnitus, and Tinnitus Handicap Inventory (THI). The results of this interesting study indicated that 435 students (46.9%) had suffered from tinnitus more than once, and 41 (4.4%) experienced it constantly. Self-perception of hearing loss, dizziness, headache, and concerns about obesity had significant differences between patients with tinnitus and those without tinnitus, whereas other stress factors did not demonstrate any difference. TAIC scores revealed statistically significant differences according to the frequency of tinnitus in children suffering from tinnitus, whereas SAIC scores did not. Annoyance, influence on daily life, disturbance of sleep, and study by tinnitus and THI scores indicated significant differences according to the frequency of tinnitus. The authors concluded that this epidemiological study supported the concept that many children know about tinnitus and that they may be susceptible to stressful environments. Interestingly, anxiety may be associated with tinnitus. Because both tinnitus and anxiety can affect the daily lives and health of children, a comprehensive protocol for the treatment of tinnitus in pediatric patients should be developed.

A. Minagar, MD

Risk of Developing Sudden Sensorineural Hearing Loss in Diabetic Patients: A Population-Based Cohort Study

Lin S-W, Lin Y-S, Weng S-F, et al (Univ of British Columbia, Vancouver, Canada; Taipei Med Univ, Taiwan, Republic of China; Chi Mei Med Ctr, Taiwan, Republic of China)

Otol Neurotol 33:1482-1488, 2012

Objectives.—To explore the risk of development of sudden sensorineural hearing loss (SSHL) among diabetes mellitus patients.

Study Design.—A retrospective cohort study.

Setting.—Population-based study of Taiwan National Health Insurance Research Database.

Patients.—Approximately 26,556 newly diagnosed diabetic patients and 26,556 comparison subjects without diabetes mellitus were selected from claims made during 2000 to 2004.

Main Outcome Measures.—The incidence of sudden sensorineural hearing loss (SSHL) at the end of 2009 was determined.

Results.—The incidence of SSHL was 1.54-fold higher in the diabetic group compared with the nondiabetic group (1.29 versus 0.78 per 1,000 person-years), and using Cox proportional hazard regressions, the adjusted hazard ratio (HR) was 1.592 (95% confidence interval [CI], 1.295–1.957). The risk of developing SSHL increased substantially to an HR of 2.060 (95% CI, 1.051–4.037), for patients who required triple antidiabetic medication compared with diabetic patients treated with a single antidiabetic drug. An increased risk of developing SSHL, with adjusted HRs of 1.574 (95% CI, 1.091–2.271) and 2.842 (95% CI, 1.880–4.295), was observed in diabetic patients with newly diagnosed comorbidities of retinopathy or retinopathy combined with renal insufficiency, which are both expected to reflect the severity of diabetes.

Conclusion.—Diabetes mellitus was significantly associated with an increased risk of developing SSHL. Coronary heart disease or retinopathy comorbidities in diabetic patients seemed to be associated with an increased risk of developing SSHL. The risk of developing SSHL increased with the severity of diabetes.

▶ Sudden sensorineural hearing loss (SSHL) is defined as a loss of more than 30 dB in 3 contiguous frequencies in less than 3 days.[1] The exact cause of SSHL remains unknown and the present proposed etiologies include various causes, such as viral infection, vascular insufficiency, compromise, rupture of the intracochlear membrane rupture, and immune-mediated inner ear disease.[2] Diabetes mellitus (DM) has been linked to chronic hearing impairment. It has been proposed that DM causes small-vessel disease and narrowing, which plays a role in chronic hearing loss.[3,4] The authors of this interesting article aimed to assess the risk of development of SSHL in patients with DM. During this retrospective, population-based, cohort study, the investigators assessed approximately 26 556 newly diagnosed diabetic patients and 26 556 comparison subjects without DM between 2000 and 2004. The authors determined the incidence of SSHL at the end of 2009 and detected that the incidence of SSHL was 1.54-fold higher in the diabetic patients compared with the individuals without DM (1.29 vs 0.78 per 1000 person-years). Using Cox proportional hazard regressions, the adjusted hazard ratio (HR) was 1.592 (95% confidence interval [CI], 1.295-1.957). Based on their findings, the risk of developing SSHL increased substantially to an HR of 2.060 (95% CI, 1.051-4.037), for patients who required triple antidiabetic medication compared with diabetic patients treated with a single antidiabetic drug. In addition, an increased risk of developing SSHL, with adjusted HRs of 1.574 (95% CI, 1.091-2.271) and 2.842 (95% CI, 1.880-4.295), was detected in diabetic patients with newly diagnosed comorbidities of retinopathy or retinopathy plus renal failure, which are both expected to reflect the severity of the underlying DM. The investigators concluded that DM was significantly associated with an increased risk of developing SSHL. Furthermore, other comorbidities, such as coronary heart disease or retinopathy, in patients with DM were associated with an increased risk of developing SSHL. Therefore, the risk of developing SSHL increased with the severity of DM. This is a very important study for clinicians who visit and examine diabetic patients on a daily basis in our clinics. The findings of this study should alert the treating physician about the possibility of this type of hearing loss in diabetic patients and again emphasizes the significance of more powerful treatment of underlying disease.

A. Minagar, MD

References

1. Hughes GB, Freedman MA, Haberkamp TJ, Guay ME. Sudden sensorineural hearing loss. *Otolaryngol Clin North Am.* 1996;29:393-405.
2. Hashisaki GT. Sudden sensory hearing loss. In: Bailey BJ, Johnson JT, Newlands SD, eds. *Head & Neck Surgery-Otolaryngology.* 4th ed. Philadelphia, PA: Lippincott Williams & Wilkins; 2006:2231-2233.

3. Dejgaard A. Pathophysiology and treatment of diabetic neuropathy. *Diabetic Med.* 1998;15:97-112.
4. Koide Y, Tajima S, Yoshida M, Konno M. Biochemical changes in the inner ear induced by insulin, in relation to the cochlear microphonics. *Ann Otol Rhinol Laryngol.* 1960;69:1083-1097.

9 Pediatric Neurology

Early-Onset Epileptic Encephalopathies: Ohtahara Syndrome and Early Myoclonic Encephalopathy

Beal JC, Cherian K, Moshe SL (Albert Einstein College of Medicine and Montefiore Med Ctr, Bronx, NY)

Pediatr Neurol 47:317-323, 2012

Ohtahara syndrome and early myoclonic encephalopathy are the earliest presenting of the epileptic encephalopathies. They are typically distinguished from each other according to specific clinical and etiologic criteria. Nonetheless, considerable overlap exists between the two syndromes in terms of clinical presentation, prognosis, and electroencephalographic signature. Newer understandings of underlying etiologies of these conditions may support the previously suggested concept that they represent a single spectrum of disease rather than two distinct disorders. We review both syndromes, with particular focus on the underlying genetics and pathophysiology and implications regarding the classification of these conditions.

▶ Ohtahara syndrome and early myoclonic encephalopathy (EME) are 2 rather common, yet unfortunate, epileptic encephalopathies in infancy. These syndromes that occur in early childhood are of particular interest to pediatric neurologists because of their very similar clinical presentations and overlapping electroencephalographic (EEG) findings. Ohtahara syndrome characteristically presents with tonic spasms, whereas EME is generally heralded by focal myoclonus and focal seizures. Both may have a burst-suppression pattern in EEG studies. However, in 50% of cases EME may evolve into a hypsarrhythmia, which is seen also when Ohtahara syndrome transitions to West syndrome. In general, children with Ohtahara syndrome have central nervous system malformations compared with patients with EME who are more likely to have metabolic disorders, such as nonketotic hyperglycinemia, other aminoacidemias, molybdenum cofactor deficiency, sulfite oxidase deficiency, Menkes disease, and Zellweger syndrome. Unfortunately, therapy for both is mainly supportive, including the use of antiepileptics and the correction of the underlying metabolic abnormality, and it does not appreciably affect the long-term neurologic prognosis for these patients.

R. Riel-Romero, MD

A Randomized, Double-Blind Study of 30 Versus 20 mg Dexmethylphenidate Extended-Release in Children With Attention-Deficit/Hyperactivity Disorder: Late-Day Symptom Control

Brams M, Turnbow J, Pestreich L, et al (Baylor College of Medicine, Houston; Westex Clinical Investigations, Lubbock, TX; US Med, East Hanover, NJ; et al)
J Clin Psychopharmacol 32:637-644, 2012

The objective of this study was to evaluate the safety and efficacy of dexmethylphenidate extended-release (d-MPH-ER) 30 versus 20 mg in children with attention-deficit/hyperactivity disorder (ADHD) in a 12-hour laboratory classroom setting. In a randomized, double-blind, 3-period × 3-treatment, crossover study, children aged 6 to 12 years with *Diagnostic and Statistical Manual of Mental Disorders, Fourth Edition*–diagnosed ADHD previously stabilized on MPH (40–60 mg/d) or D-MPH (20–Combined score from predose to 10, 11, and 12 hours postdose [Avg(10–4.47) compared with D-MPH-ER 20 mg (−2.02; $P = 0.002$). Most common adverse events (≥3% in any group) were decreased appetite (6.1%, 4.9%, and 0%), headache (4.3%, 4.3%, and 1.9%), abdominal pain (3.7%, 3.1%, and 3.1%), and tachycardia (1.2%, 3.1%, and 0.6%) for D-MPH-ER 30 mg, D-MPH-ER 20 mg, and placebo, respectively). Significantly greater improvement in ADHD symptoms was noted with D-MPH-ER 30 mg compared with D-MPH-ER 20 mg at hours 10 through 12. Tolerability was comparable between doses. Dexmethylphenidate extended-release 30-mg dose may provide further benefit to patients who do not maintain optimal symptom control later in the day with D-MPH-ER 20 mg.

▶ Attention-deficit/hyperactivity disorder (ADHD) is a very common psychiatric diagnosis in children, with an estimated prevalence of 8% to 12% worldwide. The symptoms associated with ADHD can significantly impact a child's social and academic functioning. To date, psychostimulants have been widely used to alleviate symptoms associated with ADHD. Various formulations of methylphenidate have been used. This article focuses on the comparative safety and efficacy of 2 doses of dexmethylphenidate extended release (d-MPH-ER) namely, 20 mg vs 30 mg at 10, 11, and 12 hours after dose. Using a randomized, double-blind, crossover study design with outcomes measured by the SKAMP (Swanson, Kotkin, Agler, M-Flynn, and Pelham combined rating scales) and a math test, the authors concluded that whereas both doses appeared to be effective compared with placebo 12 hours after dose, 30 mg d-MPH-ER is superior to 20 mg d-MPH-ER for controlling symptoms during the latter part of a classroom laboratory day with similar safety profile. As the authors stated, limitations of the study included potential carryover effects, as this is a crossover study; exclusion of inattentive type ADHD and the overrepresentation of females resulting in a potential sampling bias; and the lack of pharmacokinetic laboratory data to support the observations that were made.

R. Riel-Romero, MD

Glucose transporter type I deficiency syndrome: Epilepsy phenotypes and outcomes

Pong AW, Geary BR, Engelstad KM, et al (Columbia Univ, NY; Univ of Notre Dame, IN; et al)

Epilepsia 53:1503-1510, 2012

Purpose.—Glut 1 deficiency syndrome (DS) is defined by hypoglycorrhachia with normoglycemia, acquired microcephaly, episodic movements, and epilepsy refractory to standard antiepileptic drugs (AEDs). Gold standard treatment is the ketogenic diet (KD), which provides ketones to treat neuroglycopenia. Our purpose is (1) to describe epilepsy phenotypes in a large Glut 1 DS cohort, to facilitate diagnosis; and (2) to describe cases in which non-KD agents achieved seizure freedom (SF), highlighting potential adjunctive treatments.

Methods.—Retrospective review of 87 patients with Glut 1 DS (45% female, age range 3 months–35 years, average diagnosis 6.5 years) at Columbia University, from 1989 to 2010.

Key Findings.—Seventy-eight (90%) of 87 patients had epilepsy, with average onset at 8 months. Seizures were mixed in 68% (53/78): generalized tonic–clonic (53%), absence (49%), complex partial (37%), myoclonic (27%), drop (26%), tonic (12%), simple partial (3%), and spasms (3%). We describe the first two cases of spasms in Glut 1 DS. Electrophysiologic abnormalities were highly variable over time; only 13 (17%) of 75 had exclusively normal findings. KD was used in 82% (64/78); 67% (41/61) were seizure-free and 68% of seizure-free patients (28/41) resolved in <1 week and 76% (31/41) in <1 month. Seven patients achieved SF with broad agents only.

Significance.—Glut 1 DS is a genetic metabolic encephalopathy with variable focal and multifocal seizure types and electroencephalographic findings. Infants with seizures, spasms, or paroxysmal events should be tested for Glut 1 DS. Evidence is insufficient to recommend specific AEDs as alternatives to KD. Early diagnosis and initiation of KD and prevention of unnecessary AED trials in Glut 1 DS are important goals for the treatment of children with epilepsy.

▶ Glucose transporter deficiency syndrome (Glut 1 DS) is one of the causes of refractory pediatric epilepsy, characterized by hypoglycorrhachia with normoglycemia. Hallmark clinical features include microcephaly, episodic movements, and difficult-to-control seizures. Ketogenic diet (KD) is considered to be the treatment of choice. In a retrospective review of 87 patients with Glut 1 DS, the authors expanded the epilepsy phenotype to include generalized-tonic seizures; absence; complex partial seizures; myoclonic, tonic, drop, simple partial; and spasms, with 63% having a mixed seizure phenotype. Interestingly, 7 patients achieved seizure-freedom despite therapy with nonketogenic diet strategies, that is, other antiepileptic drugs, such as topiramate, valproate, and lamotrigine, suggesting that other adjunctive treatments are effective aside from KD. Another take-home message is that intractable absence seizures can be the presenting sign in Glut 1 DS, as some of these patients were treated with ethosuximide for greater than 6 years. The main drawback of this study is that it is, as the authors pointed out, retrospective in design.

R. Riel-Romero, MD

Does a Normalizing Electroencephalogram in Benign Childhood Epilepsy with Centrotemporal Spikes Abort Attention Deficit Hyperactivity Disorder?

Schneebaum-Sender N, Goldberg-Stern H, Fattal-Valevski A, et al (Dana Children's Hosp, Tel Aviv, Israel; Tel Aviv Univ, Petah Tiqva, Israel)
Pediatr Neurol 47:279-283, 2012

This retrospective study delineated the efficacy of antiepileptic drugs in preventing the need for methylphenidate in patients with benign childhood epilepsy with centrotemporal spikes and attention deficit hyperactivity disorder. Seventeen patients were identified. A reduction of electroencephalogram pathologic activity by more than 50% was achieved in some patients with the antiepileptic drugs levetiracetam, sulthiame, lamotrigine, clobazam, and valproic acid. Complete normalization was achieved in two patients with sulthiame. Improvement in attention along with the reduction of pathologic electroencephalogram activity was observed in four patients, two with sulthiame, and one each with lamotrigine and levetiracetam (which was ceased because of suicidal tendencies). However, this improvement in attention was either temporary or not significant enough to discontinue methylphenidate. Methylphenidate was eventually prescribed to all patients.

▶ Benign rolandic epilepsy, or benign epilepsy with centrotemporal spikes (BECTS), is a common pediatric epilepsy syndrome familiar to many pediatric neurologists. It is widely believed that children afflicted with this disorder do better than those with other epilepsy syndromes, with reports of spontaneous resolution of seizures during latter adolescence. However, it is increasingly being recognized as well that many patients with BECTS have subtle deficits in cognitive functioning, including visuomotor skills and attention. In this small, retrospective study of 17 patients, Schneebaum-sender et al studied whether reduction in interictal epileptiform activity by the use of antiepileptic drugs (AEDs) can also result in a corresponding improvement in cognitive functioning, perhaps obviating the need for additional treatment with stimulants such as methylphenidate. They found that, although some AEDs do cause improvement or even complete normalization of the electroencephalogram, attentional problems persisted or recurred, necessitating the eventual use of methylphenidate. This is interesting to note, as many parents often question the wisdom of using stimulant medications in children with epilepsy because these drugs reportedly exacerbate seizures. This study suggests that a 2-pronged regimen with both an AED and a stimulant may be a reasonable option to consider in children with BECTS.

R. Riel-Romero, MD

Fever and fever-related epilepsies

Cross JH (UCL-Inst of Child Health, Lingfield, UK)

Epilepsia 53:3-8, 2012

Febrile seizures are a common emergency faced by general pediatricians. They are mostly self-limiting, isolated events with no sequelae in later life. A minority are more complex. In the acute stage, there are a small number of underlying etiologies that are important to recognize in order to determine the prognosis accurately and to optimize management. There has been a long-standing debate about the relationship of early febrile seizures to the later development of epilepsy. It is now clear that this risk differs for simple and complex febrile seizures: complex febrile seizures may herald the presentation of a number of epilepsy syndromes of which febrile and illness-related seizures are part of the phenotype. This review examines the existing knowledge on febrile seizures and the various clinical phenotypes to which they are linked.

▶ Febrile seizures are a common reason for emergency room visits. This article is a review on the definitions of simple and complex febrile seizures, possible genetic underpinnings, and common encephalograph findings. It also explores the questions of how fever triggers seizures, relationship to immunizations, concept of febrile infection related epilepsy syndrome (FIRES), and the role of gastroenteritis in the genesis of seizures, as well as the relationship of febrile seizures to Dravet syndrome. A question that arises, however, is whether FIRES may simply be a form of autoimmune epilepsy. More importantly, the article addresses the issue of later epilepsy. The author cited an article by Neligan et al[1] whereby in 220 children followed up for a median of 24 years after their first febrile seizure, 68% had no further seizures. Of the 180 children followed up for 20 years or longer, 175 (97%) were seizure free. Seventeen children (7.7%) had afebrile seizures and 14 (6.4%) had epilepsy. Additionally, it was helpful for the author to discuss the current thoughts about the relationship of febrile seizures to the genesis of hippocampal sclerosis.

R. Riel-Romero, MD

Reference

1. Neligan A, Bell GS, Giavasi C, et al. Long-term risk of developing epilepsy after febrile seizures: a prospective cohort study. *Neurology*. 2012;78:1166-1170.

10 Sleep Disorders

Society for Ambulatory Anesthesia Consensus Statement on Preoperative Selection of Adult Patients With Obstructive Sleep Apnea Scheduled for Ambulatory Surgery

Joshi GP, Ankichetty SP, Gan TJ, et al (Univ of Texas Southwestern Med Ctr, Dallas; Univ of Toronto, Canada; Duke Univ Med Ctr, Durham, NC)

Anesth Analg 115:1060-1068, 2012

The suitability of ambulatory surgery for a patient with obstructive sleep apnea (OSA) remains controversial because of concerns of increased perioperative complications including postdischarge death. Therefore, a Society for Ambulatory Anesthesia task force on practice guidelines developed a consensus statement for the selection of patients with OSA scheduled for ambulatory surgery. A systematic review of the literature was conducted according to the Preferred Reporting Items for Systematic Reviews and Meta-Analyses guidelines. Although the studies evaluating perioperative outcome in OSA patients undergoing ambulatory surgery are sparse and of limited quality, they do provide useful information that can guide clinical practice. Patients with a known diagnosis of OSA and optimized comorbid medical conditions can be considered for ambulatory surgery, if they are able to use a continuous positive airway pressure device in the postoperative period. Patients with a presumed diagnosis of OSA, based on screening tools such as the STOP–Bang questionnaire, and with optimized comorbid conditions, can be considered for ambulatory surgery, if postoperative pain can be managed predominantly with nonopioid analgesic techniques. On the other hand, OSA patients with nonoptimized comorbid medical conditions may not be good candidates for ambulatory surgery. What other guidelines are available on this topic? The American Society of Anesthesiologists (ASA) practice guidelines for management of surgical patients with OSA published in 2006. Why was this guideline developed? The ASA guidelines are outdated because several recent studies provide new information such as validated screening tools for clinical diagnosis of OSA and safety of ambulatory laparoscopic bariatric surgery in OSA patients. Therefore, an update on the selection of patients with OSA undergoing ambulatory surgery is warranted. How does this guideline differ from existing guidelines? Unlike the ASA guidelines, this consensus statement recommends the use of the STOP–Bang criteria for preoperative OSA screening and considers patients' comorbid conditions in the patient selection process. Also, current literature does not support the ASA recommendations that upper abdominal procedures are not appropriate for ambulatory surgery.

Why does this guideline differ from existing guidelines? This consensus statement differs from existing ASA guidelines because of the availability of new evidence (Fig 2, Tables 1 and 6).

▶ This is a consensus statement developed by the Society for Ambulatory Anesthesia task force. This article has been included because it provides a nice summary of the latest research on screening for obstructive sleep apnea (OSA) in ambulatory surgery settings and management of these patients perioperatively and postoperatively. Table 1 reviews potential complications in OSA patients who undergo ambulatory anesthesia. The STOP-Bang screening questionnaire is a preferred screening tool (Table 6) with good sensitivity. Comorbidities, severity of OSA (if known), in addition to the likelihood of patient compliance with continuous positive airway pressure postoperatively all play important roles in decision making. Finally, the use of nonopioid analgesics for pain control in those with known OSA or presumed OSA is recommended in the ambulatory postoperative setting (Fig 2).

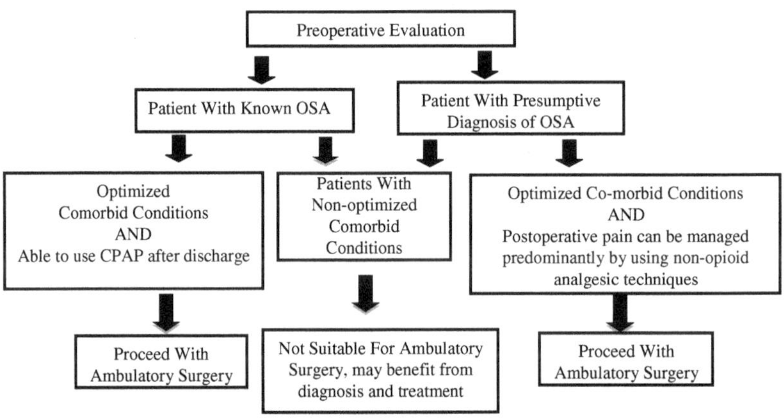

Preoperative Considerations:

- Comorbid conditions include hypertension, arrhythmias, heart failure, cerebrovascular disease, and metabolic syndrome.
- If OSA is suspected during the preoperative evaluation, one could proceed with a presumptive diagnosis of OSA albeit with caution.
- Educate surgeon, patient and family (see the text for details)

Intraoperative Considerations:

- Non-opioid analgesic techniques, when possible.

Postoperative Considerations:

- Exercise caution in OSA patients who develop prolonged and frequent severe respiratory events (e.g., sedation analgesic mismatch, desaturation, and apneic episodes) in the postoperative period.

FIGURE 2.—Decision making in preoperative selection of a patient with obstructive sleep apnea scheduled for ambulatory surgery. OSA = obstructive sleep apnea; CPAP = continuous positive airway pressure. (Reprinted from Joshi GP, Ankichetty SP, Gan TJ, et al. Society for ambulatory anesthesia consensus statement on preoperative selection of adult patients with obstructive sleep apnea scheduled for ambulatory surgery. *Anesth Analg*. 2012;115:1060-1068, with permission from International Anesthesia Research Society.)

TABLE 1.—Concerns with Obstructive Sleep Apnea Patients Undergoing Ambulatory Surgery

Intraoperative	Difficult/failed mask ventilation and/or tracheal intubation.
	Difficulty maintaining adequate oxygen saturation.
Immediate postoperative	Delayed extubation.
	Obstruction and/or desaturation after extubation.
	Postobstructive pulmonary edema.
	Need for tracheal reintubation.
	Exacerbation of cardiac comorbidities: hypertension, arrhythmias, myocardial ischemia and infarction, pulmonary hypertension, heart failure.
	Cerebrovascular disorders (e.g., stroke).
	Prolonged postanesthesia care unit stay.
	Delayed discharge home.
	Unanticipated hospital admission.
Postdischarge	Readmission after discharge.
	Hypoxic brain death and death.

TABLE 6.—STOP–Bang Questionnaire Used to Screen Patients to Determine the Risk of Obstructive Sleep Apnea (OSA)[8]

S = Snoring. Do you snore loudly (louder than talking or loud enough to be heard through closed doors)?
T = Tiredness. Do you often feel tired, fatigued, or sleepy during daytime?
O = Observed apnea. Has anyone observed you stop breathing during your sleep?
P = Pressure. Do you have or are you being treated for high blood pressure?
B = BMI > 35 kg/m^2
A = Age > 50 years
N = Neck circumference >40 cm
G = Male gender

From Hathaway, 2006.[15] Fewer than 3 questions positive = low risk of OSA; 3 or more questions positive: high risk of OSA; 5 to 8 questions positive: high probability of moderate-to-severe OSA.[11]
Editor's Note: Please refer to original journal article for full references.

Practitioners with known OSA patients and, even more importantly, patients who are at risk for OSA but not yet diagnosed need to be familiar with these guidelines.

S. Shafazand, MD, MS

Characteristics of refractory vs. medically controlled epilepsy patients with obstructive sleep apnea and their response to CPAP treatment

Li P, Ghadersohi S, Jafari B, et al (Univ at Buffalo, NY; Yale Univ School of Medicine, New Haven, CT; et al)
Seizure 21:717-721, 2012

Obstructive sleep apnea (OSA) commonly coexists with epilepsy, and treatment of OSA may decrease seizure frequency. However, it is unclear whether patients with medically refractory epilepsy have a higher incidence of OSA compared with well-controlled epilepsy patients and whether the two groups carry different risk factors.

Purpose.—This study aimed to investigate the presence of OSA in patients with refractory vs. well-controlled epilepsy and their associated risk factors. We also assessed the benefits of treatment of OSA with continuous positive airway pressure (CPAP) in refractory epilepsy patients.

Methods.—We retrospectively reviewed data from patients who presented to the Jacobs Neurological Institute Comprehensive Epilepsy Center of University at Buffalo from 2007 to 2010.

Results.—There is a tendency for much higher incidence of OSA in our epilepsy population compared with the general population (15.2% vs. 4.41%). For patients with well-controlled epilepsy, older age, male gender, and higher seizure frequency were predictors of a diagnosis of OSA. However, in medically refractory epilepsy patients, diabetes and snoring predicted a diagnosis of OSA. Treatment of OSA with CPAP in refractory epilepsy patients improved their seizure control ($p < 0.02$).

Conclusion.—This study confirms that OSA is common in epilepsy patients and treatment of OSA can improve seizure control in medically refractory cases. Patients with refractory epilepsy who have diabetes are more likely to have OSA.

▶ Sleep and epilepsy are 2 distinct neurophysiologic conditions that, heretofore, appeared to be strange bedfellows. However, more recent research suggests that both conditions are remarkably intertwined. One of the issues that has been discussed is whether improvement in sleep can also positively impact seizure control in patients with epilepsy. This article addresses this issue partially by investigating the presence of obstructive sleep apnea (OSA) in patients with well-controlled epilepsy and those with refractory seizures. Using retrospective data, the authors found that older age, male sex, and higher seizure frequency in well-controlled patients were predictive of OSA. In patients with drug-resistant epilepsy, the presence of diabetes and snoring predicted a diagnosis of OSA. Interestingly, treatment of OSA with continuous positive airway pressure in patients with medically refractory seizures improved their seizure control significantly. The mechanisms behind the latter were not fully explained, but this suggested that control of OSA in those patients with epilepsy can be a meaningful, adjunctive, nonpharmacologic mode of treatment.

R. Riel-Romero, MD

The impact of epilepsy on sleep architecture during childhood

Pereira AM, Bruni O, Ferri R, et al (Division of Neurology Hosp São Lucas PUCRS, Porto Alegre, Brazil; Sapienza Univ, Rome, Italy; Oasi Inst for Mental Retardation and Brain Aging, Troina, Italy)

Epilepsia 53,9:1519-1525, 2012

Purpose.—The effect of etiology on the relationship between epilepsy and sleep during childhood has not been studied in detail. The aim of this study was to evaluate differences in sleep structure in drug-resistant epilepsies with different underlying causes.

Methods.—We studied 31 patients with drug-resistant epilepsies with or without a structural lesion (lesional and nonlesional) and compared their sleep architecture with that of normal controls and with that of a group of children with benign epilepsy with rolandic spikes (BERS). Subjects underwent a single-night polysomnographic recording. Sleep recordings were scored according to the American Academy of Sleep Medicine (AASM) and cyclic alternating pattern (CAP) criteria.

Key Findings.—Compared to normal controls, patients with drug-resistant epilepsy showed a significant reduction of time in bed, total sleep time, rapid eye movement (REM) sleep, sleep stage N3, and sleep efficiency, and a significant increase in wake after sleep onset. The lesional subgroup showed a reduction in total sleep time and sleep latency and an increase in REM latency and wake after sleep onset. No significant differences, however, were found comparing the lesional and nonlesional subgroups. When compared to BERS, patients with drug-resistant epilepsy showed a significant reduction in sleep stage N3, REM sleep, and sleep efficiency. Regarding CAP analysis, when compared to controls, the drug-resistant group had an increased A1% and a decreased A2%, with a decrease of A1 index in N3 and a global decrease of A2 and A3 indexes. The lesional subgroup showed a slight increase of A1% with a decrease of A1 index in N3 and a global decrease of A2 and A3 indexes. Drug-resistant epilepsy, compared to benign epilepsy showed an increase of CAP rate in N2 and of A1 index in N1 and N2 but not in N3; A2 and A3 indexes were similar in both, but patients with drug-resistant epilepsy showed a significant reduction of A3 index in N1.

Significance.—Our findings suggest that the presence of structural cerebral abnormalities may play an important role in disrupting sleep architecture.

▶ Sleep and epilepsy are 2 neurophysiologic conditions that are closely intertwined. Many investigators have sought to illuminate the interface between sleep and epilepsy. This article aims to evaluate the differences in sleep architecture in medically resistant epilepsies with different underlying etiologies. A case control study design was used whereby 31 patients with drug-resistant epilepsy were compared with normal controls and patients with benign rolandic epilepsy using whole-night video polysomnographic recordings. The authors conclude that patients with drug-resistant epilepsy have significant reductions in total time in bed, total sleep time, rapid eye movement (REM) sleep, N3 stage sleep, sleep efficiency, and total increase in wake time after sleep onset compared with normal controls. Lesional patients also have an increase in REM latency and sleep latency, suggesting that the presence of a visible lesion can exacerbate sleep problems. A possible limitation would be the confounding effect on sleep architecture of the antiepileptic drugs (ie, benzodiazepines) the different patients were on at the time of the study.

R. Riel-Romero, MD

Effect of Continuous Positive Airway Pressure on the Incidence of Hypertension and Cardiovascular Events in Nonsleepy Patients With Obstructive Sleep Apnea: A Randomized Controlled Trial

Barbé F, for the Spanish Sleep and Breathing Network (IRB Lleida, Spain; et al)

JAMA 307:2161-2168, 2012

Context.—Continuous positive airway pressure (CPAP) is the first-line treatment for patients with symptomatic obstructive sleep apnea (OSA). However, its indication for all patients with sleep-disordered breathing, regardless of daytime symptoms, is unclear.

Objective.—To evaluate the effect of CPAP treatment on the incidence of hypertension or cardiovascular events in a cohort of nonsleepy patients with OSA.

Design, Setting, and Patients.—Multicenter, parallel-group, randomized controlled trial in 14 teaching hospitals in Spain. Between May 2004 and May 2006, 725 consecutive patients were enrolled who had an apnea-hypopnea index of 20 h^{-1} or greater and an Epworth Sleepiness Scale score of 10 or less (scores range from 0-24, with values <10 suggesting no daytime sleepiness). Exclusion criteria were previous cardiovascular event, physical or psychological incapacity, chronic disease, or drug or alcohol addiction. Follow-up ended in May 2009.

Intervention.—Patients were allocated to receive CPAP treatment or no active intervention. All participants received dietary counseling and sleep hygiene advice.

Main Outcome Measures.—Incidence of either systemic hypertension (taking antihypertensive medication or blood pressure greater than 140/90 mm Hg) or cardiovascular event (nonfatal myocardial infarction, nonfatal stroke, transient ischemic attack, hospitalization for unstable angina or arrhythmia, heart failure, or cardiovascular death).

Results.—Seven hundred twenty-three patients underwent follow-up for a median of 4 (interquartile range, 2.7-4.4) years (1 patient from each group did not receive allocated treatment); 357 in the CPAP group and 366 in the control group were included in the analysis. In the CPAP group there were 68 patients with new hypertension and 28 cardiovascular events (17 unstable angina or arrhythmia, 3 nonfatal stroke, 3 heart failure, 2 nonfatal myocardial infarction, 2 transient ischemic attack, 1 cardiovascular death). In the control group there were 79 patients with new hypertension and 31 cardiovascular events (11 unstable angina or arrhythmia, 8 nonfatal myocardial infarction, 5 transient ischemic attack, 5 heart failure, 2 nonfatal stroke). The hypertension or cardiovascular event incidence density rate was 9.20 per 100 person-years (95% CI, 7.36-11.04) in the CPAP group and 11.02 per 100 person-years (95% CI, 8.96-13.08) in the control group. The incidence density ratio was 0.83 (95% CI, 0.63-1.1; $P = .20$).

Conclusions.—In patients with OSA without daytime sleepiness, the prescription of CPAP compared with usual care did not result in a statistically significant reduction in the incidence of hypertension or cardiovascular events. However, the study may have had limited power to detect a significant difference.

Trial Registration.—clinicaltrials.gov Identifier: NCT00127348.

► In this well-designed, randomized controlled trial (RCT), nonsleepy patients with moderate-to-severe obstructive sleep apnea (OSA) were randomized to receive continuous positive airway pressure (CPAP) treatment or no active intervention. All participants received dietary counseling and advice about sleep hygiene. Although patients and investigators were not blinded to intervention, the outcomes of interest (incidence of either systemic hypertension [among participants who were normotensive at baseline] or cardiovascular [CV] events [among all participants]) were objectively identified by individuals not involved in the study. This study concluded that in adults with moderate-to-severe OSA and no symptoms of daytime sleepiness, CPAP therapy did not reduce incident hypertension or CV event compared with no active therapy.

Previous RCTs tend to show a small but statistically significant improvement in hypertension in OSA patients treated with CPAP. These trials do not necessarily distinguish between sleepy and nonsleepy OSA. It is possible that this study simply lacked the power to show such an association and/or the duration of follow-up was not sufficient. Lack of CPAP adherence, an important determinant on whether or not CPAP works, was not fully considered in the a priori sample size calculations. Indeed, in a post hoc analysis, those who used CPAP at least 4 hours a night had statistically (and clinically) significant reduction in blood pressure and CV events. About two-thirds of those randomized to CPAP in this study used it for > 4 hours. Furthermore, the benefits of CPAP may extend beyond reductions in CV events and include metabolic improvements in this nonsleepy group. As of yet, the benefits of CPAP cannot be discounted in the nonsleepy patient who has moderate-to-severe sleep apnea.

S. Shafazand, MD, MS

Association of Sleep-Disordered Breathing With Cognitive Dysfunction in CKD Stages 4-5

Kang EW, Abdel-Kader K, Yabes J, et al (Univ of Pittsburgh, PA; et al)
Am J Kidney Dis 60:949-958, 2012

Background.—Sleep-disordered breathing and cognitive impairment are common in patients with chronic kidney disease (CKD). Sleep-disordered breathing is known to be a risk factor for cognitive dysfunction in the general population, but this association has not been studied in patients with CKD.

Study Design.—Cross-sectional study.

Settings & Participants.—A cohort of 169 patients with CKD stages 4-5.

Predictors.—Sleep-disordered breathing; covariates included demographics, diabetes, cardiovascular disease, depression, and dialysis modality.

Outcomes.—Cognitive impairment, generally defined as a score 1.5 standard deviations or more from the age- and education level–adjusted normative cognitive test score.

Measurements.—Standardized health interview, neurocognitive assessment, sleep-related questionnaires, and polysomnography.

Results.—Sleep-disordered breathing (apnea-hypopnea index >15) was diagnosed in 83 (49.1%) individuals. This group had a significantly higher prevalence of nocturnal hypoxemia (65.8% vs 26.8%; $P < 0.001$) and excessive daytime sleepiness (38.6% vs 20.7%; $P = 0.01$). In addition, this group had significantly lower scores in tests measuring verbal memory, working memory, attention, and psychomotor speed. Sleep-disordered breathing was associated with higher risk of immediate verbal memory impairment after adjustment for known confounders (adjusted OR, 2.67; 95% CI, 1.17-6.08). However, in a subgroup analysis of older adults (aged >60 years), there were no significant differences in cognitive testing between the groups with and without sleep-disordered breathing.

Limitations.—Cross-sectional design, limited sample size.

Conclusions.—Sleep-disordered breathing is associated with cognitive impairments, especially impaired verbal memory, in patients with advanced CKD. However, the impact appeared limited in older adults. Early evaluation and management of sleep-disordered breathing in patients with CKD may provide an opportunity to improve cognitive function.

▶ This is a cross-sectional study with a small sample size and many measurements evaluating the associations among sleep-disordered breathing (SDB), end-stage renal disease (ESRD), and cognitive impairment. Despite its limitations, it highlights some important points and serves as a good starting point for future studies.

First, the study once again shows that there is a high prevalence of SDB in patients with ESRD. Given the known association of SDB with cardiovascular events, including hypertension in the general population, this high prevalence in the ESRD population suggests a need for increased efforts at screening for SDB by health providers caring for ESRD patients.

Second, there appears, even in this small sample, to be an important association between SDB and some cognitive measures. However, the association was not statistically significant in the elderly, for which the reasons are unknown. Although studies showing improvement in these impairments with treatment of SDB are pending, we can speculate about the potential impact of screening and treatment of SDB in this population with ESRD and SDB who have preexisting cognitive impairments.

S. Shafazand, MD, MS

Effect of Continuous Positive Airway Pressure Therapy on Cardiovascular Risk Factors in Patients with Type 2 Diabetes and Obstructive Sleep Apnea

Myhill PC, Davis WA, Peters KE, et al (Univ of Western Australia, Fremantle, Australia; et al)

J Clin Endocrinol Metab 97:4212-4218, 2012

Context.—Few prospective intervention studies have examined the effect of continuous positive airway pressure (CPAP) therapy on cardiovascular disease (CVD) risk factors in diabetes.

Objective.—Our objective was to determine whether CPAP improves CVD risk factors in patients with type 2 diabetes and obstructive sleep apnea (OSA).

Design and Setting.—This was a randomized parallel group intervention trial in an urban Australian community.

Patients.—Fifty-nine participants of the Fremantle Diabetes Study Phase II at high risk for OSA consented to confirmatory polysomnography followed by randomization to a 3-month CPAP intervention initiated early (<1 wk) or late (1–2 months).

Main Outcome Measures.—Patients were assessed before and 1 and 3 months after CPAP started. Tests for repeated measures were used to compare variables of interest over time.

Results.—Forty-four patients (75%) completed the study. Their mean ± SD age was 66.1 ± 8.8 yr, and 61.4% were male. Completers and noncompleters had similar age, sex, diabetes duration, apnea-hypopnea index, and Epworth Sleepiness Scale ($P \geq 0.29$). There were no differences in outcome between early and late randomization, and the data were pooled. The Epworth Sleepiness Scale decreased between entry and 1 month [−4.8 (−6.5 to −3.1), $P < 0.001$]. Blood pressure improved between entry and 3 months (from 149 ± 23/80 ± 12 to 140 ± 18/73 ± 13 mm Hg; $P \leq 0.007$). Pulse rate declined within the first month [−6 (−10 to −2) beats/min, $P = 0.002$]. Glycemic control and serum lipids, which were mostly within recommended target ranges at entry, did not change.

Conclusions.—Three months of CPAP in community-based people with type 2 diabetes significantly decreased blood pressure and pulse rate but did not influence metabolic control.

▶ This study is billed as a randomized controlled trial of early (1 week) versus later (1-2 months) continuous positive airway pressure (CPAP) therapy in type 2 diabetic patients with moderate to severe obstructive sleep apnea (OSA). There really is no control arm, and, because of a lack of difference between early versus late CPAP use, the data were combined. In effect the study is a pre-post design looking at the impact of CPAP therapy on hypertension, glycemic control, and lipids in diabetics with OSA. The compliance with CPAP is surprisingly high in this study. Also, the patients included already had reasonable diabetes control and lipid levels. So the lack of effect of CPAP on these variables may not be too surprising, as they were already medically optimized. Additionally, generalizability of the results to community cohorts of diabetic patients in the

United States may be difficult. The sample size was small and only 75% completed the study, which limits its power. Nevertheless, the study once again shows the modest improvement in blood pressure in those patients with moderate to severe OSA and on CPAP therapy. It adds to the literature by demonstrating this improvement in a specialized population (ie, diabetics) that is particularly at risk for cardiovascular events.

S. Shafazand, MD, MS

Effect of Continuous Positive Airway Pressure on C-reactive Protein Levels in Sleep Apnea: A Meta-analysis

Friedman M, Samuelson CG, Hamilton C, et al (Rush Univ Med Ctr, Chicago, IL; Advocate Illinois Masonic Med Ctr, Chicago; et al)

Otolaryngol–Head Neck Surg 147:423-433, 2012

Objective.—Evaluate the effects of continuous positive airway pressure (CPAP) on C-reactive protein (CRP) levels, reported either as a primary or secondary end point among patients with obstructive sleep apnea-hypopnea syndrome (OSAHS) based on a meta-analysis of published studies.

Data Sources.—English-language searches of PubMed, Ovid, and the Cochrane databases were completed. Reference sections of identified studies were also examined for additional relevant articles to review.

Review Methods.—Studies of adult patients with OSAHS who reported pre- and post-CPAP treatment CRP were reviewed and analyzed. Two independent reviewers extracted data from 10 peer-reviewed studies, which were combined using a random effects meta-analysis model.

Results.—The CPAP treatment was found to lead to a significant reduction in CRP levels (17.8%, $P=.002$). This corresponds to an effect size of −0.485 (−0.731, −0.240). Sensitivity analysis was done to determine the impact of study design. Both case-control studies and case-series studies yielded a significant effect. Sensitivity analysis also yielded a significant effect for studies with average body mass index <30, studies where CPAP was employed over automatic positive airway pressure, and studies treating patients ≤3 months. Analysis of publication bias, however, revealed a likelihood of "missing" studies.

Conclusion.—Although there is a significant lack of high-quality studies addressing this question, this analysis suggests that treatment with CPAP leads to a statistically significant reduction in CRP levels. However, the mean pre- and posttreatment CRP levels observed are considered "high risk" for cardiovascular morbidity. The clinical significance of this finding as it relates to cardiovascular risk reduction and the relationship between CRP and OSAHS requires further study.

▶ This meta-analysis attempts to put together the limited data that exist on the impact of continuous positive airway pressure (CPAP) therapy on C-reactive protein (CRP) levels in obese individuals with severe obstructive sleep apnea-hypopnea syndrome (OSAHS). The notable limitations are the paucity of randomized, controlled trials (RCT) looking at CPAP and CRP levels and the combination of observational case series and pre/post designs with the 2 available RCTS in this meta-analysis. As a result, the studies are widely heterogeneous. The authors also acknowledge the possibility of publication bias (small but significant negative studies may not be published) that would likely negate the positive improvement they note in CRP after at least 1 month of CPAP use. Nevertheless, this article adds to the growing data that suggest that CRP, a marker of inflammation and associated with increased risk for cardiovascular events, may indeed be associated with OSAHS independent of the effects of obesity and that CPAP therapy can reduce CRP levels modestly. It remains to be seen whether this translates on a practical level to reduced cardiovascular risk in obese, symptomatic, OSAHS patients with baseline-elevated CRP.

S. Shafazand, MD, MS

Sleep-disordered breathing in multiple sclerosis

Braley TJ, Segal BM, Chervin RD (Univ of Michigan, Ann Arbor)

Neurology 79:929-936, 2012

Background.—The objectives of this cross-sectional study were to assess the prevalence and severity of sleep apnea in patients with multiple sclerosis (MS) referred for overnight polysomnography (PSG) and to explore the radiographic and clinical features that might signal risk for undiagnosed sleep apnea.

Methods.—Apnea-hypopnea (AHI) and central apnea indices (CAI) from laboratory-based PSG among 48 patients with MS were compared with those of group A, 84 sleep laboratory—referred patients without MS matched for age, gender, and body mass index; and group B, a separate group of 48 randomly selected, referred patients.

Results.—Mean AHI was higher among patients with MS than among control groups A or B (2-way analysis of variance and multiple linear regression, $p = 0.0011$ and 0.0118, respectively). Median and mean CAI were also increased among patients with MS in comparison to control groups (Wilcoxon signed rank and multiple linear regression, $p = 0.0064$ and 0.0027, respectively). Among MS patients with available data, those with evidence of brainstem involvement, compared with groups A and B, showed particularly robust differences in AHI ($p = 0.0060$ and 0.0016) and CAI ($p = 0.0215$ and < 0.0001). In contrast, MS patients without brainstem involvement, compared with groups A and B, showed diminished differences in AHI, and CAI did not significantly differ among groups.

Conclusions.—These data suggest a predisposition for obstructive sleep apnea and accompanying central apneas among patients with MS, particularly among those with brainstem involvement.

► This is a retrospective, cross-sectional study of patients with multiple sclerosis (MS) who were specifically referred to the sleep laboratory to be evaluated for sleep apnea; as such, it cannot be representative of the population-based prevalence of sleep apnea in MS. Nevertheless, several important observations emerge from this study. Patients with MS referred for clinical sleep studies had more severe obstructive sleep apnea, as well as more severe central sleep apnea, than referred individuals without MS. Furthermore, MS patients with clinical or radiographic evidence of brainstem involvement had more severe sleep apnea. In an exploratory analysis, the use of disease-modifying therapy (DMT) was associated with fewer apnea episodes. While these data bear more study, could DMT's impact on inflammatory measures be playing a role in sleep apnea as well?

The findings of this study, if duplicated in other studies, suggest that clinicians taking care of MS patients with clinical or radiographic brainstem involvement should have a low threshold for referral for evaluation for sleep apnea.

S. Shafazand, MD, MS

Effects of Continuous Positive Airway Pressure on Neurocognitive Function in Obstructive Sleep Apnea Patients: The Apnea Positive Pressure Long-Term Efficacy Study (APPLES)

Kushida CA, Nichols DA, Holmes TH, et al (Stanford Univ, CA; et al)

Sleep 35:1593-1602, 2012

Study Objective.—To determine the neurocognitive effects of continuous positive airway pressure (CPAP) therapy on patients with obstructive sleep apnea (OSA).

Design, Setting, and Participants.—The Apnea Positive Pressure Long-term Efficacy Study (APPLES) was a 6-month, randomized, double-blind, 2-arm, sham-controlled, multicenter trial conducted at 5 U.S. university, hospital, or private practices. Of 1,516 participants enrolled, 1,105 were randomized, and 1,098 participants diagnosed with OSA contributed to the analysis of the primary outcome measures.

Intervention.—Active or sham CPAP.

Measurements.—Three neurocognitive variables, each representing a neurocognitive domain: Pathfinder Number Test-Total Time (attention and psychomotor function [A/P]), Buschke Selective Reminding Test-Sum Recall (learning and memory [L/M]), and Sustained Working Memory Test-Overall Mid-Day Score (executive and frontal-lobe function [E/F]).

Results.—The primary neurocognitive analyses showed a difference between groups for only the E/F variable at the 2 month CPAP visit, but no difference at the 6 month CPAP visit or for the A/P or L/M variables at either the 2 or 6 month visits. When stratified by measures of OSA severity (AHI or oxygen saturation parameters), the primary E/F variable and one secondary E/F neurocognitive variable revealed transient differences between study arms for those with the most severe OSA. Participants in the active CPAP group had a significantly greater ability to remain awake whether measured subjectively by the Epworth Sleepiness Scale or objectively by the maintenance of wakefulness test.

Conclusions.—CPAP treatment improved both subjectively and objectively measured sleepiness, especially in individuals with severe OSA (AHI >30). CPAP use resulted in mild, transient improvement in the most sensitive measures of executive and frontal-lobe function for those with severe disease, which suggests the existence of a complex OSA-neurocognitive relationship.

Clinical Trial Information.—Registered at clinicaltrials.gov. Identifier: NCT00051363.

▶ This is a randomized, double-blind, sham-controlled, multicenter, 6-month trial of impact of continuous positive airway pressure (CPAP) therapy on neurocognitive outcomes. It is the largest study to date and is well designed. On the surface, the finding of no difference between CPAP or sham for most neurocognitive measures is disappointing. The differences noted in the primary executive and frontal-lobe function variable were small and only observed at 2 months, not after 6 months of therapy. A secondary analysis looking only at the subset that was adherent to CPAP showed no difference at all between study arms in neurocognitive measures.

It appears that the impact of obstructive sleep apnea (OSA) on neurocognitive outcomes is a complex one. The current battery of testing, although comprehensive, may not have been sensitive enough to detect subtle changes that may be of some practical value to the individual patient. The population as a whole was highly intelligent and therefore started off with greater cognitive reserve. We may see more significant differences in those with severe OSA and low cognitive reserve at baseline. The duration of therapy may simply not be long enough, and it likely takes years to note cognitive decline resulting from OSA and frequent nighttime desaturations. Can CPAP be expected to reverse that in 6 months? This is an excellent study that has given us some valuable insight, but I believe we are capturing but one aspect of this complex relationship, especially in those with severe OSA.

S. Shafazand, MD, MS

Adaptive Servoventilation for Treatment of Sleep-Disordered Breathing in Heart Failure: A Systematic Review and Meta-Analysis

Sharma BK, Bakker JP, McSharry DG, et al (Steward Health Care System, Boston, MA; Brigham and Women's Hosp and Harvard Med School, Boston, MA; et al)

Chest 142:1211-1221, 2012

Background.—Adaptive servoventilation (ASV) has demonstrated efficacy in treating sleep-disordered breathing (SDB) in patients with heart failure (HF), but large randomized trials are lacking. We, therefore, sought to perform a systematic review and meta-analysis of existing data.

Methods.—A systematic search of the PubMed database was undertaken in March 2012. Publications were independently assessed by two investigators to identify studies of ≥1-week duration that compared ASV to a control condition (ie, subtherapeutic ASV, continuous or bilevel pressure ventilation, oxygen therapy, or no treatment) in adult patients with SDB and HF. Mean, variability, and sample size data were extracted independently for the following outcomes: apneahypopnea index (AHI), left ventricular ejection fraction (LVEF), quality of life (SF-36 Health Survey; Medical Outcomes Trust), 6-min walk distance, peak oxygen consumption ($\dot{V}O_2$) % predicted, and ventilatory equivalent ratio for CO_2 ($\dot{V}E/\dot{V}CO_2$) slope measured during exercise. Random effects meta-analysis models were applied.

Results.—Fourteen studies were identified (N = 538). Comparing ASV to control conditions, the weighted mean difference in AHI (−14.64 events/h; 95% CI, −21.03 to −8.25) and LVEF (0.40; 95% CI, 0.08-0.71) both significantly favored ASV. ASV also improved the 6-min walk distance, but not peak $\dot{V}O_2$% predicted, $\dot{V}E/\dot{V}CO_2$ slope, or quality of life, compared with control conditions.

Conclusions.—In patients with HF and SDB, ASV was more effective than control conditions in reducing the AHI and improving cardiac function and exercise capacity. These data provide a compelling rationale for large-scale randomized controlled trials to assess the clinical impact of ASV on hard outcomes in these patients.

▶ Recent technological advances in positive airway therapy for heart failure (HF) include adaptive servoventilation (ASV), which adjusts the delivered pressure support and end expiratory pressure according to the needs of the patient throughout the night. This meta-analysis explores the impact of ASV in HF on sleep-disordered breathing (SDB) severity, left ventricular ejection fraction (LVEF), exercise capacity, cardiopulmonary exercise testing, and quality of life measured greater than 1 week. ASV was more effective than control conditions (combined studies) and continuous positive airway pressure treatment (subgroup analysis) in treating SDB in HF. LVEF and exercise capacity also showed greater improvement with ASV compared with control conditions. However, there were several limitations to the meta-analysis despite good methodology used. These limitations stem from the quality of included studies. Individual sample sizes were small, most studies available were not randomized design, and did not have blinded treatment assignment. These will likely lead to increased bias in individual studies. There was between-studies heterogeneity in terms of both study design and the effect sizes of each end point. Follow-up for endpoints in individual studies were for the most part less than 6 months. Nevertheless, this meta-analysis demonstrates that ASV is likely beneficial in HF patients with SDB, and the field is ready for more robust randomized clinical trials with longer follow-up to fully understand the benefits of such therapy.

S. Shafazand, MD, MS

Cardiovascular Mortality in Obstructive Sleep Apnea in the Elderly: Role of Long-Term Continuous Positive Airway Pressure Treatment: A Prospective Observational Study

Martínez-García M-A, Campos-Rodríguez F, Catalán-Serra P, et al (La Fe Univ and Polytechnic Hosp, Valencia, Spain; Valme Univ Hosp, Seville, Spain; Requena General Hosp, Valencia, Spain; et al)

Am J Respir Crit Care Med 186:909-916, 2012

Rationale.—Obstructive sleep apnea (OSA) is a risk factor for cardiovascular death in middle-aged subjects, but it is not known whether it is also a risk factor in the elderly.

Objectives.—To investigate whether OSA is a risk factor for cardiovascular death and to assess whether continuous positive airway pressure (CPAP) treatment is associated with a change in risk in the elderly.

Methods.—Prospective, observational study of a consecutive cohort of elderly patients (≥65 yr) studied for suspicion of OSA between 1998 and 2007. Patients with an apnea–hypopnea index (AHI) less than 15 were the control group. OSA was defined as mild to moderate (AHI, 15–29) or severe (AHI, ≥30). Patients with OSA were classified as CPAP-treated (adherence ≥ 4 h/d) or untreated (adherence < 4 h/d or not prescribed). Participants were monitored until December 2009. The end point was cardiovascular death. A multivariate Cox survival analysis was used to determine the independent impact of OSA and CPAP treatment on cardiovascular mortality.

Measurements and Main Results.—A total of 939 elderly were studied (median follow-up, 69 mo). Compared with the control group, the fully adjusted hazard ratios for cardiovascular mortality were 2.25 (confidence interval [CI], 1.41 to 3.61) for the untreated severe OSA group, 0.93 (CI, 0.46 to 1.89) for the CPAP-treated group, and 1.38 (CI, 0.73 to 2.64) for the untreated mild to moderate OSA group.

Conclusions.—Severe OSA not treated with CPAP is associated with cardiovascular death in the elderly, and adequate CPAP treatment may reduce this risk (Fig 2).

► There are good longitudinal studies available that show the impact of sleep apnea on cardiovascular (CV) morbidity and mortality. Continuous positive airway pressure (CPAP) has demonstrated a positive effect on blood pressure levels and the incidence of fatal and nonfatal CV events in several observational studies in middle-aged adults (mostly men). However, it is not clear whether this beneficial effect is also seen in the elderly.

This observational prospective study followed participants with a mean age of 70 with moderate-to-severe sleep apnea for a median of 69 months. The strength of the study lies in the large numbers enrolled and the surprisingly few lost to follow-up (only 4). Laboratory polysomnography was used to make the diagnosis of sleep-disordered breathing for between 30% and 50% of this population. Almost 40% of the cohort were women, which adds to the current literature.

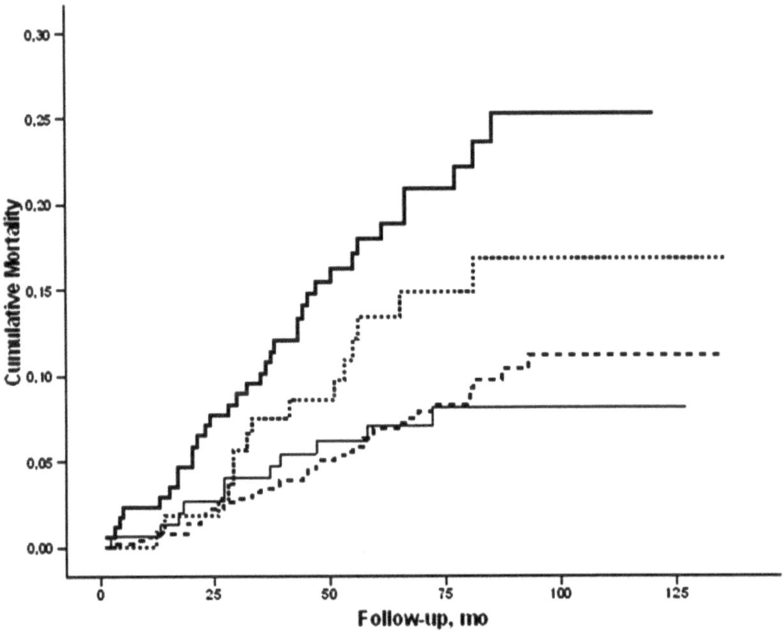

FIGURE 2.—Kaplan-Meier cardiovascular cumulative mortality curves for study. Groups: *thick solid line*, severe OSA untreated with CPAP; *dotted line*, mild to moderate OSA untreated with CPAP; *dashed line*, OSA treated with CPAP; *thin solid line*, control group (AHI, 15). Log-rank test: 11.38; $P = 0.001$ for the comparison between severe untreated OSA group and control group. Log-rank test: 3.13; $P = 0.08$ for the comparison between untreated mild to moderate OSA group and control group. Log-rank test: 0.09; $P = 0.77$ for the comparison between CPAP-treated OSA group and control group. AHI = apnea—hypopnea index; CPAP = continuous positive airway pressure; OSA = obstructive sleep apnea. (Reprinted from Martínez-García M-A, Campos-Rodríguez F, Catalán-Serra P, et al. Cardiovascular mortality in obstructive sleep apnea in the elderly: role of long-term continuous positive airway pressure treatment: a prospective observational study. *Am J Respir Crit Care Med.* 2012;186:909-916. Official Journal of the American Thoracic Society. © 2012, American Thoracic Society, http://www.ajrccm.org.)

The main findings of this study were that "in elderly patients, severe obstructive sleep apnea (OSA) not treated with CPAP was associated with an increase in cardiovascular mortality due to stroke and heart failure (but not ischemic heart disease), whereas treatment with CPAP was associated with a decrease in this excess of cardiovascular mortality to levels similar to those of patients without OSA" (Fig 2).

This is an important finding, and although it will not be possible to ascertain results in a randomized controlled study because of the ethics of withholding treatment for long periods of time, it can be argued that most of the existing body of evidence regarding CPAP and CV mortality supports this finding. This study suggests that the diagnosis and treatment of sleep apnea in the elderly should not be neglected.

S. Shafazand, MD, MS

Utility of overnight pulse oximetry and heart rate variability analysis to screen for sleep-disordered breathing in chronic heart failure

Ward NR, Cowie MR, Rosen SD, et al (Royal Brompton Hosp and Imperial College, London, UK)

Thorax 67:1000-1005, 2012

Background.—Sleep-disordered breathing (SDB) is under diagnosed in chronic heart failure (CHF). Screening with simple monitors may increase detection of SDB in a cardiology setting. This study aimed to evaluate the accuracy of heart rate variability analysis and overnight pulse oximetry for diagnosis of SDB in patients with CHF.

Methods.—180 patients with CHF underwent simultaneous polysomnography, ambulatory electrocardiography and wrist-worn overnight pulse oximetry. SDB was defined as an apnoea-hypopnoea index ≥15/h. To identify SDB from the screening tests, the per cent very low frequency increment (%VLFI) component of heart rate variability was measured with a pre-specified cutoff ≥2.23%, and the 3% oxygen desaturation index was measured with a pre-specified cutoff >7.5 desaturations/h.

Results.—173 patients with CHF had adequate sleep study data; SDB occurred in 77 (45%) patients. Heart rate variability was measurable in 78 (45%) patients with area under the %VLFI receiver operating characteristic curve of 0.50. At the ≥2.23% cutoff, %VLFI sensitivity was 58% and specificity was 48%. The 3% oxygen desaturation index was measurable in 171 (99%) patients with area under the curve of 0.92. At the pre-specified cutoff of >7.5 desaturations/h, the 3% oxygen desaturation index had a sensitivity of 97%, specificity of 32%, negative likelihood ratio of 0.08 and positive likelihood ratio of 1.42. Diagnostic accuracy was increased using a cutoff of 12.5 desaturations/h, with sensitivity of 93% and specificity of 73%.

Conclusions.—The high sensitivity and low negative likelihood ratio of the 3% oxygen desaturation index indicates that pulse oximetry would be of use as a simple screening test to rule out SDB in patients with CHF in a cardiology setting. The %VLFI component of heart rate variability is not suitable for detection of SDB in CHF (Fig 2).

▶ Sleep-disordered breathing (SDB) is prevalent in chronic heart failure (CHF) patients but is underdiagnosed. One of the reasons may be perceived difficulties in obtaining laboratory polysomnography. However, no good screening tools exist currently. The authors of this report explore 2 simple screening tools used in the general population and, not surprisingly, find that heart rate variability was not diagnostically accurate (with a sensitivity of 58%, specificity of 48%, positive likelihood ratio of 1.11, and negative likelihood ratio of 0.88 for diagnosis of SDB) (Fig 2). Pulse oximetry fared better; the 3% oxygen desaturation index had an area under the receiver operating characteristic curve of 0.92 for detection of SDB in CHF, indicating high diagnostic accuracy. At the a priori cutoff of greater than 7.5 desaturations per hour for diagnosis of SDB in CHF, there was

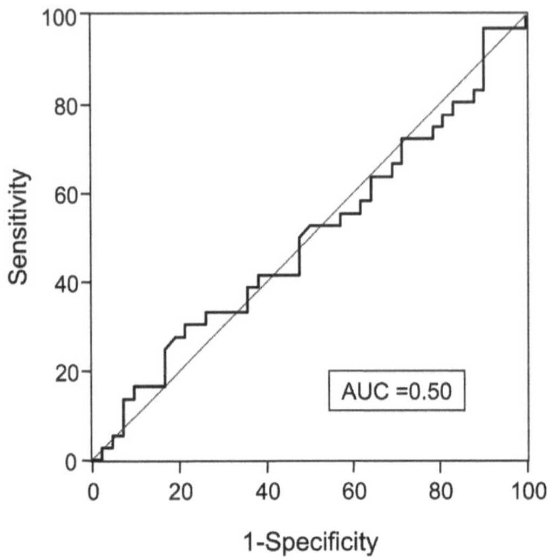

FIGURE 2.—Per cent very low frequency increment receiver-operating characteristic curve for diagnosis of sleep-disordered breathing (apnoeahypopnoea index ≥15/h) in patients with chronic heart failure. AUC, area under curve. (Reproduced from Thorax. Ward NR, Cowie MR, Rosen SD, et al. Utility of overnight pulse oximetry and heart rate variability analysis to screen for sleep-disordered breathing in chronic heart failure. *Thorax*. 2012;67:1000-1005, with permission from the BMJ Publishing Group Ltd.)

a sensitivity of 97% and negative likelihood ratio of 0.08, suggesting that pulse oximetry may be useful for ruling out SDB, not ruling it in.

It is also important to note that the CHF populations included in this study were New York Heart Association class I and II and not severe with a median ejection fraction of 40%. Additionally, only 14% had central sleep apnea. Therefore, the generalizability to a sicker, symptomatic heart failure population is limited.

Currently, the American Academy of Sleep Medicine does not recommend the use of portable sleep studies in this population with significant comorbidities and a higher-than-average prevalence of central sleep apnea. For now, cardiologists and other healthcare providers taking care of these patients should have a higher awareness of the prevalence of SDB and its clinical impact and refer early for management of SDB to sleep specialists.

S. Shafazand, MD, MS

The Associations of Insomnia With Costly Workplace Accidents and Errors: Results From the America Insomnia Survey

Shahly V, Berglund PA, Coulouvrat C, et al (Harvard Med School, Boston, MA; Univ of Michigan, Ann Arbor; Sanofi, Paris, France; et al)

Arch Gen Psychiatry 69:1054-1063, 2012

Context.—Insomnia is a common and seriously impairing condition that often goes unrecognized.

Objectives.—To examine associations of broadly defined insomnia (ie, meeting inclusion criteria for a diagnosis from *International Statistical*

Classification of Diseases, 10th Revision, DSM-IV, or Research Diagnostic Criteria/International Classification of Sleep Disorders, Second Edition) with costly workplace accidents and errors after excluding other chronic conditions among workers in the America Insomnia Survey (AIS).

Design/Setting.—A national cross-sectional telephone survey (65.0% cooperation rate) of commercially insured health plan members selected from the more than 34 million in the HealthCore Integrated Research Database.

Participants.—Four thousand nine hundred ninety-one employed AIS respondents.

Main Outcome Measures.—Costly workplace accidents or errors in the 12 months before the AIS interview were assessed with one question about workplace accidents "that either caused damage or work disruption with a value of $500 or more" and another about other mistakes "that cost your company $500 or more."

Results.—Current insomnia with duration of at least 12 months was assessed with the Brief Insomnia Questionnaire, a validated (area under the receiver operating characteristic curve, 0.86 compared with diagnoses based on blinded clinical reappraisal interviews), fully structured diagnostic interview. Eighteen other chronic conditions were assessed with medical/pharmacy claims records and validated self-report scales. Insomnia had a significant odds ratio with workplace accidents and/or errors controlled for other chronic conditions (1.4). The odds ratio did not vary significantly with respondent age, sex, educational level, or comorbidity. The average costs of insomnia-related accidents and errors ($32 062) were significantly higher than those of other accidents and errors ($21 914). Simulations

TABLE 2.—Associations of BIQ-Defined and Broadly Defined Insomnia and Costly 12-Month Workplace Accidents and Errors Among Employed AIS Respondents in the Comorbidity Subsample[a]

	OR (95% CI)		
	Accidents	Errors	Either
Presence of incidents			
Without controls for comorbidity	1.9 (1.1-3.4)[b]	1.4 (1.0-2.0)[b]	1.5 (1.1-2.1)[b]
With controls for comorbidity	1.5 (0.8-2.8)	1.3 (0.9-1.9)	1.4 (1.0-2.0)[b]
PARP of incidents, %			
Without controls for comorbidity	14.5	6.7	8.0
With controls for comorbidity	10.3	5.8	7.2
Annualized US population projections of incidents (in thousands), estimate[c]			
Without controls for comorbidity	223.3	317.0	481.6
With controls for comorbidity	158.6	274.5	433.4

Abbreviations: AIS, America Insomnia Survey; BIQ, Brief Insomnia Questionnaire; OR, odds ratio; PARP, population-attributable risk proportion.

[a]For a description of the BIQ and broadly defined insomnia, see Table 1. Only cases with a reported duration of at least 12 months at the time of interview are included in the comorbidity subsample (n = 4991). Analyses are based on a multivariate logistic regression model in which insomnia is used to predict the outcome with controls for sociodemographics and with or without controls for comorbidity.

[b]Indicates significant association between insomnia and the outcome at the .05 level, 2-sided test.

[c]These results are based on projection of the results to the total US civilian labor force using population data from the August 2010 Current Population Survey (http://www.bls.gov/cps).

estimated that insomnia was associated with 7.2% of all costly workplace accidents and errors and 23.7% of all the costs of these incidents. These proportions are higher than for any other chronic condition, with annualized US population projections of 274 000 costly insomnia-related workplace accidents and errors having a combined value of US $31.1 billion.

Conclusion.—Effectiveness trials are needed to determine whether expanded screening, outreach, and treatment of workers with insomnia would yield a positive return on investment for employers (Table 2).

▶ This article highlights the importance of insomnia in the context of occupational errors. It represents a national cross-sectional telephone survey of commercially insured health plan members selected from the more than 34 million in the HealthCore Integrated Research Database. The reports of insomnia were based on a validated questionnaire, and comorbidities that may cause insomnia were identified for the most part based on self-report and limited claims data. Reports of occupational errors and accidents were also self-reported and, therefore, likely to be underreported. Recall bias is a major limitation of this survey; however, its methodology does well in keeping with large-scale epidemiologic surveys. Given the limited data available on prevalence of insomnia in working adults and its impact on workplace errors and accidents, this study provides us with some valuable insight. After correcting for relevant comorbidities, insomnia continued to have a significant association with workplace accidents (Table 2). These errors may cause potentially important financial loss. What is now needed are trials that directly or indirectly show that improvement in insomnia symptoms improves performance and reduces errors in the workplace. That would certainly provide compelling evidence to push for widespread screening and treatment of insomnia among employees.

S. Shafazand, MD, MS

Association of Insomnia and Short Sleep Duration With Atherosclerosis Risk in the Elderly

Nakazaki C, Noda A, Koike Y, et al (Nagoya Univ Graduate School of Medicine, Japan; Chubu Univ, Kasugai, Japan)

Am J Hypertens 25:1149-1155, 2012

Background.—Short sleep duration is associated with an increased risk of cardiovascular disease and all-cause mortality, although a relationship with atherosclerosis in the elderly remains unclear.

Methods.—Eighty-six volunteers aged ≥ 65 years (mean, 73.6 ± 4.9 years) were evaluated for insomnia. Total sleep time (TST) and sleep efficiency were measured by actigraphy. Subjective symptoms were assessed with the Pittsburgh Sleep Quality Index (PSQI). Atherosclerosis was evaluated using ultrasonographic measurements of carotid intima–media thickness (IMT).

TABLE 1.—Cardiovascular and Sleep Disorder Parameters Categorized by Total Sleep Time

	All	Total Sleep Time		
		>7 h	5-7 h	≤5 h
	$n = 86$	$n = 22$	$n = 23$	$n = 41$
Age, year	73.6 ± 4.9	71.9 ± 4.0	72.7 ± 4.7	74.9 ± 5.2
Gender, % male	29.1	22.7	17.4	39.0
BMI, kg/m^2	22.3 ± 2.4	23.5 ± 2.1	21.9 ± 1.8	21.9 ± 2.7*
SBP, mm Hg	133.2 ± 15.7	135.6 ± 15.1	135.0 ± 15.3	130.9 ± 16.4
DBP, mm Hg	76.5 ± 9.3	76.5 ± 8.8	78.7 ± 8.2	75.2 ± 10.1
Hypertension, %	51.2	59.1	52.1	46.3
Hyperlipidemia, %	46.5	59.1	30.4	48.7
Diabetes, %	15.1	22.7	9.8	17.4
Current smoker, %	7.0	4.5	17.4	2.4
Current drinker, %	9.3	4.5	21.7	4.9
Total sleep time, min	328.4 ± 87.0	449.7 ± 19.5	349.4 ± 33.1*	251.5 ± 29.2*,†
Sleep efficiency,%	85.2 ± 10.3	91.0 ± 6.0	86.2 ± 9.0	81.6 ± 11.3*
PSQI	5.7 ± 2.9	5.5 ± 2.7	5.6 ± 2.6	5.8 ± 3.2
IMT, mm	1.2 ± 0.5	0.9 ± 0.3	1.2 ± 0.5	1.3 ± 0.5*
Plaque score	1.4 ± 1.5	0.7 ± 0.9	1.5 ± 1.7	1.7 ± 1.7
AHI, /h	14.9 ± 12.0	13.7 ± 12.1	17.8 ± 12.2	13.9 ± 11.9
ODI, /h	3.7 ± 4.0	3.8 ± 3.9	4.0 ± 4.3	3.6 ± 4.0
Lowest SpO_2, %	84.5 ± 6.1	83.9 ± 6.4	85.2 ± 4.6	84.6 ± 6.7
LVDd, mm	46.3 ± 6.0	48.1 ± 6.5	44.8 ± 7.5	46.1 ± 4.5
LVDs, mm	27.8 ± 5.3	29.4 ± 5.1	27.2 ± 7.9	27.3 ± 3.4
IVST, mm	8.4 ± 1.9	9.2 ± 1.9	8.6 ± 1.5	7.9 ± 1.9
LVPWT, mm	8.4 ± 2.2	8.4 ± 2.8	8.4 ± 2.3	8.4 ± 1.7
LVEF, %	71.5 ± 6.5	70.5 ± 7.1	72.0 ± 7.0	71.6 ± 5.4
LV mass/BSA, g/m^2	84.8 ± 27.0	93.9 ± 31.7	82.1 ± 33.1	81.5 ± 18.9
E/A	0.9 ± 0.9	1.0 ± 0.4	1.2 ± 1.7	0.8 ± 0.1
DcT, ms	201.7 ± 26.6	200.2 ± 18.5	200.2 ± 31.5	203.3 ± 27.9

Data are presented as mean ± SD unless otherwise indicated.

AHI, apnea–hypopnea index; BMI, body mass index; BSA, body surface area; DBP, diastolic blood pressure; DcT, deceleration time of peak E velocity; E/A, peak early systolic velocity/atrial contraction velocity; IMT, intima–media thickness; IVST, interventricular septal thickness; lowest SpO_2, lowest arterial oxyhemoglobin saturation; LVDd, left ventricular end-diastolic dimension; LVDs, left ventricular end-systolic dimension; LVEF, left ventricular ejection fraction; LVPWT, left ventricular posterior wall thickness; ODI, oxygen desaturation index; PSQI, Pittsburgh Sleep Quality Index; SBP, systolic blood pressure.

*$P < 0.05$ vs. >7 h.

†$P < 0.05$ vs. 5–7 h

Results.—IMT was significantly greater and sleep efficiency was significantly lower in subjects with TST ≤ 5 h than those with TST > 7 h (1.3 ± 0.5 vs. 0.9 ± 0.3 mm; $P = 0.009$; 91.0 ± 6.0 vs. 81.6 ± 11.3%, $P = 0.03$, respectively). IMT was also significantly greater in the insomnia group than the noninsomnia group (1.3 ± 0.5 vs. 1.1 ± 0.4 mm; $P = 0.03$). IMT was significantly correlated with systolic blood pressure (SBP), diastolic blood pressure (DBP), and TST (SBP: $r = 0.49$, $P < 0.0001$; DBP: $r = 0.33$, $P = 0.0021$; TST: $r = -0.28$, $P = 0.010$). Multiple regression analysis revealed that SBP, TST, and the PSQI were significant contributing factors for increased IMT (SBP: coefficient $\beta = 0.56$, $P = 0.0001$; TST: coefficient $\beta = -0.32$, $P = 0.005$; PSQI: coefficient $\beta = 0.22$, $P = 0.05$).

Conclusions.—High blood pressure, short sleep duration (≤5 h), poor sleep, and insomnia were associated with atherosclerosis risk leading to cardiovascular disease in the elderly (Table 1).

▶ Insomnia with objectively measured short sleep duration (< 5 h) has been associated with hypertension, catecholaminergic activity, and type 2 diabetes that may lead to increased cardiovascular events. Prevalence of insomnia is increased in the elderly. This study is a cross-sectional evaluation of the association of insomnia and objectively measured short sleep duration (actigraphy) in the elderly (mean age, 73.6 ± 4.9 years; 25 male, 61 female) and atherosclerosis (evaluated by measuring carotid artery intima-media thickness [IMT] and plaque score).

IMT was significantly greater and sleep efficiency was significantly lower in subjects with total sleep time (TST) ≤5 hours than those with TST > 7 hours, with no significant differences in hypertension, diabetes, hyperlipidemia, smoking, or alcohol consumption (Table 1). There were also no significant differences in echocardiographic findings, sleep quality, sleep apnea, oxygen desaturation index, or lowest SpO_2 among the 3 groups. Multiple regression analysis found that systolic blood pressure (SBP), TST, and the Pittsburgh Sleep Quality Index (PSQI) were significant contributing factors for increased IMT.

It is interesting that in this study, the apnea—hypopnea index (an index of sleep apnea) was not correlated with an increase in IMT. It may be that such an association does not exist in the elderly or that a subset with significant oxygen desaturation during respiratory events does indeed have increased atherosclerotic risk, but this study did not have sufficient power to demonstrate such a finding. Another noteworthy finding was that sleep duration was not associated with hypertension in this elderly population. Reasons for such a finding are unclear. A relationship has been noted for younger individuals. It remains to be seen whether interventions to improve insomnia symptoms or sleep duration in the elderly will lead to improvement in atherosclerotic risk. IMT is a surrogate marker of atherosclerosis; longitudinal studies are needed to look at these associations using objective outcomes of myocardial infarction, stroke, and mortality.

S. Shafazand, MD, MS

Sleep-disordered Breathing and Cancer Mortality: Results from the Wisconsin Sleep Cohort Study

Nieto FJ, Peppard PE, Young T, et al (Univ of Wisconsin—Madison; et al)

Am J Respir Crit Care Med 186:190-194, 2012

Rationale.—Sleep-disordered breathing (SDB) has been associated with total and cardiovascular mortality, but an association with cancer mortality has not been studied. Results from *in vitro* and animal studies suggest that intermittent hypoxia promotes cancer tumor growth.

Objectives.—The goal of the present study was to examine whether SDB is associated with cancer mortality in a community-based sample.

Methods.—We used 22-year mortality follow-up data from the Wisconsin Sleep Cohort sample (n = 1,522). SDB was assessed at baseline with full

TABLE 1.—Characteristics of the Study Population and Death Rates According to Sleep-Disordered Breathing Categories

			Sleep-Disordered Breathing (AHI Range)		
	All	Absent (<5)	Mild (5–14.9)	Moderate (15–29.9)	Severe (≥30)*
No.	1,522	1,157	222	84	59
Age, mean (SD), yr	47.5 (8.1)	46.8 (7.9)	49.8 (8.1)	50.8 (8.6)	49.4 (8.6)
BMI, mean (SD), kg/m^2	29.9 (6.6)	28.7 (5.9)	32.3 (6.5)	34.3 (7.1)	38.6 (8.4)
Alcoholic drinks/wk, mean (SD)	3.9 (6.2)	3.8 (6.1)	4.1 (6.7)	4.7 (6.4)	4.4 (7.3)
Male sex, %	55.1	50.8	64.9	72.6	78.0
Education (≤ high school), %	25.7	24.9	30.6	31.0	30.5
Smoking, %					
Current	18.1	18.5	16.7	15.5	18.6
Former	38.6	35.1	41.9	51.2	50.9
Self-rated fair/poor health, %	4.3	3.4	3.3	8.9	19.7
Severe daytime sleepiness, %	24.5	23.1	24.9	32.5	39.7
Mortality rate per 1,000 person-yr (95% CI)					
All causes	4.29 (3.54–5.17)	3.24 (2.50–4.12)	6.88 (4.45–10.2)	5.02 (2.02–10.3)	15.57 (8.72–25.7)
Cancer	1.92 (1.42–2.53)	1.54 (1.05–2.19)	1.92 (0.77–3.97)	3.58 (1.16–8,36)	7.27 (2.92–15.0)

Definition of Abbreviations: AHI = apnea-hypopnea index; CI = confidence interval.
*Includes participants who were subject to CPAP treatment during the polysomnography study (n = 9).

TABLE 2.—Adjusted Relative Hazards of Total and Cancer Mortality According to Sleep-Disordered Breathing Categories

SDB (AHI Range)	All-Cause Mortality	Cancer Mortality
Absent (<5)	1.0	1.0
Mild SDB (5–14.9)	1.8 (1.1–2.8)	1.1 (0.5–2.7)
Moderate SDB (15–29.9)	1.1 (0.5–2.5)	2.0 (0.7–5.5)
Severe SDB (≥30)*	3.4 (1.7–6.7)	4.8 (1.7–13.2)
P for trend	0.0014	0.0052

Definition of Abbreviations: AHI = apnea-hypopnea index; BMI = body mass index; CI = confidence interval; CPAP = continuous positive airway pressure; SDB = sleep-disordered breathing.

Data are presented as adjusted relative hazard (95% CI). Adjusted for age (time scale), sex, BMI, BMI^2, and smoking.

*Includes participants who were subject to CPAP treatment during the polysomnography study (n = 9).

polysomnography. SDB was categorized using the apnea-hypopnea index (AHI) and the hypoxemia index (percent sleep time below 90% oxyhemoglobin saturation). The hazards of cancer mortality across levels of SDB severity were compared using crude and multivariate analyses.

Measurements and Main Results.—Adjusting for age, sex, body mass index, and smoking, SDB was associated with total and cancer mortality in a dose–response fashion. Compared with normal subjects, the adjusted relative hazards of cancer mortality were 1.1 (95% confidence interval [CI], 0.5–2.7) for mild SDB (AHI, 5–14.9), 2.0 (95% CI, 0.7–5.5) for moderate SDB (AHI, 15–29.9), and 4.8 (95% CI, 1.7–13.2) for severe SDB (AHI ≥ 30) (*P*-trend = 0.0052). For categories of increasing severity of the hypoxemia index, the corresponding relative hazards were 1.6 (95% CI, 0.6–4.4), 2.9 (95% CI, 0.9–9.8), and 8.6 (95% CI, 2.6–28.7).

Conclusions.—Our study suggests that baseline SDB is associated with increased cancer mortality in a community-based sample. Future studies that replicate our findings and look at the association between sleep apnea and survival after cancer diagnosis are needed (Tables 1 and 2).

▶ This is a longitudinal, epidemiologic, population-based study exploring the association between sleep-disordered breathing (SDB) and cancer mortality. Biological plausibility of such an association has been previously shown in animal models, but this is the first such study in humans.

Among the 1522 participants, 365 (24%) had at least mild SDB, and 59 (4%) had severe apnea (apnea-hypopnea index ≥30 or wore continuous positive airway pressure during the sleep assessment; Table 1). Both total and cancer mortalities increased linearly and significantly with increasing SDB severity. This dose-response relationship was observed even after adjusting for age, sex, body mass index, sleep duration, waist circumference, diabetes, and smoking (Table 2).

This is the first population-based cohort study documenting an association between baseline SDB and cancer mortality over a follow-up period lasting up to 22 years. If this association is validated in further clinical and population-based studies, diagnosis and treatment of SDB in cancer patients may prolong survival.

Another interesting area of research is whether SDB increases risk for incident cancer in the population. This study was not designed to answer this question.

S. Shafazand, MD, MS

Association of multiple sclerosis with restless legs syndrome and other sleep disorders in women

Li Y, Munger KL, Batool-Anwar S, et al (Brigham and Women's Hosp and Harvard Med School, Boston, MA; Harvard School of Public Health, Boston, MA)

Neurology 78:1500-1506, 2012

Objective.—To assess the association of multiple sclerosis (MS) with concurrent restless legs syndrome (RLS) and daytime sleepiness. We also prospectively examined whether women with MS had an increased risk of developing RLS during 4 years of follow-up.

Methods.—The main analysis was based on a cross-sectional study of 65,544 women (aged 41–58 years) free of diabetes, arthritis, and pregnancy, who were participating in the Nurses' Health Study II cohort. Participants were considered to have RLS if they met 4 RLS diagnostic criteria recommended by the International Restless Leg Syndrome Study Group and had restless legs ≥ 5 times/month. MS was self-reported and confirmed by medical record review.

Results.—Among women with MS, the prevalence of RLS and severe RLS (15+ times/month) were 15.5% and 9.9% in 2005, respectively, relative to 6.4% and 2.6% among women without MS. After adjustment for potential confounders and the presence of other sleep disorders, women with MS had a higher likelihood of having RLS (odds ratio [OR] = 2.72, 95% confidence interval [CI] 1.89–3.93), severe RLS (OR = 4.12, 95% CI 2.65–6.42), and daily daytime sleepiness (OR = 2.11, 95% CI 1.31–3.42) compared with women without MS. Among the 172 women who had MS and were free of RLS in 2005, 9 developed RLS (5.2%) during a 4-year period and all had severe RLS. The adjusted relative risk of severe RLS was 3.58 (95% CI 1.53–8.35), comparing women with MS at baseline with those without MS.

Conclusion.—Women with MS had a significantly higher prevalence of RLS and daytime sleepiness and an increased risk of developing RLS in the future (Table 2).

▶ The primary aim of this study was to assess the association between multiple sclerosis (MS) and restless legs syndrome (RLS) cross-sectionally and to prospectively examine whether individuals with MS had a higher risk of RLS in a large, population-based sample of women. A total of 264 confirmed cases of MS were found in this population. Among women with MS, the prevalence of RLS and severe RLS was 15.5% and 9.9%, respectively, relative to 6.4% and 2.6%, respectively, among individuals without MS (Table 2). Women with MS

TABLE 2.—ORs and 95% CI of RLS According to MS Status in the Nurses' Health Study II in 2005[a]

	No MS (n = 65,280)	MS (n = 264)	p Value
RLS			
No. of cases	4,182	41	
Prevalence (%)	6.4	15.5	
OR (95% CI)			
Age adjusted	1	2.68 (1.92–3.74)	<0.0001
Multivariate adjusted[b]	1	2.77 (1.92–3.98)	<0.0001
Further adjusted for other sleep disorders[c]	1	2.72 (1.89–3.93)	<0.0001
Severe RLS (15+ times/month)			
No. of cases	1,722	26	
Prevalence (%)	2.6	9.9	
OR (95% CI)			
Age adjusted	1	4.01 (2.67–6.03)	<0.0001
Multivariate adjusted[b]	1	4.21 (2.71–6.53)	<0.0001
Further adjusted for other sleep disorders[c]	1	4.12 (2.65–6.42)	<0.0001

Abbreviations: CI = confidence interval; MS = multiple sclerosis; OR = odds ratio; RLS = restless leg syndrome.

[a]Compared with individuals without MS.

[b]Adjusted for age (continuous), body mass index (kg/m^2), body mass index at age 18, ancestry (Scandinavian, Southern European, other Caucasian, or others), latitude of residence at age 15 (north, middle, or south), smoking status (never smoker, past smoker, or current smoker: cigarettes/day, 1–14 or ≥15), physical activity (quintiles), alcohol intake (g/day: 0, 0.1–4.9, 5.0–9.9, 10.0–14.9, and >15), menopause status (premenopausal, no menstrual periods, or had menopause but now induced by hormones), vitamin D supplement use, ironspecific supplement use, use of antidepressant medicine, use of tranquilizers, and history of stroke, myocardial infarction, and hypertension (each yes vs no).

[c]Further adjusted for difficulty falling or staying asleep, feeling sleep inadequate, frequent snoring, sleep time (≤6, 7, or ≥8 hours/24 hours), and frequency of daytime sleepiness that affected daily activities (no, 1–3 times/week, 3–6 times/week, or almost every day).

also had a higher risk of severe RLS than those without MS during 4 years of follow-up.

Strengths of this study include the facts that it is a population-based study with a large sample size and it uses standardized questions to assess the presence of RLS. This prospective study provides evidence that MS could be a risk factor for RLS. Most women in this study were white with similar socioeconomic backgrounds, making the findings less generalizable to other races and men.

Although the exact mechanism is unknown, the demyelination in the central nervous system may have an important role in RLS pathophysiology in MS. If future studies show an improvement in daytime symptoms of fatigue when RLS is treated in MS patients, then consideration should be given for routine screening for RLS in MS populations.

S. Shafazand, MD, MS

11 Miscellaneous

American Medical Society for Sports Medicine Position Statement: Concussion in Sport

Harmon KG, Drezner J, Gammons M, et al (Univ of Washington, Seattle; Vermont Orthopaedic Clinic, Rutland; et al)
Clin J Sport Med 23:1-18, 2013

Background.—Concussion is a transient disturbance of brain function induced by trauma that develops through a complex pathophysiologic process. It is usually self-limited and considered a less severe form of brain injury. However, suffering a concussion raises the risk for another concussion. More symptoms that are more serious and last longer are associated with a longer recovery time. An estimated 3.8 million concussions occur in the United States each year during competitive sports and recreational activities, but up to 50% are never reported. Female athletes in similar sports to male athletes are more likely to suffer a concussion. In addition, certain sports, positions, and playing styles carry a greater risk of having a concussion. All sports activities can cause concussion, but the highest incidence is found in football, hockey, rugby, soccer, and basketball. Sports medicine physicians are trained to manage sports concussions comprehensively, from the time of the injury until the decision to allow the individual to return to participation. The evidence-based best practices for managing concussion resulting from sports participation were outlined.

Diagnosis.—The diagnosis is best made by a health care provider familiar with the athlete and knowledgeable about concussion. Graded symptom lists can guide the assessment and help in tracking the severity of symptoms serially. Standardized assessment tools are also helpful, although validation is limited. In sideline evaluation and management, the athlete is removed from play and assessed. Symptoms to note include cognitive function, balance, and neurologic impairment. Although disturbed balance is a specific indicator of concussion, it is not very sensitive. Balance test results can differ from baseline because of the sideline conditions, including footwear, surface, presence of ankle tape or braces, or lower extremity injury. If intracerebral bleeding is suspected, imaging is advised. No athlete diagnosed with concussion should return to play the same day. All should be monitored for changes in physical or mental status.

Athletes can be further assessed for neuropsychologic impairment using objective measures of brain-behavior relationships, but most concussions are managed without such testing. It remains unclear when to use neuropsychologic tests, how often to use them, or which type is best. Athletes with persistent symptoms or complicated courses should undergo a comprehensive neuropsychologic evaluation during the postconcussion management period. These tests should be interpreted by health care providers skilled in the specific test's procedures and limitations and should be part of a comprehensive concussion management strategy rather than an isolated assessment. Paper and pencil tests offer comprehensive assessments, test different domains, and evaluate for conditions that mimic or complicate concussion.

Treatment and Outcomes.—Athletes are treated with cognitive rest. Students may require academic accommodations, including less work and longer time for test taking, while recovering from concussion. Exercise should be avoided until all concussion symptoms have resolved. Returning to play is accomplished in a stepwise manner, with a gradual increase in physical demands, sports-specific activities, and risk for contact. Any recurrence of symptoms should halt the progression and return the athlete to the preceding symptom-free level. Medical clearance from a licensed health care provider knowledgeable about concussion is required for the athlete to return to play. If the athlete returns to play too early, there is an increased risk for slower reaction time, which can lead to increased risk of repeat concussion or other injuries and a longer period with symptoms. Head impact exposure and recurrent concussions may contribute to long-term neurologic effects, with a possible association with chronic cognitive dysfunction. Each case must be approached individually to determine if the athlete should be disqualified from further participation in sports; no evidence-based guidelines are currently available.

Prevention and Education.—The best way to prevent some injuries involves modifying and/or enforcing the rules of fair play. Impact injuries can often be prevented by the use of helmets appropriate to the sport, but helmets and mouth guards have shown no effect on the incidence or severity of concussion. Secondary preventive efforts involve appropriate return-to-play policies. In addition, legislation may provide a uniform standard for sports organizations with respect to concussion safety and management.

Athletes, parents, coaches, officials, school administrators, and health care providers should be educated about the best approaches to concussion recognition, management, and prevention. Counseling regarding the potential long-term consequences of concussion and recurrent concussion should be offered by well-prepared physicians.

Conclusions.—Further research is needed to validate the tools used to assess athletes for concussion, determine the best uses and timing of neuropsychologic tests, and improve the ability to identify those at highest risk for prolonged concussion symptoms or other complications. Possible future advances in neuroimaging or biologic markers may help to better evaluate and manage sports concussions.

▶ Sports neurology is an emerging field in the specialty of neurology, as in all other specialties. The American Medical Society for Sports Medicine has released a statement to help physicians with the evaluation and management of sports-related concussive injuries and in clarifying levels of evidence and filling knowledge gaps. This article is an extensive review of the background, pathophysiology, epidemiology, and the clinical manifestations of sports-related concussive injury. It also touches on the management of concussion preseason, on-field or sideline and postsideline, including the utility of neuropsychologic testing, particularly in return-to-play decisions. The discussion on the long-term sequelae of sports-related concussion is also particularly helpful. This article is a useful tool in future efforts to standardize the neurologic care of athletes and in the formulation of legislation and public policy pertaining to sports. It is also helpful to compare these guidelines with those of the American Academy of Neurology, also recently released, on sports-related concussive injuries.

R. Riel-Romero, MD

Advances in stem cell therapy for spinal cord injury

Mothe AJ, Tator CH (Toronto Western Hosp, Toronto, Ontario, Canada)

J Clin Invest 122:3824-3834, 2012

Spinal cord injury (SCI) is a devastating condition producing great personal and societal costs and for which there is no effective treatment. Stem cell transplantation is a promising therapeutic strategy, though much preclinical and clinical research work remains. Here, we briefly describe SCI epidemiology, pathophysiology, and experimental and clinical stem cell strategies. Research in stem cell biology and cell reprogramming is rapidly advancing, with the hope of moving stem cell therapy closer to helping people with SCI. We examine issues important for clinical translation and provide a commentary on recent developments, including termination of the first human embryonic stem cell transplantation trial in human SCI.

▶ Spinal cord injury (SCI) is a devastating neurologic condition that has a great impact at many different levels, both personal and societal. This article describes the latest experimental and clinical aspects of stem cell therapy for SCI. The use of embryonic stem cells, mesenchymal stem cells such as bone marrow–derived stromal cells, neural stem cells, or progenitor cells, and induced pluripotent cells are explained in great detail. The authors also explain the challenges inherent in the clinical translation of stem cell–based therapy for SCI. This article is important as an update on the ongoing basic science research regarding the treatment of SCI, which thus far has no clear-cut effective therapy that can potentially reverse the initial devastating injury that occurs at the molecular level.

R. Riel-Romero, MD

A pilot study of cerebral and haemodynamic physiological changes during sedation with dexmedetomidine or propofol in patients with acute brain injury

James ML, Olson DM, Graffagnino C (Duke Univ Hosp, Durham, NC)

Anaesth Intensive Care 40:949-957, 2012

Sedation for the mechanically-ventilated, brain-injured patient remains challenging. The purpose of this pilot study was to compare the cerebral physiologic effects of sedation with propofol versus dexmedetomidine in mechanically-ventilated, brain-injured patients. Using a randomised, crossover, unblinded clinical trial, we enrolled patients with severe brain injury (Glasgow Coma Score ≤ 8) from traumatic injury, subarachnoid haemorrhage or intracerebral haemorrhage undergoing multimodal monitoring (intracranial pressure, brain temperature, oximetry and microdialysis). Patients received an infusion of either propofol or dexmedetomidine for six hours and then a crossover for the subsequent six hours after sufficient washout/in. Clinical and physiological measurements were recorded hourly. In eight patients, (four traumatic injury, three subarachnoid haemorrhage and one intracerebral haemorrhage), the mean dose of propofol used was 25.5 μg/kg/minute while the mean dose of dexmedetomidine was 0.54 μg/kg/hour. All subjects were effectively sedated to a goal of Richmond Agitation Sedation Scale -2 and Bispectral Index of 50–70 throughout the study period. We did not observe any statistically significant differences between the groups in systemic or cerebral physiologic metrics. Though differences were noted in cerebral metabolic substrates (lactate/pyruvate ratio), none were statistically significant. In our pilot cohort, dexmedetomidine and propofol appear equally effective in sedating severely brain-injured patients and neither is associated with adverse physiological effects as measured by multimodal monitoring. Larger long-term studies are required to determine whether clinically favourable benefits demonstrated in the medical critical care setting also apply to this patient population.

▶ Sedation of patients with brain injury in the neurocritical care setting is of utmost importance but can be particularly difficult. On one hand, good clinical care cannot be provided without adequate sedation; on the other hand, clinical care requires periodic neurologic assessment of the patient requiring transient lifting of sedation. The authors of the pilot study compared the cerebral physiologic effects of propofol and dexmedetomidine using a randomized, crossover, unblinded clinical trial with multimodal monitoring, that is, cerebral microdialysate analysis, brain temperature, and intracranial pressure parameters. Level of sedation was assessed using the Richmond Agitation Sedation Scale and the Bispectral Index. They conclude that both agents are efficacious for adequate sedation and well tolerated. Limitations of the study included the possibility of carry-over effects of propofol beyond the initial wash-in period, as patients were on propofol before enrollment, and the lack of stratification of patients based on the type of brain injury. However, they stressed that the choice of sedation should be individualized, that is, dexmedetomidine has no antiepileptic effects, whereas propofol does.

R. Riel-Romero, MD

Complex single gene disorders and epilepsy

Merwick A, O'Brien M, Delanty N (Beaumont Hosp and Royal College of Surgeons in Ireland, Dublin)
Epilepsia 53:81-91, 2012

Epilepsy is a heterogenous group of disorders, often associated with significant comorbidity, such as intellectual disability and skin disorder. The genetic underpinnings of many epilepsies are still being elucidated, and we expect further advances over the coming 5 years, as genetic technology improves and prices fall for whole exome and whole genome sequencing. At present, there are several well-characterized complex epilepsies associated with single gene disorders; we review some of these here. They include well-recognized syndromes such as tuberous sclerosis complex, epilepsy associated with Rett syndrome, some of the progressive myoclonic epilepsies, and novel disorders such as epilepsy associated with mutations in the *PCDH 19* gene. These disorders are important in informing genetic testing to confirm a diagnosis and to permit better understanding of the variability in phenotype-genotype correlation.

▶ This article is an excellent review of the current state of knowledge about the most common complex single gene disorders frequently associated with epilepsy. Among these disorders are tuberous sclerosis, neurofibromatosis, Angelman syndrome, Rett syndrome, Unverricht-Lundborg disease, Lafora body, myoclonic epilepsy with ragged-red fibers, seizures associated with mutations in *PCD19* (protocadherin 19) on chromosome Xq22, and seizures associated with mutations in the *ARX* gene (X-linked aristaless-related homeobox gene on chromosome Xp22.13). This article provides helpful summaries of the clinical phenotypes, the various genetic mutations seen, and the current state of therapy for each of these disorders. Overall, this article is a very useful guide for the busy clinician who needs to know the salient points of each of the above complex single gene disorders and the type of epilepsy they present.

R. Riel-Romero, MD

Clinical Applications of Hybrid PET/MRI in Neuroimaging

Garibotto V, Heinzer S, Vulliemoz S, et al (Geneva Univ Hosp, Switzerland)
Clin Nucl Med 38:e13-e18, 2013

Purpose.—We tested the performance and clinical applicability of combined protocols for brain imaging studies acquired on a new whole-body hybrid PET/MR scanner.

Patients and Methods.—Fifteen patients [6 male and 9 female patients; mean (SD) age, 51 (30) y; range, 6–89 y] were scanned on a Philips Ingenuity TF PET/MR. Standard imaging protocols of both modalities were combined, using a "head coil" and contrast-enhanced fully diagnostic MR protocols. Attenuation correction of the PET images was performed using tissue segmentation of the MR image and incorporation of attenuation templates measured for coils and table.

The clinical indications evaluated are as follows: patients with cognitive disturbance of suspected neurodegenerative origin, presurgical evaluation of drug-refractory epilepsy, and brain tumor staging. For the first 2 indications, FDG PET imaging was performed, whereas for the last, fluoroethyltyrosine, an amino acid tracer, was used.

Results.—In all cases (4 patients with neurodegenerative disease, 6 patients with epilepsy, and 5 patients with high-grade tumor), we obtained full diagnostic quality of both modalities and the total duration of the examination remained within a tolerable range (<2 hours). Twelve subjects had pathological findings: 11 of which were confirmed by clinical follow-up as true positive and 1 was confirmed as a false-positive result. For the 3 normal studies, the clinical follow-up confirmed the imaging findings as true-negative.

Conclusions.—Acquiring both PET and MR in a single session on a hybrid system minimized patient discomfort while maximizing clinical information and optimizing registration of both modalities. In addition, in comparison to PET/CT, the effective dose (related to CT) was reduced, and this is particularly beneficial in the pediatric population.

▶ Although positron emission tomography (PET) and MRI are individually available techniques used in the evaluation of many neurologic conditions, including epilepsy, brain tumors, metabolic, and neurodegenerative disease, the novel idea of combining the 2 modalities, as proposed in this article, may be just as or more effective and technically easier (shorter time for acquisition for the 2 studies and less time for sedation if needed) to manage than either procedure alone. The authors studied 15 patients of whom 12 were found to have pathologic findings using PET/MRI hybrid techniques. On clinical follow-up, the PET/MRI findings were truly positive, and for the remaining patient in whom the findings were suspicious for tumor recurrence, follow-up revealed a more favorable outcome, as the tumor regressed and was eventually diagnosed to have radiation necrosis instead. There are some clear benefits to considering such hybrid techniques, but further studies on the sensitivity, specificity, positive predictive value, and negative predictive value would have to be done on more patients.

R. Riel-Romero, MD

Comparative stroke risk of antiepileptic drugs in patients with epilepsy

Hsieh C-Y, Lai EC-C, Yang Y-HK, et al (Natl Cheng Kung Univ, Tainan, Taiwan; et al)

Epilepsia 54:172-180, 2013

Purpose.—Patients with epilepsy have higher stroke-related morbidity and mortality, leading to the suspicion that the increased stroke events may be associated with antiepileptic drug (AED) exposure. We evaluated the comparative risk of stroke in adult patients with epilepsy receiving phenytoin (PHT), valproic acid (VPA), or carbamazepine (CBZ) to help determine the stroke risk for Asian patients with specific AED exposure.

Methods.—We conducted a population-based, retrospective cohort study using the Taiwan National Health Insurance Research Database (NHIRD). The cohort consists of adult patients with epilepsy who were new to PHT, CBZ, or VPA monotherapy and without prior stroke history. Patients were followed for 5 years. The event of interest was a hospitalization or emergency visit due to stroke. Cox proportional hazard models were used to estimate the comparative risk of AEDs. Subanalyses included an evaluation of different subtypes of stroke, the propensity score matched technique, the intention-to-treat approach, and stratification analyses.

Key Findings.—Patients receiving PHT had a significantly higher stroke risk (adjusted hazard ratio [HR] 1.72; 95% confidence interval [CI] 1.20–2.47), followed by VPA (adjusted HR 1.27; 95% CI 0.78–2.07), when compared with CBZ. The results of all subanalyses showed a consistent trend of higher stroke risk with PHT use. In addition, there appeared to be a dose–response relationship between stroke risk and PHT prescriptions.

Significance.—The stroke risk was higher in PHT but not significantly different in VPA as compared to CBZ. Physicians should reconsider using PHT for patients with epilepsy who already have a higher risk of stroke.

▶ This article is a population-based, retrospective, cohort study of adult patients naive to phenytoin (PHT), valproic acid (VPA), or carbamazepine (CBZ) without prior stroke history who were followed for 5 years with the aim of assessing stroke risk among patients using the aforementioned antiepileptic drugs. It is known that CBZ can increase the serum levels of total cholesterol, low-density lipoproteins, and lipoprotein(a). It is interesting to note that the authors concluded that the stroke risk for PHT was higher but not significantly different for VPA compared with CBZ, at least in the Asian patients enrolled in this study. The authors postulate that PHT or CBZ increased serum homocysteine or decreased serum folate. Moreover, enzyme inducers of the cytochrome P450 system such as PHT and CBZ can increase cholesterol synthesis and reduce feedback inhibition of the hydroxymethylglutaryl coenzyme-A reductase. On the other hand, VPA may attenuate the risk of myocardial infarction and stroke perhaps through both enzyme inhibition and ventricular remodeling. This information about comparative stroke risk can inform neurologists' choice of antiepileptic drugs in epileptic patients with risk factors for stroke.

R. Riel-Romero, MD

NEUROSURGERY

PAUL KLIMO, JR, MD, MPH

12 Brain Tumors

Endoscopic endonasal surgery for giant pituitary adenomas: advantages and limitations

Koutourousiou M, Gardner PA, Fernandez-Miranda JC, et al (Univ of Pittsburgh Med Ctr, PA)

J Neurosurg 118:621-631, 2013

Object.—Giant pituitary adenomas (> 4 cm in maximum diameter) represent a significant surgical challenge. Endoscopic endonasal surgery (EES) has recently been introduced as a treatment option for these tumors. The authors present the results of EES for giant adenomas and analyze the advantages and limitations of this technique.

Methods.—The authors retrospectively reviewed the medical files and imaging studies of 54 patients with giant pituitary adenomas who underwent EES and studied the factors affecting surgical outcome.

Results.—Preoperative visual impairment was present in 45 patients (83%) and partial or complete pituitary deficiency in 28 cases (52%), and 7 patients (13%) presented with apoplexy. Near-total resection (> 90%) was achieved in 36 patients (66.7%). Vision was improved or normalized in 36 cases (80%) and worsened in 2 cases due to apoplexy of residual tumor. Significant factors that limited the degree of resection were a multilobular configuration of the adenoma ($p = 0.002$) and extension to the middle fossa ($p = 0.045$). Cavernous sinus invasion, tumor size, and intraventricular or posterior fossa extension did not influence the surgical outcome. Complications included apoplexy of residual adenoma (3.7%), permanent diabetes insipidus (9.6%), new pituitary insufficiency (16.7%), and CSF leak (16.7%, which was reduced to 7.4% in recent years). Fourteen patients underwent radiation therapy after EES for residual mass or, in a later stage, for recurrence, and 10 with functional pituitary adenomas received medical treatment. During a mean follow-up of 37.9 months (range 1–114 months), 7 patients were reoperated on for tumor recurrence. Three patients were lost to follow-up.

Conclusions.—Endoscopic endonasal surgery provides effective initial management of giant pituitary adenomas with favorable results compared with traditional microscopic transsphenoidal and transcranial approaches.

▶ Giant pituitary tumors (> 4 cm in maximal diameter) are associated with a higher surgical risk of morbidity and mortality and often cannot be completely resected because of tumor invasion into surrounding critical structures, such as the cavernous sinus, temporal lobe, and hypothalamus. The goals of surgery are decompression of the optic apparatus and maximal tumor resection that is safely possible. Gross total resection can be attainable in some tumors that have a rounded configuration (as opposed to multilobulated) and lack invasion beyond the lateral wall of the cavernous sinus (Knosp grade D). I would agree that the endoscopic transsphenoidal approach allows us to achieve a higher extent of resection over the microscopic approach because of a better panoramic visualization and the ability to look upward toward the third ventricle, laterally in the cavernous sinuses, and inferiorly in the clivus. The nasal speculum used in the microscopic approach limits the exposure and working corridor and relies on blind curettage through a smaller dural opening. With the endoscopic approach, multiple corridors (transplanum, transtuberculum, transcavernous, and transclival) can be explored simultaneously, thereby achieving maximal tumor decompression. The visual and endocrinologic results as well as the extent of resection presented here are very favorable.

J. K. Liu, MD

Value of endoscopy for maximizing tumor removal in endonasal transsphenoidal pituitary adenoma surgery

McLaughlin N, Eisenberg AA, Cohan P, et al (John Wayne Cancer Inst at Saint John's Health Ctr, Santa Monica, CA; David Geffen School of Medicine at UCLA)
J Neurosurg 118:613-620, 2013

Object.—Endoscopy as a visual aid (endoscope assisted) or as the sole visual method (fully endoscopic) is increasingly used in pituitary adenoma surgery. Authors of this study assessed the value of endoscopic visualization for finding and removing residual adenoma after initial microscopic removal.

Methods.—Consecutive patients who underwent endoscope-assisted microsurgical removal of pituitary adenoma were included in this study. The utility of the endoscope in finding and removing residual adenoma not visualized by the microscope was noted intraoperatively. After maximal tumor removal under microscopic visualization, surgeries were categorized as to whether additional tumor was removed via endoscopy. Tumor removal and remission rates were also noted. Patients undergoing fully endoscopic tumor removal during this same period were excluded from the study.

Results.—Over 3 years, 140 patients (41% women, mean age 50 years) underwent endoscope-assisted adenoma removal of 30 endocrine-active microadenomas and 110 macroadenomas (39 endocrine-active, 71 endocrine-inactive); 16% (23/140) of patients had prior surgery. After initial microscopic removal, endoscopy revealed residual tumor in 40% (56/140) of cases and the additional tumor was removed in 36% (50 cases) of these cases. Endoscopy facilitated additional tumor removal in 54% (36/67) of the adenomas measuring ≥ 2 cm in diameter and in 19% (14/73) of the adenomas smaller than 2 cm in diameter ($p < 0.0001$); additional tumor removal was achieved in 20% (6/30) of the microadenomas. Residual tumor was typically removed from the suprasellar extension and folds of the collapsed diaphragma sellae or along or within the medial cavernous sinus. Overall, 91% of endocrine-inactive tumors were gross-totally or near-totally removed, and 70% of endocrine-active adenomas had early remission.

Conclusions.—After microscope-based tumor removal, endoscopic visualization led to additional adenoma removal in over one-third of patients. The panoramic visualization of the endoscope appears to facilitate more complete tumor removal than is possible with the microscope alone. These findings further emphasize the utility of endoscopic visualization in pituitary adenoma surgery. Longer follow-ups and additional case series are needed to determine if endoscopic adenomectomy translates into higher long-term remission rates.

► In this study, the endoscope was introduced into the operative field to inspect for any residual tumor after attempted maximal microsurgical removal of pituitary adenoma using the traditional microscopic transsphenoidal approach. Residual tumor was visualized with the endoscope in 40% (56 of 140) of cases, which resulted in additional tumor removal in 50 of these cases. Endoscopy facilitated additional removal in 54% of adenomas 2 cm or larger and in 19% of smaller adenomas less than 2 cm. This resulted in 91% of gross or near-total resection of nonfunctioning adenomas and 70% early remission of functioning adenomas. This suggests that the endoscope offers better panoramic visualization of the parasellar region than the microscope, which translates to a better extent of resection. The narrow speculum-based working corridor used in the microsurgical approach limits visualization of lateral and superior sellar compartments and the maneuverability of instruments. It is not surprising that the senior author in this study adapted a fully endoscopic binostril approach toward the end of this study. The endoscope makes a significant difference in extent of resection, especially with macroadenomas with suprasellar or lateral extension.

I have often performed fully endoscopic reoperations of pituitary macroadenomas that were initially performed elsewhere via a standard speculum-based microscopic approach where the sellar bony opening was suboptimal and the tumor was removed partially. With the fully endoscopic approach using angled endoscopes, the technique of blind curettage of tumor is now obsolete. I suspect that intraoperative MRI will not be as useful in fully endoscopic transsphenoidal operations, but more studies are needed to validate this.

J. K. Liu, MD

Hearing preservation in patients with vestibular schwannoma treated with Gamma Knife surgery

Baschnagel AM, Chen PY, Bojrab D, et al (William Beaumont Hosp, Royal Oak, MI; Michigan Ear Inst, Royal Oak; et al)
J Neurosurg 118:571-578, 2013

Object.—Hearing loss after Gamma Knife surgery (GKS) in patients with vestibular schwannoma has been associated with radiation dose to the cochlea. The purpose of this study was to evaluate serviceable hearing preservation in patients with VS who were treated with GKS and to determine if serviceable hearing loss can be correlated with the dose to the cochlea.

Methods.—Forty patients with vestibular schwannoma with serviceable hearing were treated using GKS with a median marginal dose of 12.5 Gy (range 12.5–13 Gy) to the 50% isodose volume. Audiometry was performed prospectively before and after GKS at 1, 3, and 6 months, and then every 6 months thereafter. Hearing preservation was based on pure tone average (PTA) and speech discrimination (SD). Serviceable hearing was defined as PTA less than 50 dB and SD greater than 50%.

Results.—The median cochlear maximum and mean doses were 6.9 Gy (range 1.6–16 Gy) and 2.7 Gy (range 0.7–5.0 Gy), respectively. With a median audiological follow-up of 35 months (range 6–58 months), the 1-, 2-, and 3-year actuarial rates of maintaining serviceable hearing were 93%, 77%, and 74%, respectively. No patient who received a mean cochlear dose less than 2 Gy experienced serviceable hearing loss ($p = 0.035$). Patients who received a mean cochlear dose less than 3 Gy had a 2-year hearing preservation rate of 91% compared with 59% in those who received a mean cochlear dose of 3 Gy or greater ($p = 0.029$). Those who had more than 25% of their cochlea receiving 3 Gy or greater had a higher rate of hearing loss ($p = 0.030$). There was no statistically significant correlation between serviceable hearing loss and age, tumor size, pre-GKS PTA, pre-GKS SD, pre-GKS Gardner-Robertson class, maximum cochlear dose, or the percentage of cochlear volume receiving 5 Gy. On multivariate analysis there was a trend toward significance for serviceable hearing loss with a mean cochlear dose of 3 Gy or greater ($p = 0.074$). Local control was 100% at 24 months. No patient developed facial or trigeminal nerve dysfunction.

Conclusions.—With a median mean cochlear dose of 2.7 Gy, the majority of patients with serviceable hearing retained serviceable hearing 3 years after GKS. A mean cochlear dose less than 3 Gy was associated with higher serviceable hearing preservation.

▶ This article emphasizes the importance of limiting mean cochlear dose to optimize hearing preservation rates after Gamma Knife radiosurgery of sporadic acoustic neuromas. The authors report that a mean cochlear dose of less than 3 Gy was associated with statistically better hearing preservation rates at 2 years compared with those who received more than 3 Gy (90% vs 59%, $P = .029$, see Fig 3 in the original article). No hearing loss was observed in those who received a mean cochlear dose less than 2 Gy (see Fig 2 in the original article). However, the relatively short duration of follow-up is a major limitation of this study (median audiological follow-up of 35 months). The 1-year, 2-year, and 3-year actuarial rates of maintaining serviceable hearing were 93%, 77%, and 74%, respectively. It is likely that hearing can continue to deteriorate with time, as noted in previous radiosurgical series as well as natural history studies from Denmark.[1-3] Therefore, long-term follow-up with imaging and formal audiograms is necessary to validate these results. Nevertheless, I agree with limiting the dose to the cochlea, perhaps to less than 3 Gy if technically possible, to optimize the chance of hearing preservation.

J. K. Liu, MD

References

1. Stangerup SE, Thomsen J, Tos M, Cayé-Thomasen P. Long-term hearing preservation in vestibular schwannoma. *Otol Neurotol.* 2010;31:271-275.
2. Hasegawa T, Kida Y, Kato T, Iizuka H, Kuramitsu S, Yamamoto T. Long-term safety and efficacy of stereotactic radiosurgery for vestibular schwannomas: evaluation of 440 patients more than 10 years after treatment with Gamma Knife surgery. *J Neurosurg.* 2013;118:557-565.
3. Carlson ML, Jacob JT, Pollock BE, et al. Long-term hearing outcomes following stereotactic radiosurgery for vestibular schwannoma: patterns of hearing loss and variables influencing audiometric decline. *J Neurosurg.* 2013;118:579-587.

Longitudinal analysis of hearing before and after radiosurgery for vestibular schwannoma

Yomo S, Carron R, Thomassin J-M, et al (CHU Timone, Marseille, France)
J Neurosurg 117:877-885, 2012

Object.—The aim of this study was to perform an accurate analysis of changes in hearing in patients with vestibular schwannoma (VS) who have undergone Gamma Knife surgery (GKS) and distinguish the impact of radiosurgery from the natural course of hearing deterioration due to the tumor itself.

Methods.—This study was a retrospective review of prospectively collected patient data. A group of 154 patients with unilateral nonsurgically treated VS was conservatively monitored for more than 6 months and then treated with GKS between July 1997 and September 2005. They were followed up with serial clinical examination, MRI, and audiometry. The annual hearing decrease rate (AHDR) was measured before and after radiosurgery, and the possible prognostic factors for hearing preservation were investigated.

Results.—The mean dose prescribed to the tumor margins was 12.1 Gy. The mean radiological follow-up period after GKS was 60 months (range 7–123 months). The tumor control rate was 94.8%, and 8 patients underwent subsequent intervention due to tumor progression. The mean audiological follow-up times before and after GKS were 22 and 52 months, respectively. The mean AHDRs before and after GKS were 5.39 dB/year (95% CI 3.31–7.47 dB/year) and 3.77 dB/year (95% CI 3.13–4.40 dB/year), respectively ($p > 0.05$). The mean pre- and post-GKS AHDRs in patients who initially had Gardner-Robertson (GR) Class I hearing were −0.57 dB/year (95% CI −2.95 to 1.81 dB/year) and 3.59 dB/year (95% CI 2.52–4.65 dB/year), respectively ($p = 0.007$). The mean pre- and post-GKS AHDRs in patients who initially had GR Class II hearing were 5.09 dB/year (95% CI 1.36–8.82 dB/year) and 4.98 dB/year (95% CI 3.86–6.10 dB/year), respectively ($p > 0.05$). A subgroup of 80 patients had both early and late post-intervention AHDR assessment (with early referring to the period from GKS to the assessment closest to the 2-year follow-up point and late referring to the period from that assessment to the most recent one); in these patients, the mean early post-GKS AHDR was 5.86 dB/year (95% CI 4.25–7.50 dB/year) and the mean late post-GKS AHDR was 1.86 dB/year (95% CI 0.77–2.96 dB/year) ($p < 0.001$). A maximum cochlear dose of less than 4 Gy was found to be the sole prognostic factor for hearing preservation.

Conclusions.—The present study demonstrated the absence of an increase in AHDR after radiosurgery as compared with the preoperative AHDR. There was even a trend indicating a reduction in the annual hearing loss after radiosurgery over the long term. To fully elucidate a possible protective effect of radiosurgery, longer-term follow-up with a larger group of patients will be required.

▶ In this study, the authors calculated the annual hearing decrease rate (AHDR) by dividing the difference in pure tone average by the follow-up period (in years). The mean AHDR overall was 4.05 dB per year. Before radiosurgery, the AHDR was 5.39 dB per year, and after radiosurgery, the AHDR was 3.77 dB per year ($P > .05$). In a subgroup analysis, those who had Gardner-Robertson (GR) Class I hearing, the AHDR was −0.57 dB per year before radiosurgery and 3.59 dB per year after radiosurgery. For those with Class II hearing, AHDR was 5.09 dB per year and 4.98 dB per year before and after radiosurgery, respectively. It seems as if those with better pretreatment hearing (Class I) became worse and those with worse hearing (Class II) stabilized after radiation. In a select group of 80 patients who received multiple audiograms posttreatment, the ADHR was significantly lower in the late posttreatment period (1.84 dB per year) as opposed to the early posttreatment period (5.86 dB per year). Thus, the authors have suggested that perhaps radiosurgery in some patients may slow the hearing loss process.

The major criticism I have with this study is that there is an assumption that hearing loss is linear. This is certainly not the case. Some patients may maintain good hearing that is stabilized for a period of time before abruptly losing hearing without any warning signs. Some may lose a large amount of decibels and remain at a stable low level. The other issue with this study is that there is no report of postradiosurgery hearing status in terms of GR classification. For example, there is no mention of what percentage of patients were in which GR class at the latest audiological follow-up. In addition, there is no assessment of the speech discrimination score, which is very important in assessing one's hearing status. Patients with GR Class III or IV should also be excluded from the study because these patients have no useful hearing and calculating differences in decibel change in this group can skew the results. Very few would argue that stereotactic radiosurgery offers excellent rates of tumor control for small- to medium-sized sporadic acoustic neuromas. The controversy remains in long-term hearing preservation and whether it is more or less favorable than the natural history (simply observe and do nothing). We do know from natural history studies that patients with acoustic neuromas will eventually lose hearing. The results presented here do not demonstrate a protective effect of radiosurgery on hearing loss as some may suggest. Longer-term follow-up with proper audiological assessment is warranted to determine if radiosurgery beats the natural history in terms of hearing loss. And let us be reminded in good experienced hands with proper patient selection, hearing can be preserved with surgical removal.

J. K. Liu, MD

Long-term hearing outcomes following stereotactic radiosurgery for vestibular schwannoma: patterns of hearing loss and variables influencing audiometric decline

Carlson ML, Jacob JT, Pollock BE, et al (Mayo Clinic School of Medicine, Rochester, MN)

J Neurosurg 118:579-587, 2013

Object.—The goals of this retrospective cohort study were as follows: 1) to describe the long-term prevalence and timing of hearing deterioration following low-dose (12- to 13-Gy marginal dose) stereotactic radiosurgery (SRS) for vestibular schwannoma (VS); and 2) to identify clinical variables associated with long-term preservation of useful hearing following treatment.

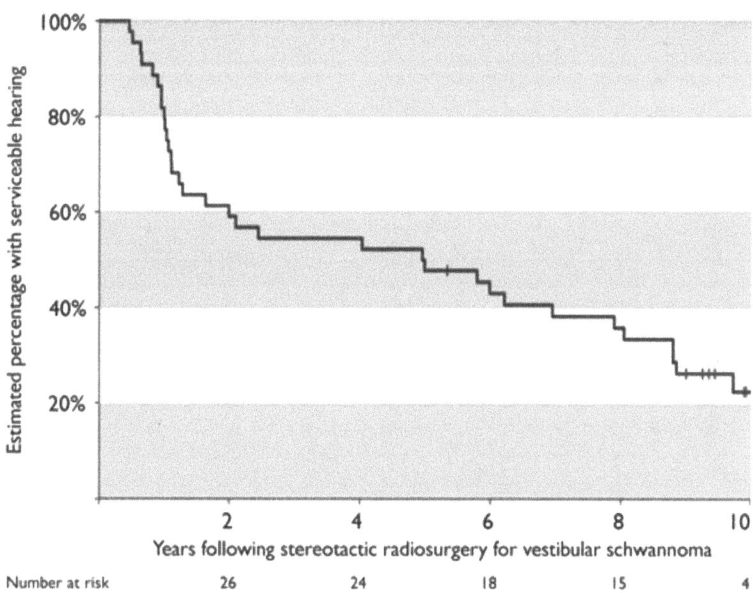

FIGURE 1.—Kaplan-Meier graph showing estimated rates of serviceable hearing among 44 patients with unilateral VS treated with low-dose SRS. (Reprinted from Carlson ML, Jacob JT, Pollock BE, et al. Long-term hearing outcomes following stereotactic radiosurgery for vestibular schwannoma: patterns of hearing loss and variables influencing audiometric decline. *J Neurosurg*. 2013;118:579-587, Copyright 2013, with permission from American Association for Neurological Surgeons, with Rockwater, Inc, http://aans.org/.)

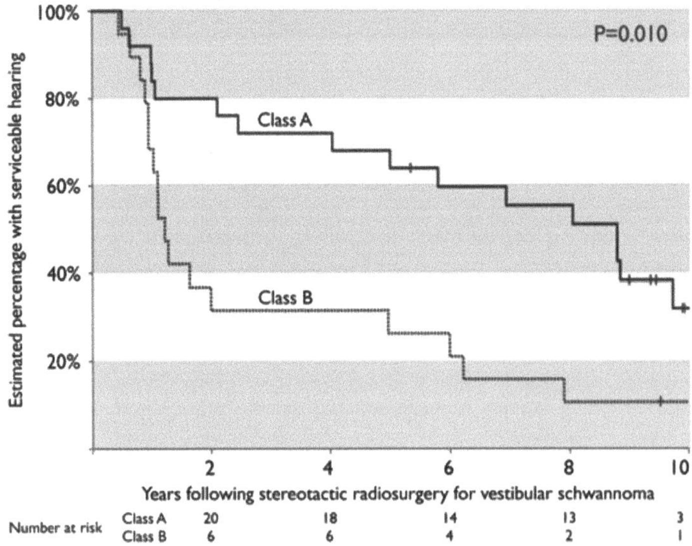

FIGURE 2.—Kaplan-Meier graph showing estimated rates of serviceable hearing comparing patients with pretreatment AAO-HNS Class A and Class B hearing. (Reprinted from Carlson ML, Jacob JT, Pollock BE, et al. Long-term hearing outcomes following stereotactic radiosurgery for vestibular schwannoma: patterns of hearing loss and variables influencing audiometric decline. *J Neurosurg.* 2013;118:579-587, Copyright 2013, with permission from American Association for Neurological Surgeons, with Rockwater, Inc, http://aans.org/.)

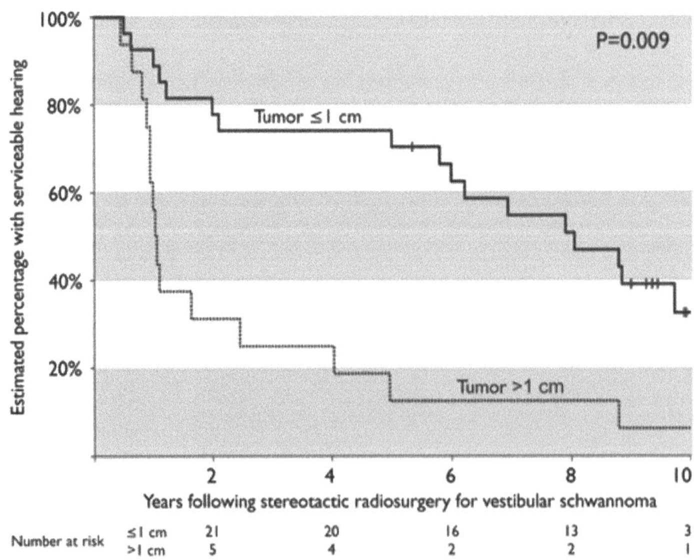

FIGURE 3.—Kaplan-Meier graph showing estimated rates of serviceable hearing comparing patients with sporadic VSs ≤ 1 cm and tumors > 1 cm. (Reprinted from Carlson ML, Jacob JT, Pollock BE, et al. Long-term hearing outcomes following stereotactic radiosurgery for vestibular schwannoma: patterns of hearing loss and variables influencing audiometric decline. *J Neurosurg.* 2013;118:579-587, Copyright 2013, with permission from American Association for Neurological Surgeons, with Rockwater, Inc, http://aans.org/.)

Methods.—Patients with serviceable hearing who underwent SRS for VS between 1997 and 2002 were studied. Data including radiosurgery treatment plans, tumor characteristics, pre- and posttreatment pure tone average, speech discrimination scores, and American Academy of Otolaryngology–Head and Neck Surgery hearing class were collected. Time to nonserviceable hearing was estimated using the Kaplan-Meier method. Univariate and multivariate associations with time to nonserviceable hearing were evaluated using Cox proportional hazards regression models.

Results.—Forty-four patients met the study criteria and were included. The median duration of audiometric follow-up was 9.3 years. Thirty-six patients developed nonserviceable hearing at a mean of 4.2 years following SRS. The Kaplan-Meier estimated rates of serviceable hearing at 1, 3, 5, 7, and 10 years following SRS were 80%, 55%, 48%, 38%, and 23%, respectively. Multivariate analysis revealed that pretreatment ipsilateral pure tone average ($p < 0.001$) and tumor size ($p = 0.009$) were statistically significantly associated with time to nonserviceable hearing.

Conclusions.—Durable hearing preservation a decade after low-dose SRS for VS occurs in less than one-fourth of patients. Variables including preoperative hearing capacity and tumor size may be used to predict hearing outcomes following treatment. These findings may assist in pretreatment risk disclosure. Furthermore, these data demonstrate the importance of long-term follow-up when reporting audiometric outcomes following SRS for VS (Figs 1-3).

▶ Although stereotactic radiosurgery has demonstrated good overall tumor control of growth, the results of long-term hearing preservation remain questionable. This article demonstrates that serviceable hearing after radiosurgery for acoustic neuroma is durable in less than 25% over long-term follow-up of 10 years. As clearly shown by the authors, serviceable hearing (American Academy of Otolaryngology Head and Neck Surgery class A or B) declines over time, even with radiosurgical treatment of these tumors (Fig 1). The authors present 44 patients with acoustic neuromas with serviceable pretreatment hearing managed with low-dose radiosurgery (12-13 Gy marginal dose) with at least 5 years of follow-up. Neurofibromatosis type 2 patients were excluded. Follow-up posttreatment audiometric data were obtained by incentivizing the patients with compensation of $60. Thirty-six patients (81.8%) deteriorated to nonserviceable hearing (class C or D) at a mean of 4.2 years. Factors affecting hearing deterioration over time included worse pretreatment hearing (class B), tumors occupying the cerebellopontine angle greater than 1 cm in size (as opposed to intracanalicular tumors), and tumors that contacted the brainstem (Figs 2 and 3). The outcomes reported here corroborate with other studies demonstrating that most patients will eventually lose their hearing as a result of either radiosurgical treatment or from natural history of the disease. The factors that appear to be associated with more favorable radiosurgical outcomes include small tumor size, fundal fluid capping (distance of lateral margin of tumor to the cochlea), and excellent pretreatment hearing status. This article underscores the importance of long-term follow-up with accurate outcomes reporting with audiometric data. These data are also important to consider when individualizing treatment strategies for patients with acoustic neuroma.

J. K. Liu, MD

Long-term safety and efficacy of stereotactic radiosurgery for vestibular schwannomas: evaluation of 440 patients more than 10 years after treatment with Gamma Knife surgery

Hasegawa T, Kida Y, Kato T, et al (Komaki City Hosp, Japan)
J Neurosurg 118:557-565, 2013

Object.—Little is known about long-term outcomes, including tumor control and adverse radiation effects, in patients harboring vestibular schwannomas (VSs) treated with stereotactic radiosurgery > 10 years previously. The aim of this study was to confirm whether Gamma Knife surgery (GKS) for VSs continues to be safe and effective > 10 years after treatment.

Methods.—A total of 440 patients with VS (including neurofibromatosis Type 2) treated with GKS between May 1991 and December 2000 were evaluable. Of these, 347 patients (79%) underwent GKS as an initial treatment and 93 (21%) had undergone prior resection. Three hundred fifty-eight patients (81%) had a solid tumor and 82 (19%) had a cystic

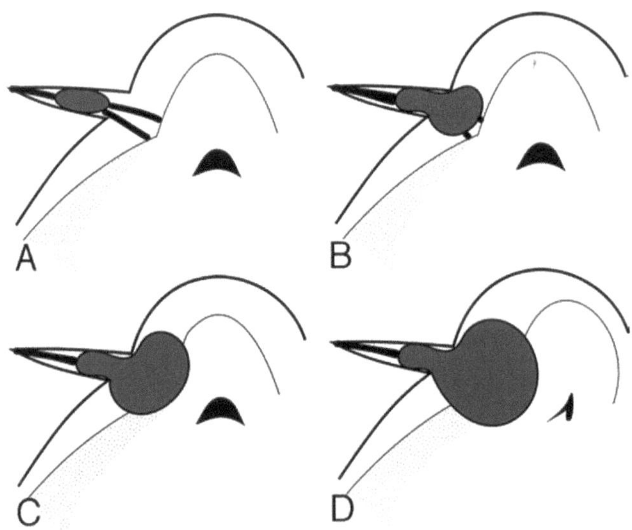

FIGURE 1.—Schematic drawings showing tumor classification depending on the location and brainstem compression. A: Type A—intracanalicular tumor. B: Type B—a cerebellopontine angle tumor without brainstem compression. C: Type C—tumor compressing the brainstem with no deviation of the fourth ventricle. D: Type D—tumor with a deviation of the fourth ventricle. (Reprinted from Hasegawa T, Kida Y, Kato T, et al. Long-term safety and efficacy of stereotactic radiosurgery for vestibular schwannomas: evaluation of 440 patients more than 10 years after treatment with Gamma Knife surgery. *J Neurosurg.* 2013;118:557-565, Copyright 2013, with permission from American Association for Neurological Surgeons, with Rockwater, Inc, http://aans.org/.)

tumor. The median tumor volume was 2.8 cm^3 and the median marginal dose was 12.8 Gy.

Results.—The median follow-up period was 12.5 years. The actuarial 5- and ≥ 10-year progression-free survival was 93% and 92%, respectively. No patient developed treatment failure > 10 years after treatment. According to multivariate analysis, significant factors related to worse progression-free survival included brainstem compression with a deviation of the fourth ventricle ($p < 0.0001$), marginal dose ≤ 13 Gy ($p = 0.01$), prior treatment ($p = 0.02$), and female sex ($p = 0.02$). Of 287 patients treated at a recent optimum dose of ≤ 13 Gy, 3 (1%) developed facial palsy, including 2 with transient palsy and 1 with persistent palsy after a second GKS, and 3 (1%) developed facial numbness, including 2 with transient and 1 with persistent facial numbness. The actuarial 10-year facial nerve preservation rate was 97% in the high marginal dose group (>13 Gy) and 100% in the low marginal dose group (≤13 Gy). Ten patients (2.3%) developed delayed cyst formation. One patient alone developed malignant transformation, indicating an incidence of 0.3%.

Conclusions.—In this study GKS was a safe and effective treatment for the majority of patients followed > 10 years after treatment. Special attention should be paid to cyst formation and malignant transformation as late adverse radiation effects, although they appeared to be rare. However, it is necessary to collect further long-term follow-up data before making conclusions about the long-term safety and efficacy of GKS, especially for young patients with VSs (Fig 1).

▶ This article represents an important contribution detailing the results of 440 patients undergoing Gamma Knife radiosurgery for acoustic neuroma with greater than 10-year follow-up. In terms of tumor control, 34% had stable tumor, 58% had partial remission (shrinkage of at least 2 mm), 1% had complete remission, and 7% had treatment failure. It is not surprising that tumor control was significantly worse for larger tumors (Fig 1). Type D tumors (tumors that compress the brainstem and displace the fourth ventricle) had an actuarial 10-year or more progression-free survival (PFS) of 76%, whereas type A (intracanalicular), type B (tumor in the cerebellopontine angle but not touching the brainstem), and type C (tumor compressing brainstem but not displacing fourth ventricle) had actuarial 10-year or more PFS of 100%, 95%, and 92%, respectively. Based on tumor volume, the actuarial 10-year PFS was 94% in small tumors (< 10 cm^3) and 77% in large tumors (≥10 cm^3). Tumor control was also worse for these larger tumors. There was no significant difference in long-term PFS between those who received a marginal dose greater than 13 Gy versus those who received 13 Gy or less. Nevertheless, the higher dose (> 13 Gy) was associated with worse facial nerve outcomes (5 permanent facial palsies) and worse hearing outcomes. The actuarial 3-year and 5-year hearing preservation rates were 71% and 64%, respectively, in patients with initial pretreatment Gardner-Robertson class I hearing, and 40% and 24%, respectively, with class II hearing. This demonstrates that those with worse hearing to begin with (class II) tend to do worse after radiosurgery. It is also important to note that hearing continues to decline with longer follow-up. When compared with the prospective natural history data published by Stangerup et al,[1] observation (watch and wait approach) appears to have better hearing preservation rates of 69% at 10 years for class I and 38% for class II. Overall, radiosurgery remains an important tool in the armamentarium for the acoustic neuroma surgeon that needs to be included in the treatment discussion with the patient along with observation and surgery, as the treatment strategy is individualized for each patient based on age, symptoms, tumor size, and risks.

J. K. Liu, MD

Reference

1. Stangerup SE, Thomsen J, Tos M, Cayé-Thomasen P. Long-term hearing preservation in vestibular schwannoma. *Otol Neurotol.* 2010;31:271-275.

Gamma Knife surgery in the treatment paradigm for foramen magnum meningiomas

Zenonos G, Kondziolka D, Flickinger JC, et al (Univ of Pittsburgh School of Medicine, PA)

J Neurosurg 117:864-873, 2012

Object.—Microsurgical management of foramen magnum meningiomas (FMMs) can be associated with significant morbidity and mortality. Stereotactic radiosurgery may be an efficient and safe alternative treatment modality for such tumors. The object of this study was to increase the documented experience with Gamma Knife surgery (GKS) for FMMs and to delineate its role in an overall management paradigm.

Methods.—The authors report on their experience with 24 patients harboring FMMs managed with GKS. Twelve patients had primary symptomatic tumors, 5 had asymptomatic but enlarging primary tumors, and 7 had recurrent or residual tumors after a prior surgery.

Results.—Follow-up clinical and imaging data were available in 21 patients at a median follow-up of 47 months (range 3—128 months). Ten patients had measurable tumor regression, which was defined as an overall volume reduction >25%. Eleven patients had no further tumor growth. Two patients died as a result of advanced comorbidities before follow-up imaging. One patient was living 8 years after GKS but had no clinical evaluation. Ten of 17 symptomatic patients with at least 6 months of follow-up had symptom improvement, and 7 remained clinically stable. Smaller tumors were more likely to regress. No patient suffered an adverse radiation effect after radiosurgery.

Conclusions.—Gamma Knife surgery was a safe management strategy for small, minimally symptomatic, or growing FMMs as well as for residual tumors following conservative microsurgical removal.

▶ The authors report their experience with Gamma Knife radiosurgery for foramen magnum meningiomas in 24 patients. Indications for radiosurgery included patients with residual (2 patients) or recurrent (5 patients) tumor after initial resection, primary treatment for newly diagnosed symptomatic tumors (12 patients), and interval growth of asymptomatic tumors (5 patients). The mean marginal dose was 13 Gy. Overall, there was stability in lesion size in 52% and tumor regression (defined as > 25% volume reduction) in 48%. However, when the data are critically analyzed, only 8 patients had greater than 5-year imaging follow-up and 6 had between 1- and 5-year imaging follow-up. It is important to weigh this against the natural history, as the majority of these meningiomas are mostly slow-growing tumors, and imaging follow-up less than 5 years after radiosurgery is not a reliable measure.

The other area of concern is the treatment of symptomatic tumors, some of which had tumor volumes ranging as high as 12 cm^3. The tumors that were greater than 3 cm^3 had worse outcomes than those that were less than 3 cm^3. Nine patients in this series had myelopathy as the presenting symptom, and 4 patients were reported as being better after radiosurgery. It is not clear in the report as to how these patients were evaluated and assessed and how their myelopathy was scored as improved after radiosurgery. Was there resolution of long tract signs? Improvement of weakness? Improvement of gait? This is not mentioned in the text. The authors also do not display any figures showing tumor regression and relief of brainstem compression after radiosurgery. In addition, only 10 patients had an actual visit to the neurosurgery office for clinical follow-up, where a detailed and reliable neurologic assessment was performed. Clinical follow-up in the remaining patients was obtained via phone calls to patients or letters from referring physicians, which clearly lacks an objective assessment by the neurosurgeon.

Aside from the above limitations of the report, I agree that radiosurgery can be considered as adjuvant therapy for recurrent tumor. Residual tumors, for the most part, can be observed until documented growth is demonstrated. However, one should be very cautious when considering radiosurgery as primary treatment for newly diagnosed tumor that exhibits radiographic brainstem or spinal cord compression, even when the patient is asymptomatic or minimally symptomatic. The natural history of these tumors is quite formidable, as patients can quickly progress to spastic quadriparesis. It doesn't take much tumor volume to cause significant displacement of cervicomedullary junction in the region of the foramen magnum. Surgical resection remains the primary mode of therapy and offers the best chance at brainstem decompression and gross total resection, if safely possible.

J. K. Liu, MD

Giant anterior clinoidal meningiomas: surgical technique and outcomes

Attia M, Umansky F, Paldor I, et al (Hebrew Univ-Hadassah Med Ctr, Jerusalem, Israel)

J Neurosurg 117:654-665, 2012

Object.—Surgery for giant anterior clinoidal meningiomas that invade vital neurovascular structures surrounding the anterior clinoid process is challenging. The authors present their skull base technique for the treatment of giant anterior clinoidal meningiomas, defined here as globular tumors with a maximum diameter of 5 cm or larger, centered around the anterior clinoid process, which is usually hyperostotic.

Methods.—Between 2000 and 2010, the authors performed 23 surgeries in 22 patients with giant anterior clinoidal meningiomas. They used a skull base approach with extradural unroofing of the optic canal, extradural clinoidectomy (Dolenc technique), transdural debulking of the tumor, early optic nerve decompression, and early identification and control of key neurovascular structures.

Results.—The mean age at surgery was 53.8 years. The mean tumor diameter was 59.2 mm (range 50–85 mm) with cavernous sinus involvement in 59.1% (13 of 22 patients). The tumor involved the prechiasmatic segment of the optic nerve in all patients, invaded the optic canal in 77.3% (17 of 22 patients), and caused visual impairment in 86.4% (19 of 22 patients). Total resection (Simpson Grade I or II) was achieved in 30.4% of surgeries (7 of 23); subtotal and partial resections were each achieved in 34.8% of surgeries (8 of 23). The main factor precluding total removal was cavernous sinus involvement. There were no deaths. The mean Glasgow Outcome Scale score was 4.8 (median 5) at a mean of 56 months of follow-up. Vision improved in 66.7% (12 of 18 patients) with consecutive neuroophthalmological examinations, was stable in 22.2% (4 of 18), and deteriorated in 11.1% (2 of 18). New deficits in cranial nerve III or IV remained after 8.7% of surgeries (2 of 23).

Conclusions.—This modified surgical protocol has provided both a good extent of resection and a good neurological and visual outcome in patients with giant anterior clinoidal meningiomas.

▶ The surgical treatment of giant anterior clinoidal meningiomas remains a formidable challenge mainly because of the tumor size, frequent involvement of the optic canal with optic nerve compression, intimate involvement of displaced neurovascular structures (such as the middle cerebral artery, internal carotid artery, posterior communicating artery, anterior choroidal artery, and cranial nerves), and invasion of the cavernous sinus. Tumor adherence to critical structures and cavernous sinus invasion usually preclude the ability to obtain a gross total (Simpson grade 1 or 2) resection.

The authors present excellent results for a very difficult tumor using a highly technical skull-base operation. The skull-base technique that is used, adapted from the original extradural–intradural exposure of the cavernous sinus as described by Vinko Dolenc, offers several advantages for attacking these tumors (see Fig 2 in the original article). One major advantage is early optic nerve decompression with extradural unroofing of the optic canal and anterior clinoidectomy. This maneuver allows identification of the clinoidal segment of the internal carotid artery and provides a landmark of the proximal segment of the carotid artery that can be followed distally (past the distal dural ring) to the intradural segment. Second, the lateral wall of the cavernous sinus is peeled away from the inner membranous layer, which allows a more complete resection of the dural attachment of these types of medial wing sphenoid meningiomas and allows the tumor to be detached from the skull base. During surgery, the falciform ligament is incised to decompress the optic nerve, and any tumor that can be dissected from the nerve is removed. These maneuvers allow safe identification of the optic nerve and internal carotid artery in the midst of these giant tumors and are associated with better postoperative visual outcomes (probably from early extradural optic nerve decompression and clinoidectomy). I have found this skull-base approach useful in the treatment of other spheno-orbital, sphenocavernous, cavernous sinus, clinoidal, and tuberculum sellae meningiomas (all of which can often present with optic canal involvement). My preference is to use a modified orbito-zygomatic approach rather than a pterional approach for these tumors because the orbital rim osteotomy provides a wider working corridor with increased angles of attack while reducing brain retraction.

J. K. Liu, MD

The role of radiotherapy following gross-total resection of atypical meningiomas

Komotar RJ, Bryan Lorgulescu J, Raper DMS, et al (The Univ of Miami Miller School of Medicine, FL; Memorial Sloan-Kettering Cancer Ctr, NY; Royal North Shore Hosp, Sydney, Australia; et al)
J Neurosurg 117:679-686, 2012

Object.—Atypical (WHO Grade II) meningiomas comprise a heterogeneous group of tumors, with histopathology delineated under the guidance of the WHO and a spectrum of clinical outcomes. The role of postoperative radiotherapy for patients with atypical meningiomas who have undergone gross-total resection (GTR) remains unclear. In this paper, the authors sought to clarify this role by reviewing their experience over the past 2 decades.

Methods.—The authors retrospectively analyzed all patients at their institution who underwent GTR between 1992 and 2011 with a final histology demonstrating atypical meningioma. Information regarding patients, tumor characteristics, and postoperative adjuvant therapy was gleaned from medical records. Time to recurrence and overall survival were analyzed using univariate, multivariate, and Kaplan-Meier survival analyses.

Results.—Forty-five patients who met the inclusion criteria underwent GTR for atypical meningiomas. By a median follow-up of 44.1 months, 22% of atypical meningiomas had recurred. There was no recurrence in 12 (92%) of 13 patients who received postoperative radiotherapy or in 19 (59%) of 32 patients who did not undergo postoperative radiotherapy ($p = 0.085$), demonstrating a strong trend toward improved local control with postoperative radiotherapy. No other factors were significantly associated with recurrence in univariate or multivariate analyses.

Conclusions.—This retrospective series supports the observation that postoperative radiotherapy likely results in lower recurrence rates of gross totally resected atypical meningiomas. Although a multicenter prospective trial will ultimately be needed to fully define the role of radiotherapy in managing gross totally resected atypical meningiomas, the authors' results contribute to a growing number of series that support routine postoperative radiotherapy as an adjuvant treatment for these lesions.

▶ When a patient undergoes incomplete removal of an atypical (World Health Organization Grade II) meningioma, the postoperative management includes adjuvant radiation therapy. However, if a complete Simpson Grade I or II gross total resection (GTR) is performed, the role of postoperative radiation therapy remains controversial.

In this study, 45 patients underwent GTR for atypical meningioma with a median follow-up of 44.1 months (range, 2.7-225.5 months), with an overall recurrence rate of 22%. Only 13 patients (28.9%) of this cohort received postoperative radiotherapy, and 12 of these 13 (92%) patients did not recur during the study period, resulting in a recurrence rate of 8% (see Figs 2 and 3 in the original article). For the remaining 32 patients who did not receive postoperative radiation therapy, the recurrence rate was 41% (13 of 32 patients). Although this was not statistically significant ($P = .085$), it did trend toward improved local control with upfront postoperative radiotherapy.

It has been postulated that an intact p53 system may confer a radiation-sensitive phenotype, which supports the role for early adjuvant radiotherapy. The majority (60%) of these tumors had convexity, which offers the best chance at GTR, as opposed to parasagittal or sphenoid, which has more of a chance of tumor adherence to critical structures, thus obviating GTR. Interestingly, of the 14 patients who demonstrated recurrence, 50% of them had convexity meningiomas. Tumor size ranged from 2.0 to 8.9 cm (median, 4.9 cm). Forty patients (88.9%) were alive at the last follow-up. Certainly, with longer follow-up, it is more likely the tumor will recur, as noted in their Kaplan-Meier analysis (median time to recurrence 24 months). However, the addition of radiation therapy (RT) may increase that time to recurrence (52.5 months in RT group vs 19.0 months in the non RT group). What is also interesting and worth investigating with longer follow-up is the group of patients who did recur and received additional treatment (RT alone, surgery plus RT, surgery alone). The cohort is small and the follow-up is relatively short, but it appears that these patients continue to survive with aggressive treatment.

What remains unclear, which is not discussed in this article, is the planned target of RT. This becomes less obvious, particularly when there is no radiographic target on postoperative imaging after complete resection. So where does one target the radiation? Does one include the surface of the brain that was in contact with tumor, or should one include the original tumor volume, or somewhere in between? Does one include the region of dural attachment even when it was completely resected? How does one tailor the field of radiation when brain shifts resolve and previously compressed brain reexpands on a delayed postoperative magnetic resonance imaging? Can smaller targets be more amenable to stereotactic radiosurgery as opposed to fractionated conventional RT? These questions remain to be answered.

J. K. Liu, MD

Cerebral revascularization and carotid artery resection at the skull base for treatment of advanced head and neck malignancies

Kalani MYS, Kalb S, Martirosyan NL, et al (St Joseph's Hosp and Med Ctr, Phoenix, AZ; et al)

J Neurosurg 118:637-642, 2013

Object.—Resection of cancer and the involved artery in the neck has been applied with some success, but the indications for such an aggressive approach at the skull base are less well defined. The authors therefore evaluated the outcomes of advanced skull base malignancies in patients who were treated with bypass and resection of the internal carotid artery (ICA).

Methods.—The authors retrospectively reviewed the charts of all patients with advanced head and neck cancers who underwent ICA sacrifice with revascularization in which an extracranial-intracranial bypass was used between 1995 and 2010 at the Barrow Neurological Institute.

Results.—Eighteen patients (11 male and 7 female patients; mean age 46 years, range 7–69 years) were identified. There were 4 sarcomas and 14 carcinomas that involved the ICA at the skull base. All patients underwent ICA sacrifice with revascularization. One patient died of a stroke after revascularization. A second patient died of the effects of a fistula between the oral and cranial cavities (surgery-related mortality rate 11.1%). Eight months after the operation, 1 patient developed occlusion of the bypass and died. Complications associated with the bypass surgery included 1 case of subdural hematoma (SDH) with blindness, 1 case of status epilepticus, and 1 case of asymptomatic bypass occlusion (bypass-related morbidity 16.7%). Complications associated with tumor resection included 3 cases of CSF leakage requiring repair and shunting, 1 case of hydrocephalus requiring shunting, 1 case of SDH, and 1 case of contralateral ICA injury requiring a bypass (tumor resection morbidity rate 33.3%). In 1 patient treated with adjuvant therapy before surgery, the authors identified only a radiation effect and no tumor on resection. In a second patient the bypass was occluded, and her tumor was not resected. The other 16 patients underwent gross-total resection of their tumor. Excluding the surgery-related deaths, the mean and median lengths of survival in this series were 13.2 and 8.3 months, respectively (range 1.5–48 months). Including the surgery-related deaths, the mean and median lengths of survival were 11.8 and 8 months, respectively (range 17 days–48 months). At last follow-up all patients had died of cancer or cancer-related causes.

Conclusions.—Despite maximal surgical intervention, including ICA sacrifice at the skull base with revascularization, patient survival was dismal, and the complication rate was significant. The authors no longer advocate such an aggressive approach in this patient population. On rare occasions, however, such an approach may be considered for low-grade malignancies.

▶ The conclusions of this article are quite interesting, and I commend the authors for critically analyzing their complication and survival rates, which has resulted in a paradigm shift in the management strategy for these difficult tumors. In short, an aggressive approach (gross-total resection, including internal carotid artery [ICA] sacrifice and bypass) to malignant disease involving the ICA has resulted in a "long run for a short slide." The mean survival for such an operation was less than 12 months, with an overall complication rate of 55.5% (10 of 18 patients incurring a postoperative complication, whether it was related to bypass or tumor resection). Only 2 patients survived longer than 24 months (overall 2-year survival rate of 11.1%). The pathologies treated were nasopharyngeal cancer, squamous cell carcinoma, osteosarcoma, rhabdomyosarcoma, adenocystic carcinoma, and medullary thyroid cancer. Subgroup analysis showed that patients with adenocystic carcinoma had longer survival. In some cases, these tumors can invade diffusely into the soft tissues of the infratemporal fossa, and achieving a negative margin resection cannot be feasible without significant collateral damage. It would be important to compare survival rates of this series with those who underwent subtotal or palliative decompression without ICA sacrifice and also to those who underwent palliative chemotherapy and radiation.

J. K. Liu, MD

Chromosomal alterations, prognostic factors, and targeted molecular therapies for malignant meningiomas

Yew A, Trang A, Nagasawa DT, et al (Univ of California Los Angeles)

J Clin Neurosci 20:17-22, 2013

Meningiomas are the second most common intracranial neoplasm in adults and originate from arachnoidal cap cells. Malignant meningiomas are resistant to conventional treatments such as surgery, chemotherapy, and radiotherapy. Unlike benign meningiomas, atypical and anaplastic tumors generally display more complex karyotypes associated with aggressive behavior. While these chromosomal anomalies are associated with greater malignancy in meningiomas, the specific genes involved remain unknown. Malignant meningiomas are characterized by increased tumor aggressiveness, rapid recurrence, local invasion, atypical histological appearance, and a high mitotic index. Potential prognostic factors include extent of resection, treatment with radiotherapy or stereotactic radiosurgery, Ki-67/MIB-1 labeling index, p53 overexpression, percentage of tumor cells in the S-phase, telomerase activity, and numerous genetic expression profiles. A greater understanding of prognostic factors and molecular markers involved in critical signaling pathways may aid in the identification of novel therapeutic targets. As such, further studies are needed to establish reliable prognostic factors and develop more effective treatments for malignant meningiomas.

▶ This article comprehensively reviewed chromosomal alterations, aberrant cellular pathways, prognostic factors, and targeted molecular therapies for malignant meningiomas in a clear and concise manner.

In addition to general prognostic factors, such as extent of surgery and tumor grade, this article covered several less commonly documented prognostic factors.

More specifically, the article included Ki-67/MIB-1 labeling index, p53 overexpression, percentage of tumors in S phase, telomerase activity, and SEMA3A. Each subsection was succinct as well as extensive.

The section on novel therapies was particularly thorough. Overall, this article successfully introduces readers to prognostic factors and novel therapies for malignant meningiomas.

I. Yang, MD

Ten years of experience with microsurgical treatment of large and giant petroclival meningiomas

Fang T, Zhu H, Yan R, et al (Capital Univ of Med Sciences, Beijing, China; Sanbo Neurosurgical Hosp, Beijing, China; et al)

J Clin Neurosci 20:238-243, 2013

During a 10-year period, 41 patients underwent surgery for resection of large or giant petroclival meningiomas. Gross total resection (GTR) was accomplished in 25 patients (61.0%), subtotal resection (STR) in 15 patients (36.6%), and partial resection in one patient (2.4%). Postoperative complications were observed in 27 patients (65.9%). Postoperative radiosurgery was administered in six patients who had residual tumors. Survival and postoperative quality of life are the goals of successful surgery on large or giant petroclival meningiomas, and the strategic surgical approach is based on the tumor location, the direction of growth, the invasion of adjacent structures, patient age and neurosurgeon expertise. Selectively pursuing STR with radiotherapy rather than GTR is a reasonable strategy.

▶ This article is a compilation of data from 41 meningioma patients treated with gross total resection (GTR), subtotal resection (STR), or partial tumor resection (PTR) at a single institution between 2001 and 2011. Based on their data, the authors suggest that pursuing less-invasive approaches may be a more reasonable therapeutic option for treatment of patients with large and giant petroclival meningiomas. Patient information, neuroradiologic evaluations, and specific surgical approaches were clearly documented in the article. Of the 41 patients reviewed, 61% received GTR, 37% received STR, and 2% received PTR.

The authors reported that 6 STR patients also underwent Gamma Knife radiosurgery. In addition, 6 patients developed recurrent tumors. Of these 6 patients, 4 underwent repeat surgery, and 2 received Gamma Knife radiosurgery. The authors documented postoperative complications, such as cranial nerve impairment, temporary hemiplegia, intracranial infection, and cerebrospinal fluid leakage. However, these complications were not broken down based on the type of resection (GTR, STR, or PTR) the patients received. Therefore, it was unclear which of these treatments was associated with the complications discussed.

The article described specific details about the authors' surgical experiences in the operating room. For example, they discussed potential advantages to the approaches they used in terms of simplicity, shorter operation time, improved safety, and decreased invasiveness. They also noted that based on their experiences, certain surgical approaches worked better with patients under a certain age who presented with tumors at a specific location.

Overall, this article described the surgical experiences of a single institution with large and giant petroclival meningioma patients, and the authors reported general results of the surgeries, descriptions of surgical approaches, and positive characteristics of less-invasive surgical approaches. Based on their experiences at this institution, the authors recommend using less-invasive approaches as opposed to aggressive and risky tumor resection. Although statistical evidence was not presented, this article proposes an interesting viewpoint on the balance between postoperative quality of life and the ability to achieve gross total resection, a key point in surgical management for petroclival meningioma patients.

I. Yang, MD

Radiation-induced meningiomas after high-dose cranial irradiation

Godlewski B, Drummond KJ, Kaye AH (WAM Univ Hosp in Lodz, Poland; The Royal Melbourne Hosp, Parkville, Victoria, Australia)

J Clin Neurosci 19:1627-1635, 2012

Radiation-induced meningiomas (RIM) are known to occur after high and low dose cranial radiation therapy. Currently, RIM are the most common form of radiation-induced neoplasm reported. We present the largest series of RIM induced by high dose radiation reported thus far and review the literature. Radiation therapy was most commonly given for childhood malignancy. We compared our group of 26 patients with RIM with previously published reports of RIM, and also with 364 patients with spontaneous meningioma (SM) treated at The Royal Melbourne Hospital between 2007 and 2011 with regard to age, gender, and histopathology. In our group of patients with RIM, the mean age at presentation was 38.5 years, in comparison to 60.1 years for patients with SM. The female-to-male ratio was 1.88:1 in RIM compared to 2.37:1 for SM. Of the RIM, 86.5% were World Health Organization (WHO) grade I and 11.5% were grade II (atypical) meningiomas. There were no anaplastic or malignant RIM. Of the SM, 91.5% were WHO grade I, 7.1% WHO grade II, and 1.4% WHO grade III meningiomas. The characteristics of RIM induced by low dose radiation therapy have been well described. It is timely to consider RIM due to high dose radiation, which is now frequently employed in the management of various childhood and other malignancies.

▶ This article presents the largest case study thus far pertaining to radiation-induced meningiomas resulting from the use of high-dose radiation from a single institution. The authors did a comprehensive job in defining what constitutes radiation-induced meningiomas through 7 specific criteria, specifying that the article regarded high dose as greater than 10 Gy, and reviewing the cellular mechanisms that lead to radiation-induced meningiomas.

Patient data were examined between 1995 and 2011; 26 were found to meet the criteria set. Initial treatment information, reason for irradiation, age, dose, tumor location, and histopathological information were extracted from a patient database. The 26 radiation-induced meningioma patients were then compared with spontaneous meningioma patients treated at the same location. The article also did a good job comparing their results with that of previously published case reports pertaining to radiation-induced meningiomas.

This case study elucidated that radiation-induced meningiomas were more prevalent at a younger age and in females. The article also determined that, of the 26 patients, 88.46% were World Health Organization (WHO) grade I and 11.53% were WHO grade II. This was compared with the 364 spontaneous meningioma patients from the same institution and to a case study from a different institution, with results suggesting the radiation-induced meningioma data were consistent and that it displayed no increase relative to spontaneous meningiomas.

The findings from this single-institutional retrospective study contribute to the literature available about radiation-induced meningiomas resulting from high-dose irradiation, which is important because of its use for the management of tumors.

I. Yang, MD

The role of radiotherapy following gross-total resection of atypical meningiomas

Komotar RJ, Bryan Lorgulescu J, Raper DMS, et al (The Univ of Miami Miller School of Medicine, FL; Memorial Sloan–Kettering Cancer Ctr; Royal North Shore Hosp, Sydney, Australia; et al)

J Neurosurg 117:679-686, 2012

Object.—Atypical (WHO Grade II) meningiomas comprise a heterogeneous group of tumors, with histopathology delineated under the guidance of the WHO and a spectrum of clinical outcomes. The role of postoperative radiotherapy for patients with atypical meningiomas who have undergone gross-total resection (GTR) remains unclear. In this paper, the authors sought to clarify this role by reviewing their experience over the past 2 decades.

Methods.—The authors retrospectively analyzed all patients at their institution who underwent GTR between 1992 and 2011 with a final histology demonstrating atypical meningioma. Information regarding patients, tumor characteristics, and postoperative adjuvant therapy was gleaned from medical records. Time to recurrence and overall survival were analyzed using univariate, multivariate, and Kaplan-Meier survival analyses.

Results.—Forty-five patients who met the inclusion criteria underwent GTR for atypical meningiomas. By a median follow-up of 44.1 months, 22% of atypical meningiomas had recurred. There was no recurrence in 12 (92%) of 13 patients who received postoperative radiotherapy or in 19 (59%) of 32 patients who did not undergo postoperative radiotherapy ($p = 0.085$), demonstrating a strong trend toward improved local control with postoperative radiotherapy. No other factors were significantly associated with recurrence in univariate or multivariate analyses.

Conclusions.—This retrospective series supports the observation that postoperative radiotherapy likely results in lower recurrence rates of gross totally resected atypical meningiomas. Although a multicenter prospective trial will ultimately be needed to fully define the role of radiotherapy in managing gross totally resected atypical meningiomas, the authors' results contribute to a growing number of series that support routine postoperative radiotherapy as an adjuvant treatment for these lesions.

▶ This article provides a comprehensive assessment of a single institution's experience with atypical meningiomas in order to further the available data analyzing the role of radiotherapy following gross total resection. Each case was appropriately evaluated for patient data, including sex, age of diagnosis, tumor size, tumor location, operative characteristics, recurrence characteristics, radiotherapy data, and follow-up dates, with proper exclusion parameters. Comprehensive univariate and multivariate statistical analyses were conducted to elucidate factors that contribute to recurrence.

The article did well in describing the World Health Organization classification, prognostic factors, various tumor location, and radiation sensitivity. The authors also acknowledged the study's limitations, including a small sample size, which is common for many case studies emanating from a single institution. Although the article analyzes a large subset of factors that could contribute to recurrence, the small sample size culminated in no statistically significant difference in the results. Despite the lack of significant findings, the article suggests from its authors for clinical therapy the use of postoperative radiotherapy after gross total resection. The article also did a concise comparison of its findings to a set of experiences from other institutions that were able to elucidate statistically significant results.

Although the article lacks a larger sample size and statistically significant results, it is an important addition to the pool of experiences from individual institutions pertaining to the role of radiotherapy following gross total resection of atypical meningiomas. It also brings to attention the need to conduct a multicentered study to better understand the benefits of radiotherapy.

I. Yang, MD

Single-Fraction Radiosurgery of Benign Intracranial Meningiomas

Pollock BE, Stafford SL, Link MJ (Mayo Clinic College of Medicine, Rochester, MN; et al)

Neurosurgery 71:604-613, 2012

Background.—Stereotactic radiosurgery (SRS) of benign intracranial meningiomas is an accepted management option for well-selected patients.

Objective.—To analyze patients who had single-fraction SRS for benign intracranial meningiomas to determine factors associated with tumor control and neurologic complications.

Methods.—Retrospective review was performed of 416 patients (304 women/112 men) who had single-fraction SRS for imaging defined (n = 252) or confirmed World Health Organization grade I (n = 164) meningiomas from 1990 to 2008. Excluded were patients with radiation-induced tumors, multiple meningiomas, neurofibromatosis type 2, and previous or concurrent radiotherapy. The majority of tumors (n = 337; 81%) involved the cranial base or tentorium. The median tumor volume was 7.3 cm^3; the median tumor margin dose was 16 Gy. The median follow-up was 60 months.

Results.—The disease-specific survival rate was 97% at 5 years and 94% at 10 years. The 5- and 10-year local tumor control rate was 96% and 89%, respectively. Male sex (hazard ratio [HR]: 2.5, $P = .03$), previous surgery (HR: 6.9, $P = .002$) and patients with tumors located in the parasagittal/falx/convexity regions (HR: 2.8, $P = .02$) were negative risk factors for local tumor control. In 45 patients (11%) permanent radiation-related complications developed at a median of 9 months after SRS. The 1- and 5-year radiation-related complication rate was 6% and 11%, respectively. Risk factors for permanent radiation-related complication rate were increasing tumor volume (HR: 1.05, $P = .008$) and patients with tumors of the parasagittal/falx/convexity regions (HR: 3.0, $P = .005$).

Conclusion.—Single-fraction SRS at the studied dose range provided a high rate of tumor control for patients with benign intracranial meningiomas. Patients with small volume, nonoperated cranial base or tentorial meningiomas had the best outcomes after single-fraction SRS.

► This article reports the results of a retrospective study of 416 patients with World Health Organization grade I meningiomas treated at a single institution from 1990 to 2008. Because many tumors cannot be fully excised without damaging critical cranial nerves or arteries, the authors propose that single-fraction stereotactic radiosurgery (SRS) is an effective alternative for patients with recurrent or residual meningiomas. Dose planning used magnetic resonance imaging (MRI) in 407 patients and stereotactic computed tomography in 9 patients. Analyses were based on data from follow-up MRIs, and clinical evaluations were obtained for each patient at 6 months, 12 months, 24 months, and biyearly after SRS.

The article successfully described the association of several key measures (disease-specific survival [DSS]; local tumor control [LTC]) of patient survival with the use of SRS. DSS was 97% and 94%, and LTC was 96% and 89% at 5-year and 10-year follow-up, respectively. Because this was a retrospective analysis of patients at a single institution, this study is limited by confounding factors and sample bias. However, the authors did well in clearly acknowledging and documenting the permanent radiation-related complications (RRCs) in 11% of the patients, including hemiparesis, new or increased seizures, facial pain, facial numbness, and diplopia. Furthermore, the article provided additional discussion on risk factors for the RRCs after SRS.

In addition, the article also touched on the importance of proper patient selection to obtain optimal results after SRS. The authors used the risk factors for RRCs to develop a clear and reasonable classification system that can provide guidance in management decisions for intracranial meningioma patients. More specifically, histologic tumor grade, tumor location, and tumor volume were the 3 factors that affected LTC after SRS. Patients in the study were ranked from 1 to 5 in terms of benign meningioma radiosurgery score, based on LTC and RRC. The study found that 84% of the patients had LTC without significant neurologic morbidity after SRS was administered.

This article successfully documented both the survival outcomes and RRC for meningioma patients with SRS. Despite the limitations of the study, the authors did well in supporting their conclusion that SRS can control tumor growth. A sound classifications scheme was developed to illustrate the likelihood of having successful SRS procedures based on the patient's tumor location, volume, and previous resection. Overall, the results of this study provide strong support for the use of single fraction SRS as an alternative therapy for meningioma patients.

I. Yang, MD

The influence of surgery on quality of life in patients with intracranial meningiomas: a prospective study

Jakola AS, Gulati M, Gulati S, et al (St Olavs Univ Hosp, Trondheim, Norway; Norwegian Univ of Science and Technology, Trondheim, Norway)

J Neurooncol 110:137-144, 2012

Meningiomas may influence both survival and neurological functions. Studies assessing the impact of surgery on health-related quality of life (HRQL) remain absent. In this prospective study we aimed to describe HRQL dynamics before and after surgery in patients with meningiomas. HRQL assessments were performed using EuroQol-5D (EQ-5D), a generic HRQL instrument. All adult patients with suspected intracranial meningioma from 2007 through 2011 were eligible for inclusion, and 54 patients were included after informed consent. All patients received a histopathological diagnosis of meningioma. The average preoperative EQ-5D index value (±SD) was 0.69 ± 0.26. The mean improvement 6 weeks after surgery was 0.06 (95% CI, −0.03 to 0.16; $p = 0.161$) and the mean long term improvement was 0.09 (95% CI, 0.00–0.17; $p = 0.040$). Surgery reduced pain/discomfort and anxiety/depression and improved the capability of performing usual activities. Clinically significant improvement at long-term assessment was noted in 25 patients (49%) while a significant deterioration was reported in 10 patients (20%). Patients who reported postoperative worsening of HRQL were also reporting better preoperative scores, suggesting a possible ceiling effect of EQ-5D in some of these patients. In our patients a modest average improvement in HRQL was seen after surgery for meningioma. About half of the patients reported a clinical important improvement at the late follow-up assessment. This improvement was mainly observed in the domains usual activities, pain/discomfort and anxiety/depression. However, one in five patients fared worse on late follow up assessment, a figure of particular importance when treating asymptomatic meningiomas.

▶ This article assesses the impact of surgery on the quality of life of meningioma patients based on the experiences of a single institution. In this prospective longitudinal study, the health-related quality of life (HRQL) of 54 patients with intracranial meningiomas was evaluated at 3 distinct time points: before the operation, 6 weeks postoperative, and long-term postoperative.

Given the subjectivity of HRQL, the article clearly explained and justified the means of evaluating HRQL. EuroQol-5D (EQ-5D) was used to evaluate 5 health-related dimensions of quality of life (mobility, self-care, usual activities, pain/discomfort, anxiety/depression) on a scale of 3 options (slight problem, no problem, major problem). Although this form of assessment is not often used in patients, (EQ-5D) is used commonly in the evaluation of glioma and other conditions. Therefore, the authors did well in using an appropriate assessment for HRQL. In addition, the article clearly documented and presented the statistical significance of each of their results. Compared with the preoperative scores, the 6 weeks postoperative scores did not show significant improvement. However, the study did report statistically significant improvement in HRQL in the long run (median follow-up time of 33 months).

Although 54 patients were included in the study, several patients were unable to be reached for follow-up. Overall, the study encountered 5 nonresponses. In these cases, the median value for the group was used to obtain the results presented in the article. Furthermore, 3 patients died during follow-up, and the article was unclear as to how their data were incorporated in the statistical tests. Based on the numbers of patients presented in each group, it appears that the 3 patients were not included in the study and the presented percentages are based on a sample size of 51 patients. In addition to incomplete HRQL data, the authors acknowledged other limitations, such as a lack of a control group and a potential positive bias from telephone administration of the (EQ-5D) questionnaire.

This was a strong article that may have underestimated the long-term benefit of surgery that cannot be measured with an (EQ-5D) questionnaire. Overall, the results of this study allow for a deeper understanding of the topic of HRQL in postoperative meningioma patients.

I. Yang, MD

Risk for leptomeningeal seeding after resection for brain metastases: Implication of tumor location with mode of resection

Ahn JH, Lee SH, Kim S, et al (Seoul Natl Univ College of Medicine, Goyang, Korea; Natl Cancer Ctr, Goyang, Korea)

J Neurosurg 116:984-993, 2012

Object.—Surgical spillage has been one of the causative factors for the development of leptomeningeal seeding (LMS) after resection of brain metastases. In this paper, the authors' goal was to define the factors related to the development of LMS and to evaluate the difference according to tumor location.

Methods.—The authors retrospectively analyzed 242 patients who had undergone resection for brain metastases. The factors investigated included tumor location with proximity to the CSF pathway (that is, contacting, involved with, or separated from the CSF pathway), the method of resection, and the use of the Cavitron Ultrasonic Surgical Aspirator (CUSA).

Results.—A total of 39 patients (16%) developed LMS at a median of 6.0 months (range 1–42 months) after resection. The risk of developing LMS was significantly higher in patients whose tumors were resected piecemeal than in those whose tumors were removed en bloc, with a hazard ratio (HR) of 4.08 ($p < 0.01$). The incidence of LMS was significantly higher in patients in whom the CUSA was used, and the HR was 2.64 ($p < 0.01$). The proximity of tumor to the CSF pathway in the involved group conferred an increased risk of LMS compared with the separated group (HR 11.36, $p < 0.01$). The risk of piecemeal resection for LMS was significant only in involved lesions ($p < 0.01$), and the use of the CUSA in both contact and involved lesions increased the incidence of LMS ($p < 0.01$ and $p < 0.03$, respectively).

Conclusions.—The authors suggest that piecemeal resection using the CUSA should be limited because of the risk of postsurgical LMS, especially when the tumor is in contact with the CSF pathway.

▶ This article characterizes the factors that are related to the development of leptomeningeal seeding (LMS) after brain metastasis treatment. The article thoroughly explores the factors that can create an increased risk of LMS, including location, treatment, and histology of the primary cancer. Additionally, the study addresses a possible increased incidence after piecemeal resection and the use of a Cavitron ultrasonic surgical aspirator (Valleylab, Boulder, CO [formerly Cavitron Inc, Stamford, CT]).

Table 2 in the original article lists and assesses the many risk factors (ie, primary cancer, age, tumor volume, location, proximity to cerebrospinal fluid [CSF] pathway, and mode of resection) that contribute to LMS. The authors suggest the incidence of LMS was much higher in a younger age group (< 60 years old) with an increased risk of LMS.

Neither the number of lesions nor the location of the tumor produced an increase incidence of LMS. The proximity of the tumor to the CSF pathway greatly affected the incidence of LMS, and the method of resection was additionally a significant risk factor. Of the patients who underwent bloc resection, 5.7% developed LMS, whereas 22% of the patients who underwent piecemeal resection developed LMS. Piecemeal resection displayed a higher incidence rate for LMS over any other type of resection.

I. Yang, MD

Systematic review of primary intracranial glioblastoma multiforme with symptomatic spinal metastases, with two illustrative patients

Shahideh M, Fallah A, Munoz DG, et al (Univ of Toronto, Ontario, Canada)

J Clin Neurosci 19:1080-1086, 2012

Glioblastoma multiforme is a malignant tumour with a universally fatal diagnosis. We report two patients with glioblastoma with symptomatic metastasis to the spinal cord and perform a systematic review all 35 reports of symptomatic glioblastoma dissemination to the spinal leptomeninges and/or intramedullary spinal axis. Our analysis of the data shows a median time to spinal metastasis of 10 months and a median time of three months from spinal metastasis to death. Treatments described include palliative laminectomies, radiotherapy and chemotherapy. No treatment strategy offered a therapeutic advantage as patients deteriorated rapidly regardless of intervention. Patients who underwent only a biopsy for intracranial glioblastoma had a shorter time to development of spinal metastasis. In addition, there may be an association between intramedullary metastasis and shorter survival. This paper highlights the importance of considering symptomatic spinal dissemination in glioblastoma multiforme. We also review the incidence and postulate mechanisms of tumour dissemination in the central nervous system. Clearly, further research into radiotherapeutic and chemotherapeutic options in this clinical setting is required.

▶ The authors of this article performed a systematic review of primary intracranial glioblastoma multiforme (GBM) with symptomatic spinal metastases, including 2 patients from their own institution. The article begins with these 2 case reports, detailing their diagnosis and treatment before discussing the systematic review culminating in the analysis of data from 37 intracranial GBM patients with spinal metastasis.

The authors effectively compiled and analyzed these data using univariate analysis. The percentages of primary surgery type (none, biopsy, sub total resection (STR), gross total resection (GTR)), type of adjuvant treatment received postsurgery, and type of spinal metastasis treatment are presented. The median length of time between primary intracranial surgery and presentation of spinal metastasis was found to be 10 months, whereas the median length of time between presentation of spinal metastasis and death was only 3 months. The data revealed that patients who solely underwent biopsies as their primary surgery developed spinal metastases sooner than those who received GTR or STR.

Patients with intramedullary spinal metastasis also had shorter survival times between development of metastasis and death. The authors performed further analysis on these associations by adjusting for the confounding variable of age at time of surgery, demonstrating good analytic technique. No significant associations were found between all other variables tested: age at surgery, gender, type of adjuvant treatment, and spine metastasis treatment.

The article gives some background on the neurological presentations for patients with disseminated GBM, sites of spinal metastasis, and potential mechanisms of dissemination. The proximity of tumor to the ventricles was not found as a risk factor for spinal dissemination in this study, yet the article mentions that this has been found as a risk factor in prior literature. Treatments for these patients, including steroids, decompressive surgery, radiation therapy, and chemotherapy, are briefly discussed.

I. Yang, MD

Retrosigmoid Approach to Cerebellopontine Angle Tumor Resection: Surgical Modifications

Heman-Ackah SE, Cosetti MK, Gupta S, et al (New York Univ School of Medicine)

Laryngoscope 122:2519-2523, 2012

Background.—About 5% to 10% of all intracranial neoplasms are tumors of the cerebellopontine angle (CPA), most commonly vestibular schwannomas, meningiomas, or epidermoid tumors. The retrosigmoid approach to tumors primarily located in the CPA and minimally entering the internal auditory canal (IAC) provides wide exposure and safety. However, this approach requires a large posterior craniotomy and cerebellar retraction to be able to clearly visualize the CPA. A craniotomy must be done first immediately posterior to the sigmoid sinus and inferior to the transverse sinus, then cerebrospinal fluid (CSF) pressure is diminished by decompressing the cistern. Retractors are used to retract the lateral cerebellum posteriorly. Modifications to the standard retrosigmoid approach are suggested to eliminate the need for cerebellar retraction and to use only native bone to reconstruct the resulting defect. Complication rates with the modified method were compared with those of the standard approach.

Method.—The modified approach was used for 197 patients (96 men and 101 women, mean age 40.7 years). First, a postauricular U-shaped anteriorly based skin and subcutaneous flap was raised in a supraperiosteal plane, then an anteriorly based periosteal flap was elevated. Simple posterior mastoidectomy was done to skeletonize the sigmoid sinus, which was carefully decompressed from the transverse sinus superiorly approaching the jugular bulb inferiorly. A small craniotomy was created posterior to the sinus, with the bone flap removed and reserved for later use. A J-shaped incision in the posterior fossa dura extends about 2 to 3 mm posterior to the sigmoid sinus and inferior to the transverse sinus. The anterior dura of the incision was securely sutured to the previously created hole in the cortical mastoid bone to retract the dura and sigmoid sinus anteriorly. Telfa strips were placed on the cerebellum for protection. Superior and inferior "saloon door" dural flaps were created over the posterior face of the petrous bone before the IAC was exposed. The IAC exposure varied depending on the size of the tumor being removed. Then petrous apex air cells in the area of the IAC drilling were obliterated using bone wax, and the saloon door flaps were sutured closed to secure the fat placed in the IAC to cover the drill-out defect., which was closed primarily in watertight fashion. The bone flap was then replaced using the patient's own bone.

Results.—Intracanalicular tumors were identified in 3.8% of patients, tumors less than 1.5 cm in 30.6%, tumors between 1.5 and 3 cm in 47.8%, and more than 3 cm in 17.7%. Complications included headache (8.1% of patients), CSF leak (6.6%), wound infection (3.5%), and other problems, including pulmonary embolus, tracheotomy, pneumonia, abdominal seroma, meningitis, seizure, stroke, and death. Forty-seven patients were evaluated for postoperative vestibular dysfunction, with one having ataxia and another dysmetria (incidence of 2.1% each). None of the patients required diuretics for cerebellar edema. Patients were out of bed a median of 2 days after surgery and ambulating within 3 days. Median length of hospital stay was 4 days.

Conclusions.—The surgical modifications permitted wide exposure of the CPA without cerebellar retraction or a large craniectomy and cranioplasty. For reconstruction of the surgical defect only native bone from the patient was used. This approach proved to be safe and effective with a low rate of complications and good intraoperative exposure.

▶ This report presents a detailed assessment of surgical modifications to the standard retrosigmoid approach to tumor resection in the cerebellopontine angle, based on a retrospective literature review of 197 patients over a 10-year period who underwent retrosigmoid tumor resections modified to provide wider exposure of the cerebellopontine angle. Demographic data, tumor pathology, and postoperative complications were appropriately recorded for each case. The authors also estimated tumor size based on radiographic estimates of tumor diameter.

The surgical techniques used were very thoroughly documented and supplemented with clear figures.

The article did well in specifically reviewing 17 relevant postoperative complications, including headaches, cerebrospinal fluid leaks, and wound infections. The authors also evaluated factors pertinent to patients' postoperative quality of life, such as median time until ambulation and median hospital stay. The article included concise comparisons between patients with specific postoperative conditions in association with the modified retrosigmoid approach and those found in the literature based on the standard approach.

The authors suggest that the retrosigmoid approach can be safely and effectively modified through decompression and anterior retraction of the sigmoid sinus.

These findings were based largely on the low documented rates of postoperative complications after the modified approach.

I. Yang, MD

Early rehabilitation after surgery improves functional outcome in inpatients with brain tumours

Bartolo M, Zucchella C, Pace A, et al (IRCCS NEUROMED Mediterranean Neurological Inst, Isernia, Italy; Regina Elena Natl Cancer Inst, Rome, Italy; et al)

J Neurooncol 107:537-544, 2012

Clinical experience suggests that application of the fundamental principles of rehabilitation medicine can improve the care of patients with cancer. Despite the high incidence of neurological and functional deficits in patients affected by brain tumours (BTs), rehabilitation treatment of this population is not as well established as it is for patients with other neurological conditions. To assess functional outcome in brain tumour inpatients who underwent early rehabilitation after surgery. 75 patients who had undergone neurosurgery for primary BTs and 75 patients affected by stroke were enrolled in a case-control study. All patients were evaluated by means of a core set of clinical scales (Functional Independence Measure, Sitting Balance score, Standing Balance score, Hauser Index, Massachusetts General Hospital Functional Ambulation Classification). Patients were evaluated before the beginning (T0) and at the end (T1) of rehabilitation treatment. The neurorehabilitation programme consisted of individual 60-min sessions of treatment, administered once a day, six days a week, for four consecutive weeks. Speech therapy was included when aphasia was diagnosed. All the measures of outcome were indicative of substantial improvements for neuro-oncological and for stroke patients ($P = 0.000$). Analysis of subgroups showed that patients affected by meningioma achieved better results (in efficiency terms) as regards independence in activities of daily living ($P = 0.02$) and mobility ($P = 0.04$) compared with patients affected by glioblastoma or stroke. Rehabilitation after surgery can improve functional outcome, justifying the delivery of rehabilitation services, even during the acute phase, to BTs inpatients, irrespective of tumour type.

▶ This study does a comprehensive job of evaluating the outcomes of early rehabilitation for patients with various brain tumor types after surgery in comparison with stroke patients. The authors were thorough in their analysis and compared the functional gains in different brain tumor types, accounted for differences in histology, tumor grade, extent of resection, and treatment, and showed that meningioma patients have better functional outcomes than glioblastoma or stroke patients.

In addition to comparing the functional independence measure for activities of daily living, mobility, and cognition; Hauser index; and Massachusetts General Hospital Functional Ambulation Classification, the study incorporated a novel set of clinical scales that allow for greater sensitivity in assessing changes in motor function, such as postural control, standing, and walking.

Follow-up information, however, was lacking in this study, because the patients were discharged and sent to other hospitals for their radiotherapy and chemotherapy treatments. Such follow-up data would be valuable in evaluating the long-term outcomes in functional gain.

Nonetheless, this study thoroughly evaluates the functional outcomes of rehabilitation for brain tumor patients after surgery and justifies the delivery of such rehabilitation services for brain tumor patients postsurgery, regardless of tumor type. Such evaluation and justification of services are important in a health system where resources are often limited.

I. Yang, MD

Chromosomal anomalies and prognostic markers for intracranial and spinal ependymomas

Yang I, Nagasawa DT, Kim W, et al (Univ of California Los Angeles)
J Clin Neurosci 19:779-785, 2012

Ependymomas are neoplasms that can occur anywhere along the craniospinal axis. They are the third most common brain tumor in children, representing 10% of pediatric intracranial tumors, 4% of adult brain tumors, and 15% of all spinal cord tumors. As the heterogeneity of ependymomas has severely limited the prognostic value of the World Health Organization grading system, numerous studies have focused on genetic alterations as a potential basis for classification and prognosis. However, this endeavor has proven difficult due to variations of findings depending on tumor location, tumor grade, and patient age. While many have evaluated chromosomal abnormalities for ependymomas as a whole group, others have concentrated their efforts on specific subsets of populations. Here, we review modern findings of chromosomal analyses, their relationships with various genes, and their prognostic implications for intracranial and spinal cord ependymomas.

► This article provides a concise review of the various chromosomal gains and losses common to ependymomas. It walks through the unique findings in specific subgroups in a manner that is easy to follow and makes their potential for prognostic significance clear. This article presents the conclusion that a gain in chromosome 1q is the most reliable genetic prognostic marker overall.

In addition, this article describes Korshunov et al's prognostic classification system for ependymomas: Group 1 tumors are classified as tumors with gains on chromosome 9, 15q, or 18, or loss of chromosome 6 without gain or CDKN2A deletion. Group 2 tumors are classified as tumors balanced for chromosome 1q, 6, 9, 15q, and 18, without a homozygous deletion of CDKN2A. Group 3 tumors are classified as tumors with 1q gain or homozygous deletion of CDKN2A. This system is more consistent and reliable than the 2007 World Health Organization classification system for ependymomas, which has been a subject of controversy.

In conclusion, this article does a good job in reviewing the current literature on chromosomal analyses, their relationship with various genes, and their prognostic implications for intracranial and spinal cord ependymomas. This is important because it addresses the potential significance of the application of current chromosomal findings for the purposes of risk stratification so that patients requiring more aggressive treatment may be identified to prevent progression and recurrence, whereas low-risk groups may benefit from reduced toxicity of unnecessarily intense adjuvant therapy.

I. Yang, MD

Imaging modalities in high-grade gliomas: Pseudoprogression, recurrence, or necrosis?

Caroline I, Rosenthal MA (Royal Melbourne Hosp, Parkville, Victoria, Australia; Univ of Melbourne, Victoria, Australia)

J Clin Neurosci 19:633-637, 2012

High grade gliomas (HGG) frequently recur regardless of treatment. Radiological detection of progressive disease (PD) is challenging due to the possibility of therapy-related MRI changes including: pseudoprogression (PP) and radiation necrosis (RN). Both may mimic PD. We undertook a literature review to examine existing data regarding imaging modalities and their ability to distinguish between PP, RN and PD. The review revealed 26 articles comparing the value of imaging modalities used to differentiate PP, RN and PD. Overall, conventional MRI and ^{18}fluorine-fluorodeoxyglucose positron emission tomography (^{18}F-FDG PET) were more sensitive, while thallium single photon emission CT (SPECT) was more specific in differentiating PD from PP and RN. However, further prospective studies comparing the clinical utility of MRI, PET, and SPECT are needed to establish the most reliable diagnostic tool for the differentiation of PP, RN and PD in HGG.

▶ This article does a very extensive job at systematically reviewing historic literature to examine existing data regarding the various imaging modalities used to distinguish between recurrence, pseudoprogression, and radiation necrosis. The discussion of imaging modalities was comprehensive, yet concise and included magnetic resonance imaging, positron emission tomography, single photon emission computed tomography, and their respective subtypes. Despite its brevity, the article was able to discuss the biology behind why certain imaging modalities were more specific and/or sensitive, allowing readers to have a greater understanding of the underlying mechanisms. Specifically, the article addresses each of the imaging modalities individually in neatly organized categories that parallel the supplementary tables in a way that is very easy to understand and includes data on specificity, sensitivity, accuracy, scan time, and pathological confirmation. In addition, the authors also did an excellent job of designing a series of tables that aggregated the existing data in a very clear, concise, and intuitive manner.

Other clinical factors that influence imaging include how radiation therapy, chemotherapy, and anti–vascular endothelial growth factor VEGF drugs may influence the radiographic outcomes, especially that many treatment protocols include concurrent irradiation and chemotherapy.

Overall, this is an excellent article that does a thorough job of reviewing the various imaging modalities in a concise manner.

I. Yang, MD

Frameless robotically targeted stereotactic brain biopsy: feasibility, diagnostic yield, and safety

Bekelis K, Radwan TA, Desai A, et al (Dartmouth-Hitchcock Med Ctr, Lebanon, NH)

J Neurosurg 116:1002-1006, 2012

Object.—Frameless stereotactic brain biopsy has become an established procedure in many neurosurgical centers worldwide. Robotic modifications of image-guided frameless stereotaxy hold promise for making these procedures safer, more effective, and more efficient. The authors hypothesized that robotic brain biopsy is a safe, accurate procedure, with a high diagnostic yield and a safety profile comparable to other stereotactic biopsy methods.

Methods.—This retrospective study included 41 patients undergoing frameless stereotactic brain biopsy of lesions (mean size 2.9 cm) for diagnostic purposes. All patients underwent image-guided, robotic biopsy in which the Surgi-Scope system was used in conjunction with scalp fiducial markers and a preoperatively selected target and trajectory. Forty-five procedures, with 50 supratentorial targets selected, were performed.

Results.—The mean operative time was 44.6 minutes for the robotic biopsy procedures. This decreased over the second half of the study by 37%, from 54.7 to 34.5 minutes ($p < 0.025$). The diagnostic yield was 97.8% per procedure, with a second procedure being diagnostic in the single nondiagnostic case. Complications included one transient worsening of a preexisting deficit (2%) and another deficit that was permanent (2%). There were no infections.

Conclusions.—Robotic biopsy involving a preselected target and trajectory is safe, accurate, efficient, and comparable to other procedures employing either frame-based stereotaxy or frameless, nonrobotic stereotaxy. It permits biopsy in all patients, including those with small target lesions. Robotic biopsy planning facilitates careful preoperative study and optimization of needle trajectory to avoid sulcal vessels, bridging veins, and ventricular penetration.

▶ In this retrospective study, the authors report their experience using frameless stereotactic brain biopsy to diagnose intracranial lesions. In a review of 41 cases, the authors had reported a diagnostic yield of 97.8% per procedure with an overall complication rate of 4%. Although a limitation of frameless stereotactic biopsy is stabilization of the instrument, a frameless approach is more agile, less distressing for the patient, and is reported to have comparable accuracy. The advent of stabilization devices and specifically robotic technology has provided benefits of stabilization, among many other qualities including precision, reliability, and accuracy all independent of the operator. Using the SurgiScope robotic frameless image guidance system, the authors demonstrated in this series a diagnostic yield of 96%, comparable to rates reported by Gralla et al (diagnostic yield of 98%).

One limitation to this study is its retrospective nature and its indirect use of historical controls (rather than including a control arm within the present study). Furthermore, Gralla et al's value of 98% was obtained from lesions greater than 15 mm, whereas the average tumor size in the present study was 28 mm. The lack of elaboration of patient selection criteria and controls necessitates caution when interpreting the present results and the claimed comparison to nonrobotic guided frameless or frame-based techniques. Caution should be taken when interpreting the safety data for similar reasons. However, the authors do provide a compelling point for further research, because a better understanding of which patient cases would benefit best from robotic image-guided brain biopsies can lead to improved means of diagnostic brain biopsies.

I. Yang, MD

13 Cerebrovascular

Long-term Results of Gamma Knife Surgery for Partially Embolized Arteriovenous Malformations

Schwyzer L, Yen C-P, Evans A, et al (Univ of Virginia, Charlottesville)

Neurosurgery 71:1139-1148, 2012

Background.—The effectiveness and risk of Gamma Knife surgery (GKS) in the management of partially embolized cerebral arteriovenous malformations (AVMs) remain to be elucidated.

Objective.—To evaluate the long-term imaging and clinical outcomes of GKS in AVM patients who had undergone previous partial embolization and compare the results with patients treated with GKS alone.

Methods.—A total of 215 embolized AVMs were analyzed. The mean patient age was 32.9 years. The mean volume of the nidus was 4.6 mL (range, 0.1-29.4 mL), and the mean prescription dose was 19.6 Gy (range, 4-28 Gy). This group was compared with 729 nonembolized AVMs.

Results.—After embolization and GKS, angiographically confirmed total obliteration of the AVMs was significantly lower (33%) compared with patients in whom GKS was used alone (60.9%; $P < .001$). However, the mean nidus size was larger and the Spetzler-Martin grade was higher for the embolized AVMs compared with the nonembolized AVMs. Radiation-induced changes occurred more often in the embolized (43.4%) than the nonembolized (33.4%) AVMs ($P = .028$). Permanent neurological deficits associated with radiation-induced changes occurred in 2.7% of the embolized compared with 1.3% of the nonembolized patients ($P = .14$).

Conclusion.—In our retrospective and historical series, the long-term results suggest that the obliteration rate is significantly lower in embolized AVMs compared with nonembolized AVMs, also because of the fact that the combined treatment is applied to higher grade AVMs; the percentage of grade III-V AVMs was 58.6% and 48.8% for nonembolized AVMs.

▶ Embolization of arteriovenous malformations (AVMs) prior to radiosurgery is a commonly employed strategy, especially in larger AVMs that require volume reduction. However, recent publications have suggested questionable benefit to this practice.[1,2] This study retrospectively characterizes the experience of embolization followed by Gamma Knife radiosurgery in 215 patients. Their data suggest that total obliteration rates are lower in the embolized group, with a great rate of radiation-induced changes (RIC) and permanent neurologic deficits. These results call into question current, common treatment practices in the management of AVMs.

Before we abandon embolization prior to radiosurgery altogether, we need to better understand the conclusions of this study. One of the reasons the embolization group rates are lower may be that visualization of the nidus is more difficult, especially after the use of Onyx as the embolizing agent. This artifact is created by the tantalum powder in Onyx. In addition, embolization may result in a previously well-defined nidus being transformed into a "Swiss-cheese" configuration, further complicating radiosurgical planning. The result is that parts of the brain that may not have otherwise received radiation are now included in the treatment plan, causing a greater incidence of RIC. Additionally, parts of the AVM that are thought to be embolized may still be patent but missed on the radiosurgical planning, resulting in lower cure rates.

Embolization prior to radiosurgery was initially developed for larger AVMs that needed to have their volume reduced to the ranges traditionally used in radiosurgery. In the embolized group from this study, the Spetzler-Martin grade and size were greater, and it is well established that more complex AVMs are harder to cure. This is one of the stated limitations of comparing embolized with nonembolized AVM groups. Although these size limits for radiosurgery are still commonly applied, current publications suggest that multistaged radiosurgery may have acceptable cure rates for larger AVMs,[3] and this merits study as an alternative to embolization.

As suggested by this and other studies, routine embolization of AVMs prior to radiosurgery may have worse outcomes. However, this technique can still be beneficial if complications are carefully limited and the embolization material is selectively targeted to certain portions of the AVM that may be at high risk to receive radiation. There also may be certain subtypes of AVMs that we do not yet fully understand in which embolization may be helpful prior to radiosurgery, and identifying these will further improve outcomes.

C. Gandhi, MD

References

1. Andrade-Souza YM, Ramani M, Scora D, Tsao MN, terBrugge K, Schwartz ML. Embolization before radiosurgery reduces the obliteration rate of arteriovenous malformations. *Neurosurgery.* 2007;60:443-451.
2. Izawa M, Chernov M, Hayashi M, Iseki H, Hori T, Takakura K. Combined management of intracranial arteriovenous malformations with embolization and gamma knife radiosurgery: comparative evaluation of the long-term results. *Surg Neurol.* 2009;71:43-52.
3. Kano H, Kondziolka D, Flickinger JC, et al. Stereotactic radiosurgery for arteriovenous malformations, Part 6: multistaged volumetric management of large arteriovenous malformations. *J Neurosurg.* 2012;116:54-65.

Validation and absolute quantification of MR perfusion compared with CT perfusion in patients with unilateral cerebral arterial stenosis

Chiu F-Y, Kao Y-H, Teng MMH, et al (Natl Yang-Ming Univ, Taipei City, Taiwan; et al)

Eur J Radiol 81:4087-4093, 2012

Objective.—The aim of the study was to assess absolute quantification of dynamic susceptibility contrast-enhanced magnetic resonance perfusion (MRP) comparing with computed tomography perfusion (CTP) in patients with unilateral stenosis.

Materials and Methods.—We retrospectively post-processed MRP in 20 patients with unilateral occlusion or stenosis of >79% at the internal carotid artery or the middle cerebral artery (MCA). Absolute quantification of MRP was performed after applying the following techniques: cerebrospinal fluid removal, vessel removal, and automatic segmentation of brain to calculate the scaling factors to convert relative cerebral blood volume (rCBV) and relative cerebral blood flow (rCBF) values to absolute values. For comparison between MRP and CTP, we manually deposited regions of interest in bilateral MCA territories at the level containing the body of the lateral ventricle.

Results.—The correlation between MRP and CTP was best for mean transit time (MTT) ($r = 0.83$), followed by cerebral blood flow (CBF) ($r = 0.52$) and cerebral blood volume (CBV) ($r = 0.43$). There was no significant difference between CTP and MRP for CBV, CBF, and MTT on the lesion side, the contralateral side, the lesion-contralateral differences, or the lesion-to-contralateral ratios ($P > 0.05$). The mean differences between MRP and CTP were as follows: CBV −0.57 mL/100 g, CBF 2.50 mL/100 g/min, and MTT −0.90 s.

Conclusion.—Absolute quantification of MRP is possible. Using the proposed method, measured values of MRP and CTP had acceptable linear correlation and quantitative agreement.

▶ Both computed tomography (CT) and magnetic resonance (MR) perfusion imaging has been increasingly available at major medical centers over the past decade. Various possible clinical applications of these imaging modalities exist and include more accurate triage of stroke intervention eligible patients. Currently, patients for possible stroke intervention are treated based on the "time since symptom onset" guidelines of 3 to 4.5 hours with intravenous tissue plasminogen activator and 6 to 8 hours with embolectomy, based on prior large studies.[1-3] Ideally, a stroke patient who could demonstrate an occluded vessel on CT or MR angiography and a perfusion deficit on CT perfusion or MR perfusion could be treated outside the current treatment windows. Conversely, patients who may be eligible for treatment based on current time window guidelines but have a fixed stroke on CT or MR and no salvageable brain on CT perfusion would not undergo a procedure that could pose other risks and not offer any improved outcomes.

Despite these exciting expectations for perfusion imaging, preliminary studies into the application of this technology have produced variable results. One of the challenges has been the lack of standardization between manufactures of the scanners. Another common question from clinicians is whether CT or MR perfusion would be the best test. This article outlines an elegant validation between MR and CT perfusion, and studies such as this are critical to a successful adoption of this technology, which has the potential to drastically change stroke care.

C. Gandhi, MD

References

1. Hacke W, Kaste M, Fieschi C, et al. Intravenous thrombolysis with recombinant tissue plasminogen activator for acute hemispheric stroke. The European Cooperative Acute Stroke Study (ECASS). *JAMA*. 1995;274:1017-1025.
2. Wahlgren N, Ahmed N, Dávalos A, et al. Thrombolysis with alteplase 3-4.5 h after acute ischaemic stroke (SITS-ISTR): an observational study. *Lancet*. 2008;372: 1303-1309.
3. Smith WS, Sung G, Saver J, et al. Mechanical thrombectomy for acute ischemic stroke: final results of the Multi MERCI trial. *Stroke*. 2008;39:1205-1212.

Safety and Efficacy of Intraoperative Angiography in Craniotomies for Cerebral Aneurysms and Arteriovenous Malformations: A Review of 1093 Consecutive Cases

Chalouhi N, Theofanis T, Jabbour P, et al (Thomas Jefferson Univ, Philadelphia, PA)
Neurosurgery 71:1162-1169, 2012

Background.—In an era of indocyanine angiography, the routine use of intraoperative angiography (IOA) in the surgical treatment of aneurysms and vascular malformations is controversial.

Objective.—To retrospectively assess the safety and efficacy of IOA and to determine predictors of surgical revision.

Methods.—Between 2003 and 2011, IOA was performed during surgical treatment of 976 aneurysms, 101 arteriovenous malformations (AVMs), and 16 arteriovenous fistulas.

Results.—In 80 of 976 aneurysms (8.2%), IOA prompted clip repositioning. The reason for readjustment was residual aneurysm in 54.7%, parent vessel occlusion in 42.9%, and both in 2.4% of cases. In multivariate analysis, increasing aneurysm size ($P < .001$), ruptured aneurysm ($P < .001$), and increasing number of vessels injected ($P < .001$) were strong predictors of clip readjustment. There was a strong trend for posterior circulation aneurysm location to predict clip repositioning ($P = .06$). IOA revealed residual nidus/fistula requiring further intervention in 9 of 101 AVMs (8.9%) and 3 of 16 arteriovenous fistulas (18.8%). Of 9 AVMs requiring a surgical revision, 2 (22.2%) were Spetzler-Martin grade II, 5 (55.6%) were grade III, and 2 (22.2%) were grade IV. Mean Spetzler-Martin grade was 3.0 in AVMs requiring surgical revision compared with 2.3 in those not requiring revision ($P = .05$). IOA-related complications were all transient or minor and occurred in 0.99% of patients; none resulted in permanent morbidity.

Conclusion.—IOA remains a valuable tool in the surgical treatment of brain vascular abnormalities, guiding surgical re-exploration in >8% of cases. Easy access to an angiographer and routine use of IOA are important factors contributing to procedural safety and efficacy.

▶ Indocyanine green (ICG) angiography has replaced traditional intraoperative diagnostic angiography (IOA) at many institutions for the evaluation of intracranial vascular lesions in the operating room. This article, from a high-volume center, highlights the differences between the 2 types of angiography and emphasizes that IOA, although an older method for evaluation, remains a very useful part of the surgeon's tools in the operating room.

ICG has both advantages and disadvantages, which must be clearly understood by the operating surgeon prior to its application in clinical situations. The technique is easy to use with a simple, fixed intravenous bolus prior to imaging. Visualization of the injected dye requires only the placement of a filter, which is available for all current microscopes. The images that are produced are not as detailed as that for IOA but can be generated quickly and, in most situations, offer the information required to alter intraoperative management if needed. The ICG dye also washes out quickly, allowing for repeat imaging if needed in a short interval, with limited complications.

One of the main disadvantages of ICG imaging is that it can only see what is directly visualized through a microscope. So, it cannot discern residual aneurysm or arteriovenous malformation if that residual is under tissue and not directly visualized. Not understanding this major limitation can cause misinterpretation of ICG in the operating room.

In contrast, IOA is more tedious to obtain and requires significant technical expertise. It also has complications similar to other diagnostic angiography procedures. The tradeoff for these small risks is that the surgeon can visualize the entire cerebrum with greater detail if needed and not only the microscopic field of view. This article confirms that in expert hands, IOA has a very low complication rate, and it altered the surgical plan in 8% of cases.

C. Gandhi, MD

Solitaire flow restoration device versus the Merci Retriever in patients with acute ischaemic stroke (SWIFT): a randomised, parallel-group, non-inferiority trial

Saver JL, for the SWIFT Trialists (Univ of California, Los Angeles; et al)

Lancet 380:1241-1249, 2012

Background.—The Solitaire Flow Restoration Device is a novel, self-expanding stent retriever designed to yield rapid flow restoration in acute cerebral ischaemia. We compared the efficacy and safety of Solitaire with the standard, predicate mechanical thrombectomy device, the Merci Retrieval System.

Methods.—In this randomised, parallel-group, non-inferiority trial, we enrolled patients from 18 sites (17 in the USA and one in France). Patients were eligible for inclusion if they had acute ischaemic stroke with moderate to severe neurological deficits and were treatable by thrombectomy within 8 h of stroke symptom onset. We used a computer-generated randomisation sequence to randomly allocate patients to receive thrombectomy treatment with either Solitaire or Merci (1:1; block sizes of four and stratified by centre and stroke severity). The primary endpoint was Thrombolysis In Myocardial Ischemia (TIMI) scale 2 or 3 flow in all treatable vessels without symptomatic intracranial haemorrhage, after up to three passes of the assigned device, as assessed by an independent core laboratory, which was masked to study assignment. Primary analysis was done by intention to treat. A prespecified efficacy stopping rule triggered an early halt to the trial. The study is registered with ClinicalTrials.gov, number NCT 01054560.

Results.—Between February, 2010, and February, 2011, we randomly allocated 58 patients to the Solitaire group and 55 patients to the Merci group. The primary efficacy outcome was achieved more often in the Solitaire group than it was in the Merci group (61% *vs* 24%; difference 37% [95% CI 19–53], odds ratio [OR] 4·87 [95% CI 2·14–11·10]; $p_{non\text{-}inferiority} < 0{\cdot}0001$, $p_{superiority} = 0{\cdot}0001$). More patients had good 3-month neurological outcome with Solitaire than with Merci (58% *vs* 33%; difference 25% [6–43], OR 2·78 [1·25–6·22]; $p_{non\text{-}inferiority} = 0{\cdot}0001$, $p_{superiority} = 0{\cdot}02$). 90-day mortality was lower in the Solitaire group than it was in the Merci group (17 *vs* 38; difference −21% [−39 to −3], OR 0·34 [0·14–0·81]; $p_{non\text{-}inferiority} = 0{\cdot}0001$, $p_{superiority} = 0{\cdot}02$).

Interpretation.—The Solitaire Flow Restoration Device achieved substantially better angiographic, safety, and clinical outcomes than did the Merci Retrieval System. The Solitaire device might be a future treatment of choice for endovascular recanalisation in acute ischaemic stroke.

▶ Great technical advances have taken place in the interventional treatment of acute stroke over the past 5 years. The most recent development is the completion of this trial, which reports on the new Solitaire stent retriever. A stent retriever is a nondetachable stent that can be deployed into an intra-arterial clot after which the stent is then pulled back into the delivery catheter, hopefully along with the clot. The control device in this study is the Mechanical Embolus Removal in Cerebral Ischemia (MERCI) device, which was the first neurointerventional device approved in 2004 in the United States for mechanical thrombectomy within the brain. Various studies have confirmed that the rate of recanalization with MERCI are at best 40% to 50%.[1] Despite this limited success rate, because of the significant length of practitioner experience with the device, it was chosen for use in the control group in this review.

The Solitaire With the Intention for Thrombectomy (SWIFT) trial is a prospective, randomized trial involving both US and European centers constructed as a noninferiority comparison between Solitaire and the MERCI devices. Patients were included for intervention if their symptoms occurred within the 8-hour time window established in the initial MERCI trial.[1] The primary endpoint was complete or near-complete recanalization of the target vessel. The results were very impressive in favor of Solitaire, and the trial was stopped early because of the significant difference in primary outcome (61% vs 24%).

More patients also had better 3-month outcomes with Solitaire (58% vs 33%), and this is probably secondary to more rapid re-establishment of blood flow. Because more patients were doing better, the 90-day mortality was lower in the Solitaire group as well.

These are very compelling results for the superiority of the stent-retriever technology in the interventional treatment of stroke. Since the SWIFT trial, there has been a rapid acceptance of stent retrievers as the primary device for thrombectomy. Soon after SWIFT, a competing trial with similarly impressive results using the Trevo stent retriever was also released,[2] further expanding the use of stent retrievers. Now that the technology has improved, it is even more critical to create well-designed trials that answer the most important clinical question: Is intra-arterial thrombectomy superior to medical management with intravenous tissue plasminogen activator? To date, no clinical trials have been able to convincingly answer that question, but trial design is currently under way.

C. Gandhi, MD

References

1. Smith WS, Sung G, Starkman S, et al. Safety and efficacy of mechanical embolectomy in acute ischemic stroke: results of the MERCI trial. *Stroke.* 2005;36: 1432-1440.
2. Nogueira RG, Lutsep HL, Gupta R, et al. Trevo versus Merci retrievers for thrombectomy revascularisation of large vessel occlusions in acute ischaemic stroke (TREVO 2): a randomised trial. *Lancet.* 2012;380:1231-1240.

Early Postmarket Results After Treatment of Intracranial Aneurysms With the Pipeline Embolization Device: A US Multicenter Experience

Kan P, Siddiqui AH, Veznedaroglu E, et al (State Univ of New York, Buffalo; Stroke and Cerebrovascular Ctr of New Jersey, Trenton; et al)

Neurosurgery 71:1080-1088, 2012

Background.—The Pipeline embolization device (PED) is the latest technology available for intracranial aneurysm treatment.

Objective.—To report early postmarket results with the PED.

Methods.—This study was a prospective registry of patients treated with PEDs at 7 American neurosurgical centers subsequent to Food and Drug Administration approval of this device. Data collected included clinical presentation, aneurysm characteristics, treatment details, and periprocedural events. Follow-up data included degree of aneurysm occlusion and delayed (>30 days after the procedure) complications.

Results.—Sixty-two PED procedures were performed to treat 58 aneurysms in 56 patients. Thirty-seven of the aneurysms (64%) treated were located from the cavernous to the superior hypophyseal artery segment of the internal carotid artery; 22% were distal to that segment, and 14% were in the vertebrobasilar system. A total of 123 PEDs were deployed with an average of 2 implanted per aneurysm treated. Six devices were incompletely deployed; in these cases, rescue balloon angioplasty was required. Six periprocedural (during the procedure/within 30 days after the procedure) thromboembolic events occurred, of which 5 were in patients with vertebrobasilar aneurysms. There were 4 fatal postprocedural hemorrhages (from 2 giant basilar trunk and 2 large ophthalmic artery aneurysms). The major complication rate (permanent disability/death resulting from perioperative/delayed complication) was 8.5%. Among 19 patients with 3-month follow-up angiography, 68% (13 patients) had complete aneurysm occlusion. Two patients presented with delayed flow-limiting in-stent stenosis that was successfully treated with angioplasty.

Conclusion.—Unlike conventional coil embolization, aneurysm occlusion with PED is not immediate. Early complications include both thromboembolic and hemorrhagic events and appear to be significantly more frequent in association with treatment of vertebrobasilar aneurysms.

▶ The Pipeline embolization device (PED) is a novel stent with a braided design and a much greater density of metal stent struts, allowing for a diversion of flow away from the aneurysm and, ideally, aneurysm thrombosis. This type of device is now commonly referred to as a *flow-diverter* and was approved by the US Food and Drug Administration in 2011. This device was developed to be used on large and giant wide-necked cerebral aneurysms located within the internal carotid artery. These larger aneurysms have a poor natural history and a very high rate of recanalization with standard endovascular coil embolization techniques.[1]

This report by Kan et al is an early postmarket analysis of the PED from a consortium of experienced neurointerventionalists. Sixty-two procedures were performed with 123 stents placed (it is common to place more than one PED to achieve aneurysm thrombosis). Of the 6 thromboembolic complications, 5 were within the vertebrobasilar system with 50% of the fatal hemorrhages (2 of 4) in this location as well. The overall major complication rate was 8.5%, and at 3-month follow-up 68% of patients had complete aneurysm occlusion.

These results must be analyzed while remembering the poor natural history of these particularly challenging intracranial aneurysms and also the high rate of recurrence with standard coiling. A 3-month occlusion rate of 68% is significantly better than any prior attempt at these lesions. More recently, 6-month follow-up has become the standard period of follow-up angiography, and the rates of occlusion are even more impressive. Both early thromboembolic and hemorrhagic complications were noted, but most of these were in the posterior circulation. Since this publication, most neurointerventionalists have limited their use of PED to the anterior circulation, except in rare situations.

The PED is another technology in the arsenal of neurointerventional surgery for the treatment of a small niche of complex intracranial aneurysms.

C. Gandhi, MD

Reference

1. Murayama Y, Nien YL, Duckwiler G, et al. Guglielmi detachable coil embolization of cerebral aneurysms: 11 years' experience. *J Neurosurg*. 2003;98:959-966.

A Comparison of Radiation Exposure between Diagnostic CTA and DSA Examinations of Cerebral and Cervicocerebral Vessels

Manninen A-L, Isokangas J-M, Karttunen A, et al (Oulu Univ Hosp, Finland)

AJNR Am J Neuroradiol 33:2038-2042, 2012

Background and Purpose.—While the number of CTA examinations is continually increasing compared with DSA examinations, there is little comparative dose information about the different imaging techniques. We compared patient radiation exposure resulting from diagnostic CTA and DSA examinations for both cerebral and cervicocerebral vessels.

Materials and Methods.—An anthropomorphic phantom was irradiated by using typical diagnostic CTA and DSA setups and imaging parameters. For both imaging techniques, the imaging area of cerebral vessels included intracranial vessels only, while the imaging area of cervicocerebral vessels included both cervical and intracranial vessels from the aortic arch to the vertex. The effective dose was determined by using RPLDs. The DSA examination was simulated by using a biplane angiography system, and the CTA examination, by using a 64-row multidetector CT scanner.

Results.—For the imaging of cerebral vessels, the effective dose according to ICRP 103 was 0.67 mSv for CTA and 2.71 mSv for DSA. For the imaging of cervicocerebral vessels, the effective dose was 4.85 mSv for CTA and 3.60 mSv for DSA. The maximum absorbed dose (milligray) for skin, brain, salivary glands, and eyes was 166.2, 73.5, 35.6, and 21.8 mGy for DSA and 19.0, 16.9, 20.4, and 14.8 mGy for CTA, respectively. The conversion factors from DAP and DLP to effective dose were calculated.

Conclusions.—The effective dose for CTA assessment of cerebral vessels was approximately one-fifth the dose compared with DSA. In the imaging of cervicocerebral vessels, the effective dose for CTA was approximately one-third higher compared with DSA.

▶ The use of noninvasive imaging such as computed tomography angiography (CTA) to aid in visualizing both the cervical and cerebral vasculature has increased dramatically over the last decade. The ease by which CTAs can be obtained at most major hospitals is one of the factors that has led to the dramatic increase in these studies being performed compared with the more invasive digital subtraction angiography (DSA) studies. Other studies have confirmed that the accuracy of CTA is rapidly approaching that of DSA in critical clinical situations.[1] However, there has been little published regarding the difference in radiation doses for these modalities. This is becoming a more common line of discussion with our better understanding of the long-term risks of imaging studies in the formation of both benign and malignant tumors of the brain and other locations.

In this study, phantom models were irradiated using common clinical scanning and fluoroscopy parameters. The results conclude that for routine clinical situations, the radiation exposure and the absorbed dose were significantly lower for CTA compared with DSA. However, in the real-world situation, clinicians will have to realize that this benefit will rapidly be lost if a patient undergoes multiple CTA studies.

C. Gandhi, MD

Reference

1. Hoh BL, Cheung AC, Rabinov JD, Pryor JC, Carter BS, Ogilvy CS. Results of a prospective protocol of computed tomographic angiography in place of catheter angiography as the only diagnostic and pretreatment planning study for cerebral aneurysms by a combined neurovascular team. *Neurosurgery.* 2004;54:1329-1340. discussion 1340-2.

Endovascular Therapy after Intravenous t-PA versus t-PA Alone for Stroke

Broderick JP, for the Interventional Management of Stroke (IMS) III Investigators (Univ of Cincinnati Academic Health Ctr, OH; et al)

N Engl J Med 368:893-903, 2013

Background.—Endovascular therapy is increasingly used after the administration of intravenous tissue plasminogen activator (t-PA) for patients with moderate-to-severe acute ischemic stroke, but whether a combined approach is more effective than intravenous t-PA alone is uncertain.

Methods.—We randomly assigned eligible patients who had received intravenous t-PA within 3 hours after symptom onset to receive additional endovascular therapy or intravenous t-PA alone, in a 2:1 ratio. The primary outcome measure was a modified Rankin scale score of 2 or less (indicating functional independence) at 90 days (scores range from 0 to 6, with higher scores indicating greater disability).

Results.—The study was stopped early because of futility after 656 participants had undergone randomization (434 patients to endovascular therapy and 222 to intravenous t-PA alone). The proportion of participants with a modified Rankin score of 2 or less at 90 days did not differ significantly according to treatment (40.8% with endovascular therapy and 38.7% with intravenous t-PA; absolute adjusted difference, 1.5 percentage points; 95% confidence interval [CI], −6.1 to 9.1, with adjustment for the National Institutes of Health Stroke Scale [NIHSS] score [8−19, indicating moderately severe stroke, or ≥20, indicating severe stroke]), nor were there significant differences for the predefined subgroups of patients with an NIHSS score of 20 or higher (6.8 percentage points; 95% CI, −4.4 to 18.1) and those with a score of 19 or lower (−1.0 percentage point; 95% CI, −10.8 to 8.8). Findings in the endovascular-therapy and intravenous t-PA groups were similar for mortality at 90 days (19.1% and 21.6%, respectively; $P = 0.52$) and the proportion of patients with symptomatic intracerebral hemorrhage within 30 hours after initiation of t-PA (6.2% and 5.9%, respectively; $P = 0.83$).

Conclusions.—The trial showed similar safety outcomes and no significant difference in functional independence with endovascular therapy after intravenous t-PA, as compared with intravenous t-PA alone. (Funded by the National Institutes of Health and others; ClinicalTrials.gov number, NCT00359424.)

▶ The IMS-3 trial results featured in this article, along with the recently published MR RESCUE[1] and SYNTHESIS Expansion[2] trial results, have sparked much debate over the efficacy of interventional therapy for acute stroke. All 3 of these trials concluded that endovascular therapy was not superior to medical management. However, a more critical analysis finds significant limitations that may drastically alter the interpretation of the results.

The technology of interventional stroke therapy is rapidly evolving, and one of the major limitations of these trials is the applicability to the real-world scenario. For example, it is well known that endovascular therapy is reserved for large vessel occlusion. However, neither the IMS-3 nor SYNTHESIS Expansion trials excluded patients without large vessel occlusions. In addition, both IMS-3 and MR RESCUE allowed patients to be randomly assigned to the treatment group without the actual intended treatment occurring, and, if it did occur, it was commonly performed with outdated devices.

The IMS-3 trial looked at 656 patients, and only 33% of those patients underwent a computed tomography (CT) angiogram. This is in contradistinction to most medical centers that perform this therapy, where most patients undergo CT angiography to determine whether they do have a large vessel occlusion. By not performing a CT angiogram in most patients, 20% of patients that were randomly assigned to the treatment arm of intervention actually underwent only a diagnostic angiogram and then were deemed not to improve with intervention. In reality, no intervention was performed in these cases. These interventional arm patients also received a lower dose of intravenous tissue plasminogen activator compared with what they would have received in the medical arm of the study. In a subgroup analysis presented recently, looking only at those patients with a large vessel occlusion, a significant difference was seen.[3] This is the group that most neurointerventional surgeons are taking care of in modern practice. The other significant limitation of this study is the choice of devices utilized for intra-arterial intervention. The primary device in this study was the Merci Retriever, which is outdated and has a much lower published rate of vessel recanalization when compared with current aspiration-based or stent-based devices.

Review of this trial suggests that it may be very premature to assume that interventional therapy is not beneficial in patients with acute stroke. A handful of new stroke trials are being designed to minimize some of the glaring shortcomings of the current batch of trials. Awaiting those results and critically considering the recent data are paramount to a thoughtful paradigm with which to treat this group of patients who have a very poor natural history.

C. Gandhi, MD

References

1. Kidwell CS, Jahan R, Gornbein J, et al. A trial of imaging selection and endovascular treatment for ischemic stroke. *N Engl J Med.* 2013;368:914-923.
2. Ciccone A, Valvassori L, Nichelatti M, et al. Endovascular treatment for acute ischemic stroke. *N Engl J Med.* 2013;368:904-913.

3. Demchuk AM; IMS III Investigators. IMS III: comparison of outcomes between IV and IV/IA treatment in baseline CTA confirmed ICA, M1, M2 and basilar occlusions. International Stroke Conference; Honolulu, Hawaii, February 6–8, 2013.

Does Stent Implantation Improve the Result of Repeat Embolization in Recanalized Aneurysms?

Cho YD, Lee JY, Seo JH, et al (Seoul Natl Univ Hosp, Korea; et al)
Neurosurgery 71:ons253-ons259, 2012

Background.—Although endovascular technique and related devices continue to improve, recanalization of embolized aneurysm remains a pitfall of this approach. The problem of how to treat the recanalized aneurysm needs to be addressed.

Objective.—To determine the outcomes of patients undergoing repeat embolization for recanalized intracranial aneurysms and to evaluate the impact of stent implantation on subsequent recanalization.

Methods.—Between September 2001 and September 2011, we performed endovascular retreatment in 162 patients with a total of 197 recanalized intracranial aneurysms. Stent implantation was performed in 68 aneurysms during the retreatment. Clinical and morphological outcomes were assessed at 6 months or more after repeat embolization.

Results.—Procedure-related complications, including asymptomatic thromboembolism, occurred with 15 aneurysms (7.6%) without permanent neurological sequelae. Follow-up imaging of 172 aneurysms documented stable occlusion in 96 of the lesions (55.8%), minor recanalization in 17 (9.9%), and major recanalization in 59 (34.3%) during the mean follow-up period of 26.0 ± 18.0 months. In multiple logistic regression analysis, stent implantation was shown to reduce the major recanalization rate at 6 months after retreatment (odds ratio: 0.161; 95% confidence interval:, 0.038-0.670; $P = .012$) and thereafter (odds ratio: 0.226; 95% confidence interval: 0.088-0.581; $P = .002$).

Conclusion.—Stent implantation, as well as compact coil packing, at the time of repeat embolization seems beneficial in reducing rates of further recanalization (Fig 2).

▶ Aneurysm recanalization remains a significant challenge (Fig 2) and has been attributed to various factors, including aneurysm size and morphology, coil type and caliber, and the packing density of coils placed within the aneurysm. Recent neuroendovascular advances have attempted to reduce this rate of recanalization by modifying the thrombogenicity of the coils, increasing packing density, employing low-viscosity liquid embolic agents (ie, Onyx HD-500), and using "flow-diverting" stents (ie, Pipeline Embolization Device) across the neck of the aneurysm. The long-term efficacy of these new technologies is still being characterized.

This article reviews a significant experience with older, but more commonly used, stent technology. The Neuroform and Enterprise stents discussed here are low radial-force stents meant primarily to offer a buttress for coils at the

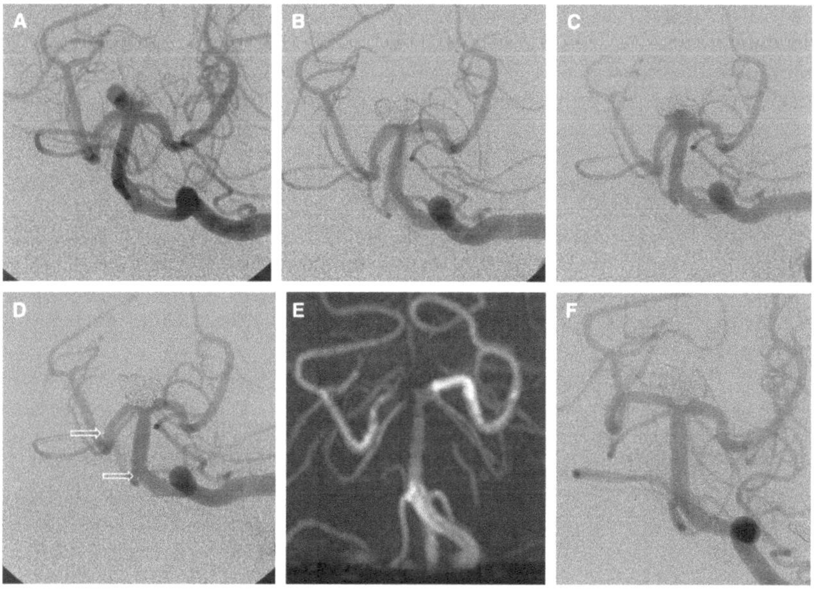

FIGURE 2.—A, cerebral angiography of a patient with headache revealed a small basilar tip aneurysm. B, the aneurysm was treated successfully with coils. C, at 4-year followup, conventional angiography showed major recanalization. D, additional coil embolization was performed, and the aneurysm was occluded satisfactorily using the stent protection technique (arrow indicates the end of the stent). E, 6-month follow-up magnetic resonance angiography showed no evidence of recanalization, but it was impossible to estimate recurrence exactly because of stent artifact. F, conventional angiography performed 12 months later showed the aneurysm to be visibly occluded. (Reprinted from Cho YD, Lee JY, Seo JH, et al. Does stent implantation improve the result of repeat embolization in recanalized aneurysms? Neurosurgery. 2012;71:ons253-ons259, the Congress of Neurological Surgeons.)

neck of the aneurysm so that the coils cannot herniate into the critical parent vessels. This allows placement of more coils within an aneurysm and increases the coil-packing density. Stents are especially useful in aneurysms that have a wider neck, which is an aneurysm morphology that has a greater chance of recurrence.

One of the other properties of stents is that, although they are porous, they do divert blood flow down the barrel of the stent and away from the aneurysm. Experts estimate that each of these types of stents diverts blood flow by about 11% per stent in a linear segment. This is the phenomenon that is being employed in the newer flow-diverting stents, such as the Pipeline, where the porosity has been reduced and the amount of diversion is much higher.

This article objectively examines the efficacy of using stents in cases where the aneurysm requires retreatment. There seems to be a measurable stability provided by stents in these cases and merits further discussion in the endovascular community.

C. Gandhi, MD

Distinctive flow pattern of wall shear stress and oscillatory shear index: similarity and dissimilarity in ruptured and unruptured cerebral aneurysm blebs

Kawaguchi T, Nishimura S, Kanamori M, et al (Aomori Prefectural Central Hosp, Japan)

J Neurosurg 117:774-780, 2012

Object.—The difference in the hemodynamics of wall shear stress (WSS) and oscillatory shear index (OSI) between ruptured and unruptured aneurysms is not well understood. The authors investigated the hemodynamic similarities and dissimilarities in ruptured and thin-walled unruptured aneurysm blebs.

Methods.—Magnetic resonance imaging–based fluid dynamics analysis was used to calculate WSS and OSI, and hemodynamic and intraoperative findings were compared. The authors also compared ruptured and unruptured thinwalled blebs for the magnitude of WSS and OSI.

Results.—Intraoperatively, 13 ruptured and 139 thin-walled unruptured aneurysm blebs were identified. Twelve of the ruptured (92.3%) and 124 of the unruptured blebs (89.2%) manifested low WSS and high OSI. The degree of WSS was significantly lower in ruptured (0.49 ± 0.12 Pa) than in unruptured (0.64 ± 0.15 Pa; $p < 0.01$) blebs.

Conclusions.—Ruptured and unruptured blebs shared a distinctive pattern of low WSS and high OSI. The degree of WSS at the rupture site was significantly lower than in the unruptured thin-walled blebs.

▶ The urgent treatment of ruptured aneurysms has been well established for many decades. However, the management of unruptured aneurysms remains controversial, and with the vast improvements and increased utilization of noninvasive diagnostic testing (CT angiography or MR angiography), it is an increasingly common clinical question. Currently, our understanding of unruptured aneurysms is based on trials that attempt to characterize the natural history of the aneurysm, looking at size, location, morphology, and various other factors.[1] These strategies have answered some questions, but an objective method by which to predict the rupture potential of any intracranial aneurysm remains elusive.

This study is a very nice demonstration of ongoing work in computational fluid dynamics applied to intracranial aneurysms. Through analysis of 152 aneurysms that were either ruptured or unruptured, the authors are able to mathematically demonstrate that there is an objective difference between the wall shear stress and oscillatory shear index in these 2 groups (see Fig 2 in the original article). Ideally, if this type of analysis could be conducted on a larger scale, perhaps we may be able to more accurately prospectively predict the rupture potential for any unruptured intracranial aneurysm. If this could be accomplished, it would dramatically alter the way we currently manage these lesions.

C. Gandhi, MD

Reference

1. Unruptured intracranial aneurysms: risk of rupture and risks of surgical intervention. International Study of Unruptured Intracranial Aneurysms Investigators. *N Engl J Med*. 1998;339:1725-1733.

Subarachnoid Hemorrhage Incidence in the United States Does Not Vary with Season or Temperature

McDonald RJ, McDonald JS, Bida JP, et al (Mayo Clinic, Rochester, MN)

AJNR Am J Neuroradiol 33:1663-1668, 2012

Background and Purpose.—Previous studies have suggested seasonal variations in rates of spontaneous rupture of intracranial aneurysms, leading to potentially devastating SAH. In an effort to identify a seasonal effect, variation in SAH incidence and in-hospital mortality rates were examined as they relate to admission month, temperature, and climate using HCUP's Nationwide Inpatient Sample.

Materials and Methods.—Cases of nontraumatic SAH and subsequent in-hospital mortality were extracted from the 2001–2008 NIS and associated with month of occurrence, local average monthly temperatures, and USDA climate zone. Multivariate regression analysis was used to study how admission month, temperature, and climate affected SAH admission and mortality rates.

Results.—Among 57,663,486 hospital admissions from the 2001–2008 NIS, 52,379 cases of spontaneous SAH (ICD-9-CM 430) and 13,272 cases of subsequent in-hospital mortality were identified. SAH incidence and in-hospital mortality rates were not significantly correlated with a monthly/seasonal effect (incidence, $\chi^2 = 2.94$, $P = .99$; mortality, $\chi^2 = 6.91$, $P = .81$). However, SAH incidence significantly varied with climate ($P < .0001$, zones 11 and 7) but not with temperature ($P = .1453$), whereas average monthly temperature and climate had no significant correlation with in-hospital mortality (temperature, $P = .3005$; climate, $P = .0863$).

Conclusions.—We identified no significant monthly or temperature-related effect in the incidence of SAH. Our data suggest that certain climate zones within the United States may be associated with significantly different SAH incidence, but the origins of these differences remain unclear and are probably unrelated to meteorologic variables (Figs 1 and 3).

▶ It has been a long-standing belief among neurosurgeons that the incidence of aneurysmal subarachnoid hemorrhage (aSAH) varies in the United States based on seasons (Fig 1). In the past this has been based on anecdotal evidence of the phenomena. However, more recently, objective attempts to define the validity of this occurrence have had differing results.[1,2] This study offers one of the largest attempts to clarify this debate.

Over a 7-year period, almost 53 000 cases of aSAH in the US were studied. The endpoints were aSAH incidence and in-hospital mortality relative to overall and average monthly climate and temperature (Fig 3). After a complex multivariate

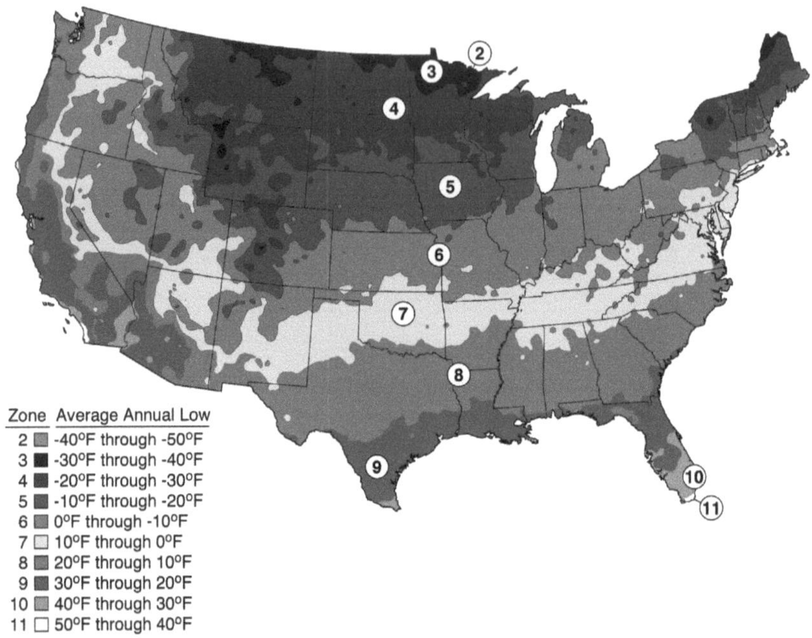

FIGURE 1.—USDA hardiness zone map. Used with permission from the Arbor Day Foundation (http://www.arborday.org/media/zones.cfm). (Reprinted from McDonald RJ, McDonald JS, Bida JP, et al. Subarachnoid hemorrhage incidence in the United States does not vary with season or temperature. *AJNR Am J Neuroradiol.* 2012;33:1663-1668, Copyright 2012, by the American Society of Neuroradiology.)

analysis, season, temperature, and climate were not found to be significant risk factors for aSAH mortality. Climate may be a risk factor for aSAH incidence, but the association was very weak. The infrequent variations were so small in the dataset that they could be caused by other complex, poorly understood factors.

A few points should be understood about the limitations of the dataset that was used. Many patients with aSAH die prior to coming to a hospital center, and this large group was not accounted for in this study. In addition, daily weather patterns were beyond the ability of the dataset, and only monthly averages were reported. This can significantly limit an analysis of more subtle variations in the incidence of aSAH. Other random errors, such as in coding, could also alter the data. Regardless of these limitations, this is a very robust dataset, and further subgroup analysis may offer more clarity. One of the questions raised by this study is whether climate and temperature are only secondary surrogates of the actual factor that surgeons perceive alters aSAH incidence. Because aSAH is multifactorial, perhaps other relationships to aSAH incidence and mortality exist and are yet to be characterized.

C. Gandhi, MD

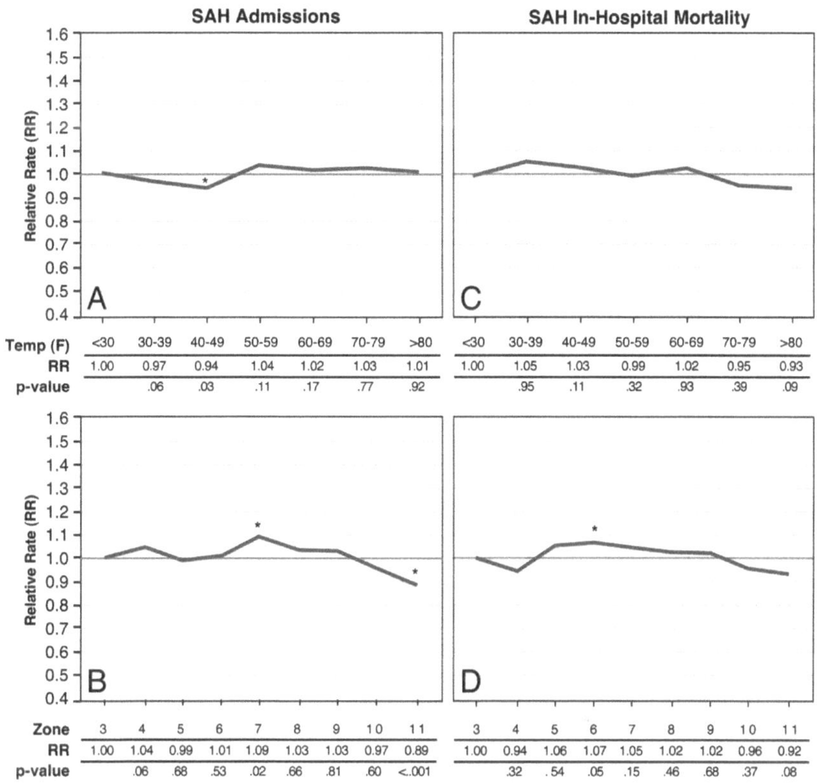

FIGURE 3.—Temperature (*A, C*) and climate (*B, D*) stratified relative rates for (*A, B*) admission frequency and (*D, E*) in-hospital mortality after admission for SAH. Relative rates of SAH admission and in-hospital mortality, stratified by temperature and climate, were determined from regression models. RRs greater than 1.0 suggest that the event (admission or death) is more likely to occur relative to the reference variable (temperature strata [<30°F]; climate strata [USDA zone 3]), whereas RRs less than 1.0 suggest the event is less likely to occur relative to the reference variable. Significant differences relative to the reference temperature stratum or zone are represented by an asterisk (*). (Reprinted from McDonald RJ, McDonald JS, Bida JP, et al. Subarachnoid hemorrhage incidence in the United States does not vary with season or temperature. *AJNR Am J Neuroradiol.* 2012;33:1663-1668, Copyright 2012, by the American Society of Neuroradiology.)

References

1. Bederson JB, Connolly ES Jr, Batjer HH, et al. Guidelines for the management of aneurysmal subarachnoid hemorrhage: a statement for healthcare professionals from a special writing group of the Stroke Council, American Heart Association. *Stroke.* 2009;40:994-1025.
2. Setzer M, Beck J, Hermann E, et al. The influence of barometric pressure changes and standard meteorological variables on the occurrence and clinical features of subarachnoid hemorrhage. *Surg Neurol.* 2007;67:264-272.

Surgical results of the Carotid Occlusion Surgery Study

Grubb RL Jr, for the Carotid Occlusion Surgery Study Investigators (Washington Univ School of Medicine in St Louis, MO; et al)

J Neurosurg 118:25-33, 2013

Object.—The Carotid Occlusion Surgery Study (COSS) was conducted to determine if superficial temporal artery–middle cerebral artery (STA-MCA) bypass, when added to the best medical therapy, would reduce subsequent ipsilateral stroke in patients with complete internal carotid artery (ICA) occlusion and an elevated oxygen extraction fraction (OEF) in the cerebral hemisphere distal to the occlusion. A recent publication documented the methodology of the COSS in detail and briefly outlined the major findings of the trial. The surgical results of the COSS are described in detail in this report.

Methods.—The COSS was a prospective, parallel-group, 1:1 randomized, open-label, blinded-adjudication treatment trial. Participants, who had angiographically demonstrated complete occlusion of the ICA causing either a transient ischemic attack or ischemic stroke within 120 days and hemodynamic cerebral ischemia indicated by an increased OEF measured by PET, were randomized to either surgical or medical treatment. One hundred ninety-five patients were randomized: 97 to the surgical group and 98 to the medical group. The surgical patients underwent an STA-MCA cortical branch anastomosis.

Results.—In the intention-to-treat analysis, the 2-year rates for the primary end point were 21% for the surgical group and 22.7% for the medical group ($p = 0.78$, log-rank test). Fourteen (15%) of the 93 patients who had undergone an arterial bypass had a primary end point ipsilateral hemispheric stroke in the 30-day postoperative period, 12 within 2 days after surgery. The STA-MCA arterial bypass patency rate was 98% at the 30-day postoperative visit and 96% at the last follow-up examination. The STA-MCA arterial bypass markedly improved, although it did not normalize, the level of elevated OEF in the symptomatic cerebral hemisphere. Five surgically treated and 1 nonsurgically treated patients in the surgical group had a primary end point ipsilateral hemispheric stroke after the 30-day postoperative period. No baseline characteristics or intraoperative variables revealed those who would experience a procedure-related stroke.

Conclusions.—Despite excellent bypass graft patency and improved cerebral hemodynamics, STA-MCA anastomosis did not provide an overall benefit regarding ipsilateral 2-year stroke recurrence, mainly because of a much better than expected stroke recurrence rate (22.7%) in the medical group, but also because of a significant postoperative stroke rate (15%). Clinical trial registration no.: NCT00029146.

▶ Symptomatic atherosclerosis resulting in internal carotid artery occlusion carries a 10% to 25% risk of transient ischemic attached CKS and ischemic strokes with a previously described failure of medical therapy in 10% to 15% of cases.

However, the negative results of the extracranial—intracranial (ED-IC) bypass trial in 1985, although commonly debated, diminished the enthusiasm for the use of a superficial temporal artery to middle cerebral artery (STA-MCA) bypass to treat these patients. One of the criticisms of the EC-IC bypass trial was that there was not an adequate subgroup analysis of patients with embolic strokes and hypoperfusion-related strokes. It was argued that the latter group would potentially benefit from STA-MCA bypass, whereas the former group would likely not benefit.

The Carotid Occlusion Surgery Study (COSS) trial was designed to test the hypothesis that STA-MCA bypass combined with best medical therapy would reduce the risk of ipsilateral ischemic stroke compared with best medical therapy alone in the study of patients with hemodynamic ischemia. It was a multicenter blindly adjudicated trial, and positron emission tomography was used to identify cases of cerebral vascular insufficiency with increased oxygen extraction. The study was composed of 195 patients, largely evenly split between the surgery and control arms, who were followed for the primary endpoint of recurrent stroke. The trial was terminated early for futility. The 2-year rates of ipsilateral recurrent strokes in both groups were similar (21.0% vs 22.7%), but the 30-day rates for ischemic stroke were 14.4% in the surgery group and only 2.0% in the medical arm.

The 2 major reasons that this trial failed were that the medically treated group had notably lower risk of stroke than what historical controls had suggested (22.7% vs 40%), and there was a significant (15%) postoperative stroke rate. It has been theorized that improvements in medical therapy, such as the aggressive use of statins, blood pressure control, and smoking cessation, may account for some of this lower risk. When looking at the surgical morbidity, 12 of 14 patients have a postoperative stroke within 2 days after surgery, and only 2 of 14 have a stroke after 30 days. The COSS trial also demonstrated that once a patient was out of the preoperative period (30 days), there was a clear benefit noted in the bypass arm with marked improvement in the oxygen extraction fraction, suggesting that perhaps reducing the surgical morbidity may be the key to demonstrating efficacy.

C. Gandhi, MD

Stroke After Carotid Stenting and Endarterectomy in the Carotid Revascularization Endarterectomy Versus Stenting Trial (CREST)

Hill MD, for the CREST Investigators (Univ of Calgary, Alberta, Canada; et al)

Circulation 126:3054-3061, 2012

Background.—Stroke occurs more commonly after carotid artery stenting than after carotid endarterectomy. Details regarding stroke type, severity, and characteristics have not been reported previously. We describe the strokes that have occurred in the Carotid Revascularization Endarterectomy versus Stenting Trial (CREST).

Methods and Results.—CREST is a randomized, open-allocation, controlled trial with blinded end-point adjudication. Stroke was a component of the primary composite outcome. Patients who received their assigned treatment within 30 days of randomization were included. Stroke

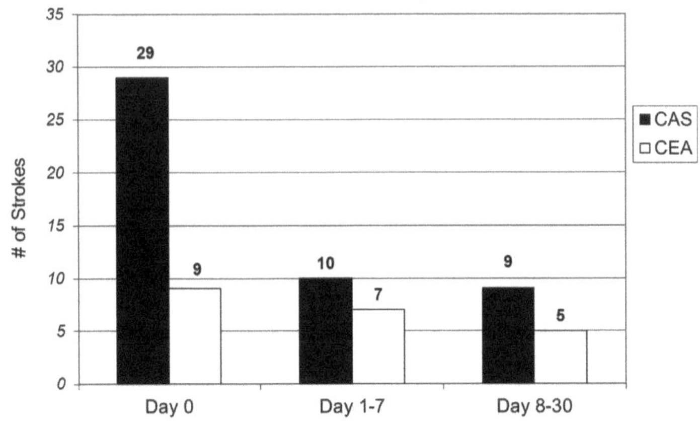

FIGURE 2.—Timing of stroke after carotid revascularization. CAS indicates carotid artery stenting; CEA, carotid endarterectomy. (Reprinted from Hill MD, for the CREST Investigators. Stroke after carotid stenting and endarterectomy in the carotid revascularization endarterectomy versus stenting trial (CREST). *Circulation.* 2012;126:3054-3061, Copyright 2012, with permission from American Heart Association, Inc.)

was adjudicated by a panel of board-certified vascular neurologists with secondary central review of clinically obtained brain images. Stroke type, laterality, timing, and outcome were reported. A periprocedural stroke occurred among 81 of the 2502 patients randomized and among 69 of the 2272 in the present analysis. Strokes were predominantly minor (81%, n = 56), ischemic (90%, n = 62), in the anterior circulation (94%, n = 65), and ipsilateral to the treated artery (88%, n = 61). There were 7 hemorrhages, which occurred 3 to 21 days after the procedure, and 5 were fatal. Major stroke occurred in 13 (0.6%) of the 2272 patients. The estimated 4-year mortality after stroke was 21.1% compared with 11.6% for those without stroke. The adjusted risk of death at 4 years was higher after periprocedural stroke (hazard ratio, 2.78; 95% confidence interval, 1.63–4.76).

Conclusions.—Stroke, particularly severe stroke, was uncommon after carotid intervention in CREST, but stroke was associated with significant morbidity and was independently associated with a nearly 3-fold increased future mortality. The delayed timing of major and hemorrhagic stroke after revascularization suggests that these strokes may be preventable (Fig 2).

▶ The CREST trial was the largest, randomized, multicenter trial to date that compared the outcomes in both symptomatic and asymptomatic patients with carotid stenosis who underwent either Carotid endarterectomy (CEA) or Carotid artery stenting (CAS).[1] The significant conclusions of the trial were that CAS was not inferior to CEA (the gold standard) in regard to overall outcomes. However, CAS was associated with a higher rate of periprocedural strokes, and CEA was associated with a higher rate of myocardial infarction (MI). This study is a follow up to the original CREST study, and it attempts to better characterize the strokes that did occur during the trial.

In the current analysis, strokes occurred in 69 of 2272 patients (3% risk), with 81% of the strokes being categorized as minor by the independent review panel of neurologists. Most strokes occurred on the day of the procedure in the CAS group, but the timing was variable in the CEA group (Fig 2). In addition, 90% were ischemic, 94% in the anterior circulation, and 88% in the territory of the vessel being treated. In the strokes that were hemorrhagic, 5 of 7 patients died. In the patients who had a stroke during the procedure, the adjusted risk of death at 4 years' follow-up was nearly 3-fold greater.

Previously performed analysis has suggested that stroke is associated with a poorer quality of life than MI.[1] This article further clarifies that, although most strokes were minor, the mortality risk after a carotid revascularization procedure is significant and should be considered in counseling patients and choosing a treatment option.

C. Gandhi, MD

Reference

1. Brott TG, Hobson RW 2nd, Howard G; CREST Investigators. Stenting versus endarterectomy for treatment of carotid-artery stenosis. *N Engl J Med.* 2010; 363:11-23.

14 Pediatric Neurosurgery

Craniocervical fusions in children

Menezes AH (Univ of Iowa Carver College of Medicine)

J Neurosurg Pediatr 9:573-585, 2012

The surgical management of craniovertebral junction (CVJ) instability in pediatric patients presents unique challenges. As compared with the adult patient, the anatomical variations of the CVJ in the pediatric patient are significant, complicate the approach, and limit the use of internal fixation. Diminutive osseous and ligamentous structures and syndromic craniovertebral abnormalities complicate the issue. Advances in imaging analysis and instrumentation have improved the armamentarium for managing the pediatric patient who requires craniocervical stabilization. In this paper, the author's experience of performing more than 850 pediatric CVJ fusions is reviewed. This work includes the indications for atlantoaxial arthrodesis and occipitocervical fusion. Early atlantoaxial fusions were performed using interlaminar rib graft fusion, and more recently using either transarticular screw fixation in the older patient, or lateral mass screws at C-1 and rod fixation with either C-2 pars interarticular screw fixation or pedicle screw fixation. A C-2 translaminar screw fixation is also described. Occipitocervical fusions are performed with rib grafts in patients younger than 6 years of age. Subsequently, above that age, contoured loop fixation was performed, and in the past 8–10 years, screw and rod fixation was used. Abnormal spine growth was not observed in children who underwent craniocervical stabilization below the age of 5 years (clearly the bone grew with the patient). However, no deleterious effects were noted in the children treated with rigid instrumentation. The success rate for bone fusion alone was 98%. The author's success rate with rigid instrumentation is nearly 100%. A detailed review of the technique of fusion is presented, as well as the indications and means of avoidance of complications, their prevention, and management.

▶ Craniocervical instrumentation and fusion techniques have undergone remarkable evolution. This article is a detailed description of a master neurosurgeon's experience in treating almost 900 children with complicated craniocervical pathology. His results are exemplary, achieving an almost 100% fusion rate. Such a large collection of patients is truly remarkable. As the author reflects on his "very gratifying" career with this review article, we all benefit greatly from the immeasurable contributions this author has given to the field of pediatric cranio-cervical surgery.

P. Klimo, Jr, MD, MPH

Image-guided cerebrospinal fluid shunting in children: catheter accuracy and shunt survival

Levitt MR, O'Neill BR, Ishak GE, et al (Univ of Washington School of Medicine, Seattle; Univ of Colorado School of Medicine, Denver)

J Neurosurg Pediatr 10:112-117, 2012

Object.—Cerebrospinal fluid shunt placement has a high failure rate, especially in patients with small ventricles. Frameless stereotactic electromagnetic image guidance can assist ventricular catheter placement. The authors studied the effects of image guidance on catheter accuracy and shunt survival in children.

Methods.—Pediatric patients who underwent placement or revision of a frontal ventricular CSF shunt were retrospectively evaluated. Catheters were placed using either anatomical landmarks or image guidance. Preoperative ventricular size and postoperative catheter accuracy were quantified. Outcomes of standard and image-guided groups were compared.

Results.—Eighty-nine patients underwent 102 shunt surgeries (58 initial, 44 revision). Image guidance was used in the placement of 56 shunts and the standard technique in 46. Shunt failure rates were not significantly different between the standard (22%) and image-guided (25%) techniques ($p = 0.21$, log-rank test). Ventricular size was significantly smaller in patients in the image-guided group ($p < 0.02$, Student t-test) and in the surgery revision group ($p < 0.01$). Small ventricular size did not affect shunt failure rate, even when controlling for shunt insertion technique. Despite smaller average ventricular size, the accuracy of catheter placement was significantly improved with image guidance ($p < 0.01$). Shunt accuracy did not affect shunt survival.

Conclusions.—The use of image guidance improved catheter tip accuracy compared with a standard technique, despite smaller ventricular size. Failure rates were not dependent on shunt insertion technique, but an observed selection bias toward using image guidance for more at-risk catheter placements showed failure rates similar to initial surgeries.

▶ This is a retrospective cohort study in which 2 groups of patients were followed in time after undergoing either an initial or revision shunt surgery, with the primary outcome being proximal shunt failure. One group used image guidance to place the proximal catheter; the other group did not. Although the accuracy of catheter placement improved in the image-guidance group, with the target being the foramen of Monro, shunt survival between the 2 groups was similar (22% in the standard group and 25% in the image-guidance group).

Unless infected, the primary reason for early shunt revision surgery (within 6 months of index surgery) is proximal catheter malfunction, and of these, malposition is one cause. In my opinion, image guidance should decrease the early revision rate, contrary to the authors' findings. Balance between the 2 groups is critical, and I wonder whether this might be the reason why there was no observed benefit. For example, there are shunt patients who are more complex than others. These are the patients who make pediatric neurosurgeons cringe when they hear their names. These are typically patients with myelomeningocele, postinfection, or posthemorrhagic etiologies as compared with others such as aqueductal stenosis. Although the authors present some baseline characteristics between the groups, were they truly balanced? We already know that patients in the image-guidance group had smaller ventricles than those in the standard group. Does this mean that the image-guidance group harbored more of these problematic patients? The authors are correct in stating that one of their study limitations is small sample size. More patients would allow us to statistically correct for imbalances between the 2 groups on one or more key variables to make the comparison as accurate as possible.

P. Klimo, Jr, MD, MPH

Optimal timing of autologous cranioplasty after decompressive craniectomy in children

Piedra MP, Thompson EM, Selden NR, et al (Oregon Health & Science Univ, Portland)

J Neurosurg Pediatr 10:268-272, 2012

Object.—The object of this study was to determine if early cranioplasty after decompressive craniectomy for elevated intracranial pressure in children reduces complications.

Methods.—Sixty-one consecutive cases involving pediatric patients who underwent autologous cranioplasty after decompressive craniectomy for raised intracranial pressure at a single academic children's hospital over 15 years were studied retrospectively.

Results.—Sixty-one patients were divided into early (<6 weeks; 28 patients) and late (≥6 weeks; 33 patients) cranioplasty cohorts. The cohorts were similar except for slightly lower age in the early (8.03 years) than the late (10.8 years) cranioplasty cohort ($p < 0.05$). Bone resorption after cranioplasty was significantly more common in the late (42%) than the early (14%) cranioplasty cohort ($p < 0.05$; OR 5.4). No other complication differed in incidence between the cohorts.

Conclusions.—After decompressive craniectomy for raised intracranial pressure in children, early (<6 weeks) cranioplasty reduces the occurrence of reoperation for bone resorption, without altering the incidence of other complications.

▶ This is a well-conducted, clean, and provocative study. Although cranioplasty is not typically thought of as a complex or highly morbid operation, the authors have demonstrated an overall complication rate of 39%, with the late cohort having more than double the rate compared with the early cohort (52% vs 25%). Postcranioplasty bone resorption was the most frequent complication in both groups. Bone resorption seems to occur more frequently in children than in adults. The only predictor found in this study of children 18 years of age or less was time to cranioplasty. The development of postcranioplasty hydrocephalus, a potential risk or causative factor for bone resorption, was no different between the cohorts. The authors defined bone resorption as being a defect requiring reoperation. It would have been of interest to know whether they had patients who developed bone resorption that was not severe enough to warrant reoperation. I personally have several young children who I am following until they are old enough to undergo implantation of a prosthesis. The findings of this study demand a prospective cohort study, which would best be a multicenter effort to accrue the greatest number of patients over a reasonable time period. Ultimately, this could be a question definitively answered by a randomized trial.

P. Klimo, Jr, MD, MPH

Treatment of choroid plexus tumors: a 20-year single institutional experience

Bettegowda C, Adogwa O, Mehta V, et al (The Johns Hopkins Univ School of Medicine, Baltimore, MD; Vanderbilt Univ School of Medicine, Nashville, TN; Univ of Southern California, Los Angeles, CA)

J Neurosurg Pediatr 10:398-405, 2012

Object.—Choroid plexus tumors (CPTs) are rare intracranial neoplasms that constitute approximately 2%–5% of all pediatric brain tumors. Most of these tumors present with severe hydrocephalus. The optimal perioperative management and oncological care remain a matter of debate. The authors present the epidemiological and clinical features of CPTs from a 20-year single-institutional experience.

Methods.—A total of 39 consecutive patients with pathologically proven CPTs (31 choroid plexus papillomas [CPPs] and 8 choroid plexus carcinomas [CPCs]) were included in this series. Patient demographics, clinical presentation, comorbidities, indications for surgery, radiological studies, tumor location, and all operative variables were reviewed for each case. Multivariate regression analysis was performed to identify independent predictors of tumor recurrence and survival.

Results.—The overall mean age (±SD) was 13.13 ± 19.59 years (15.27 ± 21.10 years in the CPP group and 3.66 ± 3.59 years in the CPC group). Hydrocephalus was noted at presentation in 34% of patients. The most common presenting symptoms were headache (32%) and nausea/vomiting (26%). Gross-total resection (GTR) was achieved in 86% of CPPs and in 71% of CPCs ($p = 0.57$). There was 100% survival in patients with CPPs observed at the 5- and 10-year follow-up and 71% survival in patients with CPCs at the 5-year follow-up. In a multivariate regression analysis, a diagnosis of papilloma, preoperative vision changes, or hydrocephalus; right ventricle tumor location; and GTR were all independently associated with a decreased likelihood of tumor recurrence at last follow-up.

Conclusions.—The authors' study suggests that patients with CPCs are more likely to experience local recurrence and metastasis; hence, GTR with chemotherapy and radiotherapy, particularly for CPCs, is pivotal in preventing recurrence and prolonging survival. While GTR was important for local control following resection of CPPs, it had a minimal effect on prolonging survival in this patient cohort.

▶ This is a single-institution review of the authors' experience treating choroid plexus tumors. Several points need to be made. First, there were very few choroid plexus carcinoma (CPC) patients (N = 7), so it would be hard to make any firm statements regarding treatment management. The authors stated that a reason for the better survival in their patients with CPC compared with other series' was because 71% underwent a gross-total resection. This is likely true. As is the case for other small, blue-cell tumors, namely medulloblastoma, the extent of resection is the most powerful predictor of survival. Second, the authors point out that adjuvant treatment had no impact on recurrence or survival in patients with CPC. I would not have made this claim with so few patients. Adjuvant therapy clearly does have an impact on other malignant pediatric tumors, such as medulloblastoma, high-grade gliomas, and ependymomas. Third, the authors state that although the extent of resection is important for survival in patients with CPC, it did not seem to be the case for choroid plexus papillomas. Of course not. I view CPC similar to other low-grade pathologies such as pilocytic astrocytoma. For that tumor, you would not expect a difference in the 5-year survival based on resection (gross total vs subtotal). Extent of resection is critical for local recurrence (which is the better outcome at 5 years) and likely survival, but you would need 10-year, 15-year, or longer data to determine this.

P. Klimo, Jr, MD, MPH

Internal cranial expansion surgery for the treatment of refractory idiopathic intracranial hypertension

Ellis JA, Anderson RC, O'Hanlon J, et al (Columbia Univ Med Ctr; NY)
J Neurosurg Pediatr 10:14-20, 2012

Object.—Idiopathic intracranial hypertension (IIH) may be refractory to available medical and surgical therapies. Patients with this condition may suffer from intractable headaches, experience visual deterioration, or have other symptoms related to elevated intracranial pressure. Internal cranial expansion (ICE) is a novel surgical procedure that the authors have developed for the treatment of patients with this condition. Here, they describe ICE and present their initial experience in using this surgical procedure for the treatment of patients with refractory IIH.

Methods.—The authors conducted a retrospective review of 10 consecutive patients who underwent ICE for the treatment of IIH during a 5-year period. Preoperative and postoperative clinical parameters including patient symptoms, presence of papilledema, and available ICP or CSF opening pressures were compared. Procedural details and complications were noted. Intracranial volume increases were calculated using available pre- and postoperative CT scans.

Results.—Follow-up for the 10 patients in this series ranged from 1 to 39.6 months (mean 15.5 months). Technically successful ICE was performed in all patients within the cohort. Surgical complications included a single postoperative seizure in one patient and a sagittal sinus tear with no clinical sequelae in another patient. At the time of last follow-up, 7 (70%) of 10 patients were either symptomatically improved or asymptomatic. Six (67%) of 9 patients with preoperative headaches had reduction or resolution of this symptom, and all patients (4 of 4) with preoperative papilledema had a reduction in or complete resolution of this sign. Postoperative ICP or CSF opening pressures were normal in all patients (4 of 4) tested. Postoperative intracranial volume expansion ranged between 3.8% and 12%.

Conclusions.—Internal cranial expansion is a safe and effective surgery for the treatment of patients with refractory IIH. This surgery expands the intracranial volume and thus promotes ICP normalization, which may lead to the reduction or complete resolution of the signs and symptoms of IIH. Internal cranial expansion may be used as part of a multidisciplinary management approach in the treatment of refractory IIH.

▶ There are few diagnoses that instill more trepidation in the heart of a neurosurgeon than pseudotumor cerebri. These patients are notoriously difficult to manage, with the most feared complication of the disease being visual loss. These patients often have chronic headaches and morbid obesity. Placement and survival of a supratentorial shunt is challenging because of small, slit-like ventricles; lumboperitoneal shunting also has high malfunction rates and can frequently induce a Chiari malformation. To control their intracranial pressure, one has to either limit cerebrospinal fluid (CSF) production (carbonic anhydrase inhibitor), remove CSF (shunt), or give the brain more room by expanding the cranial vault.

These authors present their surgical technique for the latter. A 4-quadrant craniotomy is performed with each bone flap split so as to increase the cranial volume (see Fig 1 in the original article). I'm not sure why the authors preserved the coronal suture strut, particularly in a teenage patient who had already achieved maximal head growth. They present their results in a small series of patients with good results. The increase in the intracranial volume and resulting improvement in ventricular size and subarachnoid space is striking (see Fig 4 in the original article). With these results, I wonder whether this treatment should be considered earlier in these patients.

P. Klimo, Jr, MD, MPH

Follow-up imaging to detect recurrence of surgically treated pediatric arteriovenous malformations

Lang S-S, Beslow LA, Bailey RL, et al (Univ of Pennsylvania Med Ctr, Philadelphia; Children's Hosp of Philadelphia, PA)

J Neurosurg Pediatr 9:497-504, 2012

Object.—The true postoperative incidence of arteriovenous malformation (AVM) recurrence in the pediatric population remains largely unreported. Some literature suggests that delayed imaging studies should be obtained at 6 months to 1 year after negative findings on a postoperative angiogram. The aim of this study was to describe the timing of AVM recurrences after resection and the neuroimaging modalities on which the recurrences were detected.

Methods.—This study was performed in a retrospective cohort of all pediatric patients treated surgically for AVM resection by a single neurosurgeon between 2005 and 2010. Patients were followed after resection with MR angiography (MRA) or conventional angiography, when possible, at various time points. A visual scale for compactness of the initial AVM nidus was used, and the score was correlated with probability of recurrence after surgery.

Results.—A total of 28 patients (13 female, 15 male) underwent an AVM resection. In 18 patients (64.3%) an intraoperative angiogram was obtained. In 4 cases the intraoperative angiogram revealed residual AVM, and repeat resections were performed immediately. Recurrent AVMs were found in 4 children (14.3%) at 50, 51, 56, and 60 weeks after the initial resection. Recurrence risk was 0.08 per person-year. No patient with normal results on an angiogram obtained at 1 year developed a recurrence on either a 5-year angiogram or one obtained at 18 years of age. All patients with recurrence had a compactness score of 1 (diffuse AVM); a lower compactness score was associated with recurrence ($p = 0.0003$).

Conclusions.—All recurrences in this cohort occurred less than 15 months from the initial resection. The authors recommend intraoperative angiography to help ensure complete resection at the time of the surgery. Follow-up vascular imaging is crucial for detecting recurrent AVMs, and conventional angiography is preferred because MRA can miss smaller AVMs. One-year follow-up imaging detected these recurrences, and no one who had negative results on an angiogram obtained at 1 year had a late recurrence. However, not all of the patients have been followed for 5 years or until 18 years of age, so longer follow-up is required for these patients. A lower compactness score predicted recurrent AVM in this cohort.

▶ Pediatric arteriovenous malformations (AVMs) are a challenge to treat. They are more often located deep or in the posterior fossa and have a well-known propensity to recur, even after an initial angiographic cure. This article adds to the growing literature on the need to follow these patients for much longer than would be typical for an adult patient. They had 4 recurrences that occurred at 50, 51, 56, and 60 weeks' postresection, all of them with a postresection angiogram without residual nidus or early draining vein. All of these patients harbored a diffuse-type AVM. The authors used a compactness score introduced by Du et al,[1] which I had not heard of before but is something that should be used in the same sentence as the Spetzler-Martin grade when describing an AVM in a child (see Fig 1 in the original article).

I have published an article on the University of Utah's experience with pediatric AVMs.[2] That study also found that patients with diffuse-type AVMs were the ones who were at greatest risk for having a postoperative residual and delayed recurrence. Recurrences have been reported to occur even many years after the initial resection. The authors in this current study were not entirely clear about their postresection angiogram protocol. Almost all of their patients had their first postresection angiogram within 1 year, then a follow-up angiogram was done at 5 years' postresection or when the patient reached 18 years of age, whichever occurred later. Although reasonable, I would argue that these patients should have been followed for 10 years, and my typical angiogram schedule is 1, 5, and 10 years after surgery (or other treatment modality), with noninvasive imaging done 3 to 6 months after treatment and in between the angiograms.

P. Klimo, Jr, MD, MPH

References

1. Du R, Keyoung HM, Dowd CF, Young WL, Lawton MT. The effects of diffuseness and deep perforating artery supply on outcomes after microsurgical resection of brain arteriovenous malformations. *Neurosurgery.* 2007;60:638-648.
2. Klimo P Jr, Rao G, Brockmeyer D. Pediatric arteriovenous malformations: a 15-year experience with an emphasis on residual and recurrent lesions. *Childs Nerv Syst.* 2007;23:31-37.

Programmable shunt valve affected by exposure to a tablet computer

Strahle J, Selzer BJ, Muraszko KM, et al (Univ of Michigan, Ann Arbor)
J Neurosurg Pediatr 10:118-120, 2012

Object.—The authors investigated the effect of a tablet computer on performance-level settings of a programmable shunt valve.

Methods.—Magnetic field strength near the tablet computer with and without a cover was recorded at distances between 0 and 100 mm. Programmable valves were exposed to the tablet device at distances of less than 1 cm, 1–2.5 cm, 2.5–5 cm, 5–10 cm, and greater than 10 cm. For each distance tested, the valves were exposed 100 times to the tablet with the cover, resulting in 500 total valve exposures. The tablet alone, without the cover, was also tested at distances of less than 1 cm for 30 valve exposures. Changes in valve performance-level settings were recorded.

Results.—The maximum recorded magnetic flux density of a tablet with a cover was 17.0 mT, and the maximum recorded magnetic flux density of the tablet alone was 7.6 mT. In 100 exposures at distances between 0 and 1 cm, 58% of valves had different settings following exposure. At distances greater than 1 cm but less than 2.5 cm, 5% of valves in 100 exposures had setting changes. Only a single setting change was noted in 100 exposures at

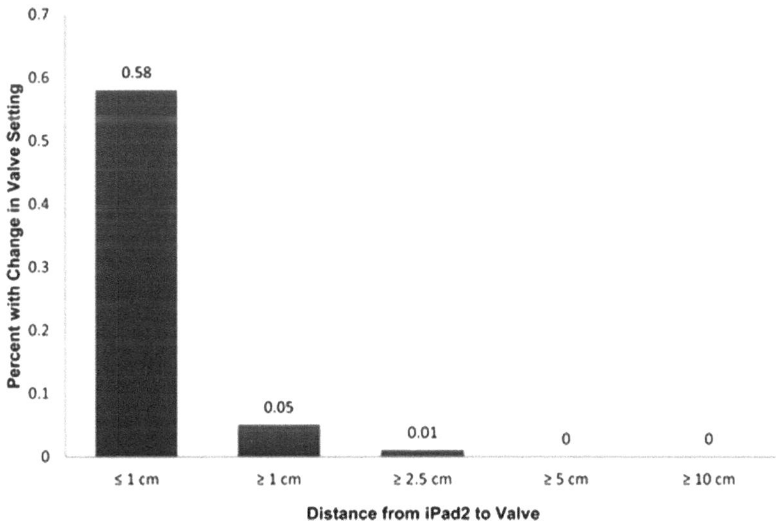

FIGURE 3.—Bar graph illustrating percent (in decimals) of valves with a change in performance level following exposure to the iPad 2 at increasingly greater distances. (Reprinted from Strahle J, Selzer BJ, Muraszko KM, et al. Programmable shunt valve affected by exposure to a tablet computer. *J Neurosurg Pediatr.* 2012;10:118-120, Copyright 2012, with permission from American Association for Neurological Surgeons, with Rockwater, Inc, http://aans.org/.)

distances greater than 2.5 cm but less than 5 cm. No setting changes were noted at distances greater than 5 cm, including 100 exposures between 5 and 10 cm, and 100 exposures of more than 10 cm. For the 30 valve exposures to the tablet without a cover, 20 valve performance-level changes (67%) were noted.

Conclusions.—Based on these results, exposure to tablet devices may alter programmable shunt valve settings (Fig 3).

▶ This short article was one of the most talked about articles in the pediatric neurosurgery literature for 2012. The authors demonstrated a high risk (up to 58%) of inadvertent changes to the valve performance-level setting. They tested Medtronic's Strata Valve, which is one of the most common, if not the most common, implanted programmable valves. When the iPad 2 was placed at distances of less than 1 cm to the valve, it changed the valve setting a shocking 58% of the time (Fig 3). Although it is unlikely that adults will be placing an iPad directly onto their valve, it is easy to imagine a mother using an iPad while holding her infant or children placing the iPad next to their shunt as they play with the device. Anybody who places programmable valves in children needs to be aware of this risk. I use the information from this study every time I counsel parents of a child who will get a programmable shunt.

P. Klimo, Jr, MD, MPH

Nonprogrammable and programmable cerebrospinal fluid shunt valves: a 5-year study

Hatlen TJ, Shurtleff DB, Loeser JD, et al (Univ of Washington School of Medicine, Seattle)

J Neurosurg Pediatr 9:462-467, 2012

Object.—Programmable valves (PVs) for shunting CSF have increasingly replaced nonprogrammable valves (NPVs). There have been only a few longer-term studies (≥5 years) conducted that have compared the effectiveness of NPVs with that of PVs for children with hydrocephalus, and only 1 study has reported NPVs as being favorable over PVs. The objective of this retrospective study was to compare the long-term survival of these 2 types of shunt valves.

Methods.—The authors collected data for all patients who underwent CSF shunt insertion or revision between January 1, 2000, and December 31, 2008. Patients underwent follow-up for a minimum of 2 years postoperatively. Statistical analyses were done using chi-square, Kaplan-Meier survival curve, and multivariate analyses.

Results.—A total of 616 valves were implanted, of which 313 were PVs and 303 were NPVs. Of these, 253 were original shunt implantations and 363 were revisions. The proportion of 5-year survival for NPVs (45.8%) was significantly higher than that for PVs (19.8%) ($p = 0.0005$, log-rank). The NPVs that survived longer than 6 months also survived through the 5th year better than the PVs ($p = 0.0001$).

Conclusions.—The authors' data suggest that NPVs survive longer than PVs in children, but there is a need for prospective, case-control studies to confirm these data (Fig).

▶ This is a well-conducted retrospective cohort study to examine the survival of programmable valves (PVs) compared with nonprogrammable valves (NPVs). The authors found a significant difference in the proportion of valves that were

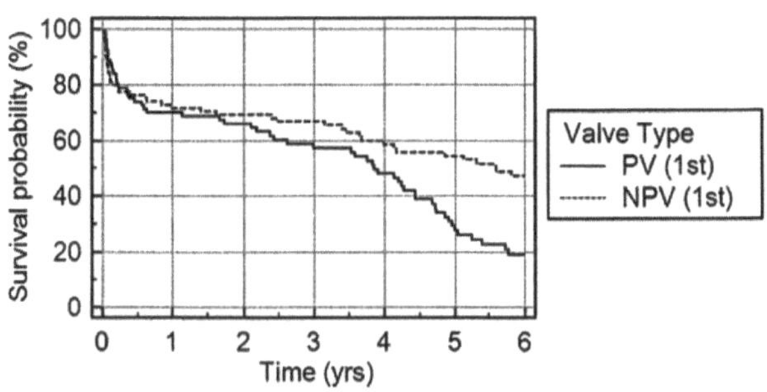

FIGURE.—Kaplan-Meier survival curve for PVs and NPVs including those that were first-insertion cohorts at our institution and underwent follow-up for a minimum of 2 years. (Reprinted from Hatlen TJ, Shurtleff DB, Loeser JD, et al. Nonprogrammable and programmable cerebrospinal fluid shunt valves: a 5-year study. *J Neurosurg Pediatr.* 2012;9:462-467, Copyright 2012, with permission from American Association for Neurological Surgeons, with Rockwater, Inc, http://aans.org/.)

still "alive" at 5 years: 45% for NPVs vs 19.8% for PVs (Fig 1). There were no major differences between the 2 cohorts in their baseline characteristics. This is the first major study that I know of that calls into question the efficacy of PVs. A cost-analysis aspect to this article would have been helpful. I strongly agree that a prospective study is warranted.

P. Klimo, Jr, MD, MPH

The use of abdominal binders to treat over-shunting headaches

Sklar FH, Nagy L, Robertson BD (Children's Med Ctr Dallas, TX)

J Neurosurg Pediatr 9:615-620, 2012

Object.—Headaches are common in children with shunts. Headaches associated with over-shunting are typically intermittent and tend to occur later in the day. Lying down frequently makes the headaches better. This paper examines the efficacy of using abdominal binders to treat over-shunting headaches.

Methods.—Over an 18-year period, the senior author monitored 1027 children with shunts. Office charts of 483 active patients were retrospectively reviewed to identify those children with headaches and, in particular, those children who were thought to have headaches as a result of over-shunting. Abdominal binders were frequently used to treat children with presumed over-shunting headaches, and these data were analyzed.

Results.—Of the 483 patients undergoing chart review, 258 (53.4%) had headache. A clinical diagnosis of overshunting was made in 103 patients (21.3% overall; 39.9% of patients with headache). In 14 patients, the headaches were very mild (1–2 on a 5-point scale) and infrequent (1 or 2 per month), and treatment with an abdominal binder was not thought indicated. Eighty-nine patients were treated with a binder, but 19 were excluded from this retrospective study for noncompliance, interruption of the binder trial, or lack of follow-up.

The remaining 70 pediatric patients, who were diagnosed with over-shunting headaches and were treated with abdominal binders, were the subjects of a more detailed retrospective study. Significant headache improvement was observed in 85.8% of patients. On average, the patients wore the binders for approximately 1 month, and headache relief usually persisted even after the binders were discontinued. However, the headaches eventually did recur in many of the patients more than a year later. In these patients, reuse of the abdominal binder was successful in relieving headaches in 78.9%.

Conclusions.—The abdominal binder is an effective, noninvasive therapy to control over-shunting headaches in most children. This treatment should be tried before any surgery is considered. It is suggested that the abdominal binder may modulate abnormally increased intracranial pulse pressures associated with over-shunting. Interactions with the cerebrovascular bed are suspected to account for persistent headache relief after the binder is discontinued.

▶ Most neurosurgeons have patients in whom shunt overdrainage complications develop. There are several clinical presentations, including postural headaches, that are better when supine and intermittent symptoms are suggestive of a shunt malfunction (headaches, emesis), the so-called "slit-ventricle syndrome." Treatment usually involves medical management initially followed by a shunt revision for persistent symptoms. Options at the time of surgery include adding an antisiphon device, converting to a flow-regulated valve (Orbis-Sigma), or placing a programmable valve.

Sklar et al have provided substantial evidence for another treatment option—the use of an abdominal binder. Intuitively, it does make sense to me. Increasing the intraabdominal pressure with the binder will result in less cerebrospinal fluid siphoning. I have used it, more as a diagnostic test and prelude to a shunt revision rather than as a stand-alone treatment. Although there are significant limitations to this study because of its retrospective nature, the take-home messages are: (1) abdominal binders are an excellent treatment for most patients who are suspected of having overdrainage symptoms, (2) the benefit can last for some time even after discontinuation of the binder, and (3) reapplication of the binder for recurrent symptoms is also effective. It is interesting to note that patients who eventually have overdrainage headaches had them at a mean age of 9.5 years but had received their initial shunt at an average of 1.21 years. Binders were worn at all times for an average of 4.7 weeks. Recurrent symptoms did develop in a significant number of patients after the binder was discontinued, but it took an average of 1.54 years! The authors' attempt at explaining why the binder works is as plausible as any other theory but somewhat confusing to me. This is clearly a question that could be better evaluated in a prospective manner. The advantage of this study is that it is based on a single surgeon's experience that spans almost 20 years.

P. Klimo, Jr, MD, MPH

Choroid plexus coagulation for hydrocephalus not due to CSF overproduction: a review

Zhu X, Di Rocco C (Chinese Univ of Hong Kong, Shatin, People's Republic of China)

Childs Nerv Syst 29:35-42, 2013

Objective.—This study aims to review the role of choroid plexus coagulation (CPC) for hydrocephalus not due to CSF overproduction.

Methods.—The literatures covering CPC/cauterization/extirpation and ablation searched through PubMed were reviewed.

Results.—The history of CPC goes back to early 1900s by open surgery. It has evolved to mainly an endoscopic surgery since 1930s. With the development of other treatment methods and the understanding of CSF dynamics, the application of CPC dramatically decreased by 1970s. In late 2000, there was a resurgence of CPC in combination with endoscopic third ventriculostomy (ETV) performed in Africa.

Conclusions.—CPC remains one of the options for the treatment of hydrocephalus in selected cases. CPC might provide a temporary reduction in CSF production to allow the further development of CSF absorption in infant. Adding CPC to ETV for infants with communicating hydrocephalus may increase the shunt independent rate thus avoiding the consequence of late complication related to the shunt device. This is important for patients who are difficult to be followed up, due to geographical and/or socioeconomic constrains. Adding CPC to ETV for obstructive hydrocephalus in infant may also increase the successful rate. Furthermore, CPC may be an option for cases with high chance of shunt complication such as hydranencephaly. In addition, CPC may act as an adjunct therapeutic measure for complex cases such as multiloculated hydrocephalus. In comparison with the traditional treatment of CSF shunting, the role of CPC needs to be further evaluated in particular concerning the neurocognitive development.

▶ Choroid plexus coagulation (CPC) is a hot topic these days within pediatric neurosurgery. Until 2005, it was a procedure that was rarely performed or discussed and was essentially relegated to the history books. In 2005, Dr Ben Warf published the first of several papers detailing his experience with this procedure as an adjunct to endoscopic third ventriculostomy in African children who suffered from hydrocephalus of various etiologies. Although his experience has generated much discussion, CPC is far from being universally accepted in North America. At a recent pediatric neurosurgery meeting, Pat McCallister, a leading basic science hydrocephalus researcher, asked the audience whether anyone was concerned with the fact that CPC destroys an organ that provides nourishment to the brain and removes harmful byproducts. The silence was palpable. As I await further studies, CPC has not found a role in my practice. This is an excellent study that provides a thorough review of the history and outcomes of this procedure, and it should be required reading for all pediatric neurosurgery residents and fellows.

P. Klimo, Jr, MD, MPH

Shunt survival after failed endoscopic treatment of hydrocephalus

Warf BC, Bhai S, Kulkarni AV, et al (Children's Hosp Boston, MA; Harvard Med School, Boston, MA; Hosp for Sick Children and Univ of Toronto, Ontario, Canada; et al)

J Neurosurg Pediatr 10:463-470, 2012

Object.—It is not known whether previous endoscopic third ventriculostomy (ETV) affects the risk of shunt failure. Different epochs of hydrocephalus treatment at the CURE Children's Hospital of Uganda (CCHU)—initially placing CSF shunts in all patients, then attempting ETV in all patients, and finally attempting ETV combined with choroid plexus cauterization (CPC) in all patients—provided the opportunity to assess whether prior endoscopic surgery affected shunt survival.

Methods.—With appropriate institutional approvals, the authors reviewed the CCHU clinical database to identify 2329 patients treated for hydrocephalus from December 2000 to May 2007. Initial ventriculoperitoneal (VP) shunt placement was performed in 900 patients under one of three circumstances: 1) primary nonselective VP shunt placement with no endoscopy (255 patients); 2) VP shunt placement at the time of abandoned ETV attempt (with or without CPC) (370 patients); 3) VP shunt placement subsequent to a completed but failed ETV (with or without CPC) (275 patients). We analyzed time to shunt failure using the Kaplan-Meier method to construct survival curves, Cox proportional hazards regression modeling, and risk-adjusted analyses to account for possible confounding differences among these groups.

Results.—Shunt failure occurred in 299 patients, and the mean duration of follow-up for the remaining 601 was 28.7 months (median 18.8, interquartile range 4.1–46.3). There was no significant difference in operative mortality ($p = 0.07$ by log-rank and $p = 0.14$ by Cox regression adjusted for age and hydrocephalus etiology) or shunt infection ($p = 0.94$, log-rank) among the 3 groups. There was no difference in shunt survival between patients treated with primary shunt placement and those who underwent shunt placement at the time of an abandoned ETV attempt (adjusted hazard ratio [HR] 1.14, 95% CI 0.86–1.51, $p = 0.35$).

Those who underwent shunt placement after a completed but failed ETV (with or without CPC) had a lower risk of shunt failure ($p = 0.008$, log-rank), with a hazard ratio (adjusted for age at shunting and etiology) of 0.72 (95% CI 0.53–0.98), $p = 0.03$, compared with those who underwent primary shunt placement without endoscopy; but this was observed only in patients with postinfectious hydrocephalus (PIH) (adjusted HR 0.55, 95% CI 0.36–0.85, $p = 0.007$), and no effect was apparent for hydrocephalus of noninfectious etiologies (adjusted HR 0.98, 95% CI 0.64–1.50, $p = 0.92$). Improved shunt survival after failed ETV in the PIH group may be an artifact of selection arising from the inherent heterogeneity of ventricular damage within that group, or a consequence of the timing of shunt placement. The anticipated benefit of CPC in preventing future ventricular catheter obstruction was not observed.

Conclusions.—A paradigm for infant hydrocephalus involving intention to treat by ETV with or without CPC had no adverse effect on mortality or on subsequent shunt survival or infection risk. This study failed to demonstrate a positive effect of prior ETV or CPC on shunt survival.

▶ This is another article that details Dr Warf's experience in treating hydrocephalus in a challenging environment (Uganda) from 2000 to 2007. He and the other authors sought to determine the possible role of prior endoscopic third ventriculostomy (ETV) or choroid plexus coagulation (CPC) on subsequent shunt survival. The improvement in shunt survival was limited to those children who had postinfectious hydrocephalus, a finding the authors felt was a result of selection bias. The evidence that prior ETV or CPC may improve subsequent shunt survival is very weak. It is not an observation I have heard during my training or at meetings. In this article, the authors reference only 2 previous papers in which this observation was suggested. The authors thought that a persistently patent ETV might decrease shunt dependence over time, and that decreased choroid plexus in the ventricle following CPC might reduce the risk of future ventricular catheter obstruction; both reasonable thoughts but something other pediatric neurosurgeons would have observed over the years if they were true. Thus, do not be surprised by the negative findings in this article. Nonetheless, the authors richly deserve our compliments for addressing a devastating health care problem in a part of the world that has very limited resources.

P. Klimo, Jr, MD, MPH

Second impact syndrome in football: new imaging and insights into a rare and devastating condition

Weinstein E, Turner M, Kuzma BB, et al (Indiana Univ School of Medicine, Indianapolis; Northwest Radiology Network, Indianapolis, IN)

J Neurosurg Pediatr 11:331-334, 2013

Premature return to play for the concussed pediatric athlete may result in devastating neurological injury. Identification of at-risk patients and ideal management of the concussed athlete remain challenging for the pediatrician. The authors review a case of second impact syndrome in which neuroimaging was obtained between the first and second impacts, a circumstance which to their knowledge has not been previously reported. This case offers new insights into the underlying pathophysiology of this disease process and potential risk factors for its development.

► Second impact syndrome is the most feared complication of sports-induced concussion. It is strictly a pediatric phenomenon and occurs when an athlete has suffered a concussion and sustains another hit while still being symptomatic from the first. Although the second hit often occurs during the same game as the first hit, it may take place several days later during another game or practice session, like the patient in this case report. The hallmark of this devastating injury is malignant global cerebral edema. The mortality of second impact syndrome is an astonishing 50%. Although extremely rare, it is the injury that tends to make headlines locally and nationally. In 2006, Zachary Leystadt was playing in a middle school football game when he sustained this devastating injury. As a result, Washington was the first state to pass legislation that prohibits a player from continuing to participate in a game in which he or she has sustained a concussion. That player can return to play only when cleared by a medical professional. Similar laws have been passed in almost all 50 states, including my own state a few weeks ago at the time of this writing.

This excellent case report documents in detail the events that led to second impact syndrome in a 17-year-old football player. He survived an unbelievably complicated hospital course, both from his cranial injury and other organ systems.

They provide imaging at every step in this patient's history, from his initial negative head computed tomography (CT) (see Fig 1 in the original article), to the CT and magnetic resonance imaging (MRI) that showed the edema and acute effects of intracranial hypertension (see Fig 2 in the original article), and the MRI 2 months after his injury (see Fig 3 in the original article). It is a must read for any neurosurgeon who cares for children who sustain sports-related concussions. The one aspect of the case report that was lacking was a detailed description of the current neurocognitive status of the patient. They simply stated that the patient lives at home and has "regained limited verbal, motor, and cognitive skills." With widespread legislation, it is our hope that this devastating neurologic injury will be all but eradicated.

P. Klimo, Jr, MD, MPH

15 Spine

Interrater and Intrarater Reliability of the Kuntz et al New Deformity Classification System

Thaler M, Lechner R, Gstöttner M, et al (Med Univ Innsbruck, Austria; et al)
Neurosurgery 71:47-56, 2012

Background.—Kuntz et al recently introduced a new system for classifying spinal deformities. This classification of spinal deformity was developed from age-dependent deviations from the neutral upright spinal alignment.

Objective.—To determine the interobserver and intraobserver reliabilities of the new Kuntz et al system for classifying scoliosis.

Methods.—Fifty consecutive patients were evaluated. Three observers independently assigned a major structural curve, minor structural curve, curve type, apical vertebral rotation, spinal balance, and pelvic alignment to each curve following the guidelines described by Kuntz et al. Assignment of the curves was repeated 4 weeks later, with the curves presented in a different blinded order. The Kendall W and Holsti agreement coefficients were used to determine the interobserver and intraobserver agreement.

Results.—The intraobserver value of agreement for all parameters was 0.85 (range, 0.28-1.0), and the mean Kendall W coefficient was 0.89 (range, 0.5-0.97), demonstrating perfect reliability. The interobserver agreement averaged 0.7 (range, 0.251-1.0). The mean Kendall W coefficient was 0.67 (range, 0.19-1.0), demonstrating substantial reliability. The average time for classification of 1 curve was approximately 8.4 minutes.

Conclusion.—The new Kuntz et al deformity classification system is comparable to the Lenke et al system in terms of reliability. However, the Kuntz et al classification system provides no recommendations for surgical interventions. It is more complex and time-consuming and therefore may be of limited value in daily clinical practice.

▶ Kuntz et al described a classification system for spinal deformities in 2008. This system is based on neutral upright spinal alignment measurements in asymptomatic patients. The Kuntz classification system is very ambitious because it attempts to include all patients. It applies to all types of spinal deformities and applies to patients of all ages.

Thaler et al note that the reliability of many other scoliosis classification systems have been measured (ie, Coonrad, Lenke, King, Scoliosis Research Society, Schwab). The reliability of the Kuntz system has not previously been measured.

Testing interobserver and intraobserver reliability of the Kuntz classification system is the main goal of this article.

Three orthopedic surgeons reviewed preoperative scoliosis x-rays of 50 patients who later underwent surgery for scoliosis. Spinal deformity consists of "at least 20% to 30%" of the daily clinical practice of these 3 surgeons. "Each surgeon independently evaluated every set of radiographs twice, on 2 separate occasions with a time interval of 4 weeks. All observers were blinded to their prior measurements and to the other observers."

Statistical analysis showed perfect intraobserver reliability and substantial interobserver reliability. Based on these statistics, the authors conclude the Kuntz classification system is more reliable than the King system and as reliable as the Lenke classification system. The excellent reliability of the system along with its ability to classify all spinal deformities in patients of all ages are the strengths of the Kuntz system.

The authors also point out the weaknesses of the system. As one would expect, because the system is all encompassing, it is also very time consuming. It took one of the surgeons 8.4 minutes per case. The authors note that their ability to classify a curve with the Lenke system takes a maximum of 1 minute. They also note that although the Lenke system helps the surgeon make treatment decisions, the Kuntz system does not.

The authors do a nice job outlining the considerable strengths and weaknesses of the Kuntz system. Deformity surgeons will need to decide if this system helps their own clinical practice.

R. Riesenburger, MD

Cervical decompression and reconstruction without intraoperative neurophysiological monitoring

Traynelis VC, Abode-Iyamah KO, Leick KM, et al (Rush Univ Med Ctr, Chicago, IL; Univ of Iowa Hosps and Clinics, Iowa City)

J Neurosurg Spine 16:107-113, 2012

Object.—The primary goal of this study was to review the immediate postoperative neurological function in patients surgically treated for symptomatic cervical spine disease without intraoperative neurophysiological monitoring. The secondary goal was to assess the economic impact of intraoperative monitoring (IOM) in this patient population.

Methods.—This study is a retrospective review of 720 consecutively treated patients who underwent cervical spine procedures. The patients were identified and the data were collected by individuals who were not involved in their care.

Results.—A total of 1534 cervical spine levels were treated in 720 patients using anterior, posterior, and combined (360°) approaches. Myelopathy was present preoperatively in 308 patients. There were 185 patients with increased signal intensity within the spinal cord on preoperative T2-weighted MR images, of whom 43 patients had no clinical evidence of myelopathy. Three patients (0.4%) exhibited a new neurological deficit postoperatively. Of these patients, 1 had a preoperative diagnosis of radiculopathy, while the other 2 were treated for myelopathy. The new postoperative deficits completely resolved in all 3 patients and did not require additional treatment. The Current Procedural Terminology (CPT) codes for IOM during cervical decompression include 95925 and 95926 for somatosensory evoked potential monitoring of the upper and lower extremities, respectively, as well as 95928 and 95929 for motor evoked potential monitoring of the upper and lower extremities. In addition to the charge for the baseline [monitoring] study, patients are charged hourly for ongoing electrophysiology testing and monitoring using the CPT code 95920. Based on these codes and assuming an average of 4 hours of monitoring time per surgical case, the savings realized in this group of patients was estimated to be $1,024,754.

Conclusions.—With the continuing increase in health care costs, it is our responsibility as providers to minimize expenses when possible. This should be accomplished without compromising the quality of care to patients. This study demonstrates that decompression and reconstruction for symptomatic cervical spine disease without IOM may reduce the cost of treatment without adversely impacting patient safety.

▶ These authors retrospectively reviewed 720 patients treated with cervical spine operations from December 2000 to May 2007. Patients who had surgery for neoplasms or focal cervical deformities greater than 45 degrees over 1 segment or greater than 60 degrees over 2 segments were excluded from the study. Patients with multilevel global cervical deformities were included, and 308 of these patients presented preoperatively with myelopathy.

All 720 patients underwent cervical spine surgery without intraoperative neurophysiological monitoring, and 0.4% (3 patients) developed a postoperative neurological deficit. These deficits ultimately resolved in all 3 patients. Based on this, the authors suggest that monitoring would probably not have helped improve outcomes in this series. I want to remind the reader that this study did not include patients with cervical neoplasms or high-grade deformity and, therefore, the conclusions cannot be applied to that population.

The authors then performed an analysis of the costs that would have been involved in performing motor-evoked potentials and somatosensory-evoked potentials monitoring in the 720 patients. Using Current Procedural Terminology codes, Medicare reimbursement fees, and assuming 4 hours of monitoring per case, they estimate the costs would have been $1 024 754.

This article justifies performing most cervical operations without neurophysiological monitoring. I do not, however, think that centers that believe strongly in monitoring cervical cases should have to completely stop this practice. I do think that these centers should probably reconsider their monitoring algorithm and review their results to see what subgroups of patients may have benefited from intraoperative monitoring. Perhaps these centers will find that monitoring is only warranted in certain subsets of patients undergoing cervical surgery.

R. Riesenburger, MD

Surgical management of unknown primary tumors metastatic to the spine

Aizenberg MR, Fox BD, Suki D, et al (The Univ of Nebraska Med Ctr, Omaha; The Univ of Texas M D Anderson Cancer Ctr, Houston)

J Neurosurg Spine 16:86-92, 2012

Object.—Patients presenting with spinal metastases from unknown primary tumors (UPTs) are rare. The authors reviewed their surgical experience to evaluate outcomes and identify predictors of survival in these patients.

Methods.—This study is a retrospective analysis of patients undergoing surgery for metastatic spine disease from UPTs between June 1993 and February 2007 at The University of Texas M. D. Anderson Cancer Center.

Results.—Fifty-one patients undergoing 52 surgical procedures were identified. The median age at spine surgery was 60 years. The median survival from time of diagnosis was 15.8 months (95% CI 8.1–23.6) and it was 8.1 months (95% CI 1.6–14.7) from time of spine surgery. Postoperative neurological function (Frankel score) was the same or improved in 94% of patients. At presentation, 77% had extraspinal disease, which was associated with poorer survival (6.4 vs 18.1 months; $p = 0.041$). Multiple sites (vs a single site) of spine disease did not impact survival (12.7 vs 8.7 months; $p = 0.50$). Patients with noncervical spinal disease survived longer than those with cervical disease (11.8 vs 6.4 months, respectively; $p = 0.029$). Complete versus incomplete resection at index surgery had no impact on survival duration ($p > 0.5$) or local recurrence ($p = 1.0$). Identification of a primary cancer was achieved in 31% of patients.

Conclusions.—This is the first reported surgical series of patients with an unknown source of spinal metastases. The authors found that multiple sites of spinal disease did not influence survival; however, the presence of extraspinal disease had a negative impact. The extent of resection had no effect on survival duration or local recurrence. With an overall median survival of 8.1 months following surgery, aggressive evaluation and treatment of patients with metastatic disease of the spine from an unknown primary source is warranted.

▶ This retrospective study analyzed 51 patients with spinal metastases of unknown primary tumor origin who underwent spinal surgery. All patients were treated at University of Texas M. D. Anderson between June 1993 and February 2007. This article is useful because there is very little literature on this topic. I have had a hard time making treatment recommendations to patients with spinal metastases with an unknown primary because it is difficult to predict their future survival. This article presents useful information that is helpful in treating this group of patients.

The median survival from the time of diagnosis was 15.8 months, whereas the median survival from the time of surgery was 8.1 months. In my opinion, this median survival supports offering surgery to selected patients with neurological deterioration from thecal sac compression as a result of a metastasis. Patients should be counseled on this median survival data.

As expected, the complication rate following surgery was high (33%). The majority of these complications were either infectious, systemic, or related to poor wound healing.

Additional work-up and pathological review of the resected metastases led to a definitive diagnosis of a primary tumor in 16 (31%) of patients. The authors write that "the median survival in the group of patients in whom a primary cancer was determined was 24.1 months. In patients in whom a primary cancer was never found, the median survival was 8 months. The difference suggested a trend toward significance ($P = .09$)."

Finally, the authors point out that 9 of the 16 patients (56%) in which a primary tumor diagnosis was made had lung cancer. This serves as a reminder that we should maintain a "heightened suspicion for lung cancer" in patients with an unknown primary tumor.

R. Riesenburger, MD

Results and complications after 2-level axial lumbar interbody fusion with a minimum 2-year follow-up

Marchi L, Oliveira L, Coutinho E, et al (Univ of California, San Diego)

J Neurosurg Spine 17:187-192, 2012

Object.—Axial lumbar interbody fusion (AxiaLIF) is a minimally invasive presacral surgical technique that damages neither the anulus fibrosus nor the anterior or posterior longitudinal ligaments. The technique was initially designed and used for L5–S1 interbody fusions and recently was extended to 2-level fusions (L4–5 and L5–S1). Until now, only biomechanical and radiological studies have discussed the feasibility of this new indication, and no clinical study has been published. The purpose of this article is to report results and complications associated with 2-level presacral AxiaLIF with a minimum of 24 months of follow-up.

Methods.—In this prospective, nonrandomized, single-center study, 27 patients underwent presacral AxiaLIF surgery at the L4–5 and L5–S1 levels. Clinical outcomes were assessed using the visual analog scale for back and leg symptoms and the Oswestry Disability Index. Radiographic parameters, such as disc height, segmental lordosis, and bone fusion, were analyzed using radiographs and CT scans. Complications and revision surgeries were recorded as needed. The minimum follow-up was 24 months (up to 72 months).

Results.—There were no intraoperative complications. One major complication was observed: a patient developed septicemia that resolved after proper care. Clinical outcomes scores showed overall improvement in pain and physical function. During follow-up, the following complications were observed in the construct: screw breakage (14.8%), proximal/distal transsacral rod detachment (11.1%), radiolucency around the transsacral rod (52%), and cephalic rod migration (24%). Disc height gain was reported early after surgery, but at the 24-month follow-up the disc space was diminished in comparison with the preoperative status. Compared with preoperative values, the 24-month results showed loss of segmental lordosis. Only 22% of all treated levels were considered to have solid fusion at the 24-month radiological evaluation.

Conclusions.—Patients undergoing presacral 2-level AxiaLIF experienced satisfactory short-term clinical outcomes; however, complications were commonly seen on imaging studies obtained 24 months postoperatively. Additional studies are required to better understand the 2-level indications for this technique.

▶ Axial lumbar interbody fusion (AxiaLIF) has been a controversial procedure since being introduced almost a decade ago. The initial description of the AxiaLIF procedure was for use in L5-S1 fusion. More recently, some have extended this to L4-S1 fusion operations. These authors report on 27 presacral AxiaLIFs done for fusion at both the L4-5 and L5-S1 levels. The most common indication for this surgery was "symptomatic 2-level lumbosacral degenerative disc disease at L4-5 and L5-S1." All of these AxiaLIF procedures were supplemented by posterior pedicle screw instrumentation.

The average patient in this cohort was clinically improved 2 years after surgery. The mean preoperative Oswestry Disability Index was 51.7 ± 21.8. This improved to 31.4 ± 19.2 at 2-year follow-up.

The complication rate, however, was extremely high; 18.5% of the patients required revision surgery for a variety of reasons, including malpositioned anterior rods, posterior pedicle screw fracture, or the need for a posterior decompressive operation. One patient sustained a bowel perforation that resulted in septicemia from a caudally migrated AxiaLIF rod 14 months after surgery. Two years after surgery, imaging studies showed rostral migration of the AxiaLIF rod into the L3-4 disc space, causing disc space collapse (see Fig 3 in the original article). At 2-year follow-up, solid fusion was seen at both L4-5 and L5-S1 in only 8% of patients! Given the high complication rate and high pseudarthrosis rate, I cannot think of a scenario in which I would ever recommend this operation to a patient.

R. Riesenburger, MD

Unilateral surgical approach for lumbar disc herniation with contralateral symptoms

Akdeniz T, Kaner T, Tutkan I, et al (Küçükyalı Delta Hosp, Istanbul, Turkey; Pendik State Hosp, Istanbul, Turkey; Fatih Sultan Mehmet Education and Training Hosp, Istanbul, Turkey; et al)

J Neurosurg Spine 17:124-127, 2012

Object.—In most cases of lumbar disc herniation, the primary problem is usually limited to radicular pain due to nerve compression on the herniated side, which is generally limited to the side of operation. The aim of this study was to reevaluate the side of the surgical approach in a selected group of patients with leg pain and contralateral lumbar disc herniation.

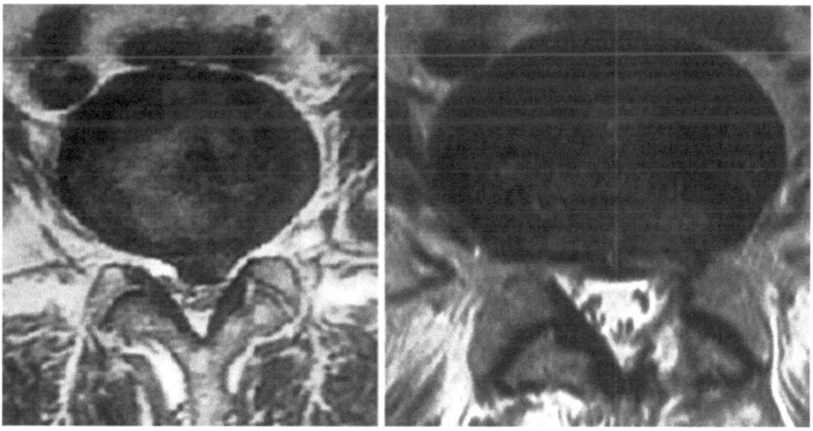

FIGURE 1.—Case 1. Preoperative and immediate postoperative images of the herniation level obtained in a 57-year-old woman with right leg pain. Surgery was conducted via the symptomatic side only. (Reprinted from Akdeniz T, Kaner T, Tutkan I, et al. Unilateral surgical approach for lumbar disc herniation with contralateral symptoms. *J Neurosurg Spine*. 2012;17:124-127, Copyright 2012, with permission from American Association for Neurological Surgeons, with Rockwater, Inc, http://aans.org/.)

Methods.—Included in this study were a total of 5 patients with lumbar disc herniations who presented with contralateral symptoms and neurological signs. In all cases, patients underwent a microdiscectomy from the side ipsilateral to the herniated lumbar disc, the side contralateral to the motor deficits and leg pain.

Results.—The symptoms and signs, to some extent, resolved during the immediate postoperative period. There were no postoperative complications.

Conclusions.—The findings confirm that performing a laminotomy via the side of the herniation is sufficient for this group of patients (Fig 1).

▶ A patient with radiculopathy in 1 leg with a contralateral disc herniation is difficult to manage. In my opinion, attributing radicular pain to a contralateral disc herniation should be a diagnosis of exclusion. In my practice, I tend to put these patients through several tests to be sure I am not missing any other diagnosis. I admittedly have never operated on a patient with this presentation because of concern that surgery would not help and the leg pain may be caused by a process other than a contralateral disc herniation.

This article provides evidence that this clinical scenario exists and that these patients may benefit from surgery. The authors report on 5 such patients, and show images for 3 of these patients (Fig 1 shows case 1 of 5). Each patient failed at least 4 weeks of nonoperative treatment. The 5 patients in the study also "had intolerable sciatica, or had severe neurological loss (progressive motor deficits). In addition, the symptoms had to be obviously attributable to a single intervertebral disc level." All 5 patients underwent a unilateral laminotomy with herniated disc removal on the side of the disc herniation only. In other words, the symptomatic side was not explored. All 5 patients improved clinically in the postoperative period.

The authors theorize that this clinical scenario may occur when "more dural attachments on the posterior longitudinal ligament than usual could cause the fixing and trapping of the contralateral side of the nerve root." They properly admit that the "factors responsible for symptoms contralateral to a lumbar disc herniation are still unclear." Nonetheless, this article supports operative management when these patients fail nonoperative treatment and no alternative diagnosis is present.

R. Riesenburger, MD

Outcomes of instrumented fusion in the pediatric cervical spine

Hwang SW, Gressot LV, Rangel-Castilla L, et al (Baylor College of Medicine, Houston, TX)

J Neurosurg Spine 17:397-409, 2012

Object.—The most common cause of cervical spine arthrodesis in the pediatric population is instability related to congenital or traumatic pathology. Instrumenting the cervical spine can be challenging given smaller anatomical structures, less ossified bone, and future growth potential and development. Studies in adult patients have suggested that using screw constructs results in improved outcomes with lower rates of instrumentation failure. However, the pediatric literature is limited to small retrospective series. Based on a review of the literature and their own patient series, the authors report that instrumenting the pediatric cervical spine with screw constructs may be safer and more effective than using wiring techniques.

Methods.—The authors reviewed the existing pediatric cervical spine arthrodesis literature and contributed 31 of their own cases from September 1, 2007, to January 1, 2011. They reviewed 204 abstracts from January 1, 1966, to December 31, 2010, and 80 manuscripts with 883 total patients were included in the review. They recorded demographic, radiographic, and outcomes data—as well as surgical details—with a focus on fusion rates and complications.

Patients were then grouped into categories based upon the procedure performed: 1) patients who underwent fusions bridging the occipitocervical junction and 2) patients who underwent fusion of the cervical spine that did not include the occiput, thus including atlantoaxial and subaxial fusions. Patients were further subdivided according to the type of instrumentation used—some had posterior cervical fusion with wiring (with or without rod implantation); others had posterior cervical fusion with screws.

Results.—The entire series comprised 914 patients with a mean age of 8.30 years. Congenital abnormalities were encountered most often (in 55% of cases), and patients had a mean follow-up of 32.5 months. From the entire cohort, 242 patients (26%) experienced postsurgical complications, and 50 patients (5%) had multiple complications. The overall fusion rate was 94.4%.

For occipitocervical fusions ($N = 285$), both screw and wiring groups had very high fusion rates (99% and 95%, respectively, $p = 0.08$). However, wiring was associated with a higher complication rate. From a sample of 252 patients, 14% of those treated with screw instrumentation had complications, compared with 50% of patients treated with wiring ($p < 0.05$).

In cervical fusions not involving the occipitocervical junction (N = 181), screw constructs had a 99% fusion rate, whereas wire instrumentation only had an 83% fusion rate ($p < 0.05$). Similarly, patients who underwent screw fixation had a lower complication profile (15%) when compared with those treated with wiring constructs (54%, $p < 0.05$).

Conclusions.—The results of this study are limited by variations in construct design, use of orthoses, follow-up duration, and newer adjuvant products promoting fusions. However, a literature review and the authors' own series of pediatric cases suggest that instrumentation of the cervical spine in children may be safer and more efficacious using screw constructs rather than wiring techniques.

▶ The authors of this study performed an extensive search of the literature on cervical spinal instrumentation in pediatric patients. They reviewed 883 patients from 80 articles and added their own series of 31 patients. Patients were subdivided into 2 groups: patients in which fusion incorporated the occiput and cervical spinal fusions that did not involve the occiput.

Of the patients in which the occiput was involved, the authors noted a very high fusion rate with both wiring and with screw fixation. The complication rates in both groups, however, were very different. Of 252 occipitocervical (OC) fusion patients, 50% treated with wiring had complications, whereas only 14% treated with screws had complications. I found it interesting that the authors report all cerebrospinal fluid (CSF) leaks in the screw group were intraoperative and did not require revision surgery, whereas "several of the reported CSF leaks in the OC wire group required reoperation, including, in 2 cases, implantation of a lumboperitoneal shunt." My own observations are completely in line with this. I recall several problematic CSF leaks in my residency when we typically passed cables via occipital burr holes. There was no great way of repairing these leaks during the initial operation. In contrast, in my current practice, all intraoperative CSF leaks encountered while drilling pilot holes in the occiput are immediately stopped by screw placement. This one factor alone has considerably helped reduce the morbidity of this operation.

Of the pediatric cervical fusions that did not incorporate the occiput (181 patients), screw constructs had a higher fusion rate (99%) compared with the wiring group (83%). The authors theorize that this may be because "screw instrumentation constructs have superior biomechanical stabilization compared with wiring techniques." The authors further report on complications in this group. The wiring group had a 54% complication rate vs 15% treated with screw fixation. They also report that the neurological complications reported with wiring techniques tended to be more severe than with screw fixation techniques. Because this report incorporates many patients from many studies, the authors appropriately did not propose a reason for this. I imagine it is most likely from injuries to the spinal cord while passing wires or cables under the lamina. This sublaminar technique is avoided in screw constructs.

This article shows a much lower complication rate when screw constructs are used for pediatric cervical spine fusion compared with wire constructs. This supports the general trend of using screw constructs when possible in this patient population.

R. Riesenburger, MD

2012 Young Investigator Award Winner: The Distribution of Body Mass as a Significant Risk Factor for Lumbar Spinal Fusion Postoperative Infections

Mehta AI, Babu R, Karikari IO, et al (Duke Univ Med Ctr, Durham, NC)
Spine 37:1652-1656, 2012

Study Design.—A retrospective review.

Objective.—The purpose of this study was to determine the role in body habitus and weight distribution on developing a surgical site infection (SSI).

Summary of Background Data.—SSI after lumbar spine surgery remains a significant cause of morbidity. The literature demonstrates an increased risk of postoperative infections associated with obesity, diabetes, and multilevel surgeries.

Methods.—A retrospective review was performed on a consecutive cohort of 298 adult patients who underwent lumbar spine fusion surgeries

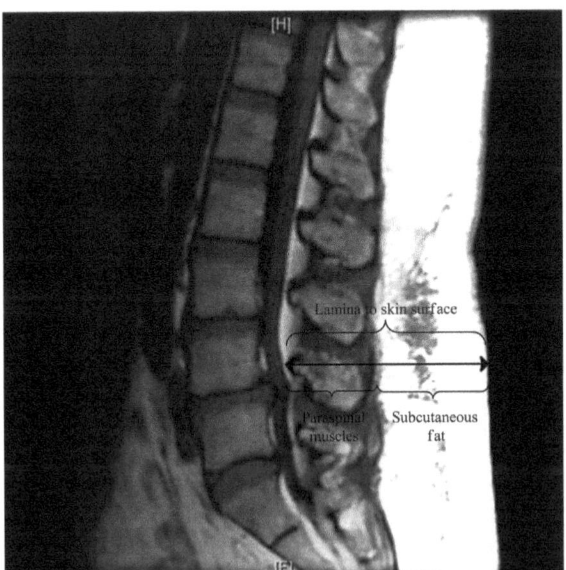

FIGURE 1.—The measurements of paraspinal muscle, subcutaneous fat, and lamina at skin surface at the level of L4 using sagittal views was determined on T2 weighted MRI (Fig 1). (Reprinted from Mehta AI, Babu R, Karikari IO, et al. 2012 young investigator award winner: the distribution of body mass as a significant risk factor for lumbar spinal fusion postoperative infections. *Spine*. 2012;37:1652-1656, with permission from Lippincott Williams & Wilkins.)

between 2006 and 2008 at the Duke University Medical Center. Previously identified risk factors (*i.e.*, number of levels, diabetes, body mass index [BMI]) were collected, as well as the horizontal distance from the lamina to the skin surface (measured at L4) and thickness of subcutaneous fat at the surgical site.

Results.—Among the 298 patients, 24 (8%) had postoperative infections. Of the previously identified risk factors, number of levels ($P = 0.0078$) was found to be significantly associated with infections, whereas BMI ($P = 0.16$) and diabetes ($P = 0.13$) were found not to be statistically significant. Obesity (BMI $\geq$ 30) ($P = 0.025$), skin to lamina distance ($P = 0.046$), and thickness of the subcutaneous fat ($P = 0.035$) were found to be significant risk factors for SSI.

Conclusion.—Our findings suggest that in obese patients, the distribution of body mass is more predictive of SSI than the absolute BMI and deserves attention in preoperative evaluation (Fig 1).

▶ It is well known that obesity is a major public health issue. Studies often use body mass index (BMI) to measure obesity. However, BMI can be high in patients with increased fat mass or in patients with increased muscle mass. More recently, authors are attempting to measure obesity in other ways.

In this article, the authors examine the relationship of several risk factors with postoperative infections after lumbar spinal fusion operations. A total of 298 patients were included in this retrospective study. Of these, 24 (8%) developed a surgical site infection (SSI).

Twelve percent of patients in the SSI group had a BMI of greater than 30, whereas only 5% had a BMI greater than 30 in the noninfected control group. This result was statistically significant. However, there was no statistically significant difference when looking at mean BMI alone. The mean BMI in the SSI group was 30.9, whereas the mean BMI in the control group was 28.9.

The authors then also looked at different markers of body habitus. At the L4 level, they measured distance from the lamina to the skin surface, thickness of the subcutaneous fat, and thickness of the paraspinal muscles (Fig 1). The thickness of the paraspinal musculature was not a risk factor for SSI. Greater lamina to skin distance and greater thickness of the subcutaneous fat were both clear risk factors for the development of a surgical site infection. The mean lamina to skin distance in the SSI group was 74.8 mm versus 67.4 mm in the control group ($P = .046$). The thickness of subcutaneous fat in the SSI group was 30.2 mm versus 23.9 mm in the control group ($P = .035$).

In this study, the authors showed that a greater lamina to skin distance and greater subcutaneous fat at the L4 level are better predictors of SSI than BMI measurements. These 2 new variables should be used in guiding lumbar spinal fusion patients on their risk of SSI.

R. Riesenburger, MD

An Injectable Nucleus Pulposus Implant Restores Compressive Range of Motion in the Ovine Disc

Malhotra NR, Han WM, Beckstein J, et al (Univ of Pennsylvania, Philadelphia; et al)

Spine 37:E1099-E1105, 2012

Study Design.—Investigation of injectable nucleus pulposus (NP) implant.

Objective.—To assess the ability of a recently developed injectable hydrogel implant to restore nondegenerative disc mechanics through support of NP functional mechanics.

Summary of Background Data.—Although surgical intervention for low back pain is effective for some patients, treated discs undergo altered biomechanics and adjacent levels are at increased risk for accelerated degeneration. One potential treatment as an alternative to surgery for degenerated disc includes the percutaneous delivery of agents to support NP functional mechanics. The implants are delivered in a minimally invasive fashion, potentially on an outpatient basis, and do not preclude later surgical options. One of the challenges in designing such implants includes the need to match key NP mechanical behavior and mimic the role of native nondegenerate NP in spinal motion.

Methods.—The oxidized hyaluronic acid gelatin implant material was prepared. *In vitro* mechanical testing was performed in mature ovine bone-disc-bone units in 3 stages: intact, discectomy, and implantation versus sham. Tested samples were cut axially for qualitative structural observations.

Results.—Discectomy increased axial range of motion (ROM) significantly compared with intact. Hydrogel implantation reduced ROM 17% ($P < 0.05$) compared with discectomy and returned ROM to intact levels (ROM intact 0.71 mm, discectomy 0.87 mm, postimplantation 0.72 mm). Although ROM for the hydrogel implant group was statistically unchanged compared with the intact disc, ROM for sham discs, which received a discectomy and no implant, was significantly increased compared with intact. The compression and tension stiffness were decreased with discectomy and remained unchanged for both implant and sham groups as expected because the annulus fibrosus was not repaired. Gross morphology images confirmed no ejection of NP implant.

Conclusion.—An injectable implant that mimics nondegenerate NP has the potential to return motion segment ROM to normal subsequent to injury.

▶ Investigators such as Malhotra et al continue to test implants to restore or rejuvenate degenerated discs. In this study, the authors tested oxidized hyaluronic acid gelatin implant material.

Bone-disc-bone units at L4-L5 from 20 cadaveric sheep were potted and studied. The 20 specimens were divided into an experimental group (n = 10) and a control group (n = 10). Instron testing of axial range of motion was performed on all specimens. Each specimen underwent 3 tests. The experimental specimens first underwent testing in the intact state. A right posterior discectomy was performed, and the specimens were then tested for a second time. The oxidized hyaluronic acid gelatin implant was injected into the "nucleus pulposus cavity through the annular opening created during discectomy with a blunt 21-gauge needle." The mean volume injected was 0.26 mL. The specimens were then tested for a third time after undergoing this implantation.

The control specimens were tested first in the intact state and again after a right posterior discectomy. The 21-gauge needle was then placed in the discectomy cavity, "but no material was injected" (ie, sham surgery). The control specimens were then tested for a third time.

Range of motion significantly increased after discectomy in both groups. The range of motion in the experimental group after injection of the gelatin implant was unchanged statistically compared with the intact, prediscectomy state. Range of motion in the specimens that underwent sham surgery remained significantly increased.

This study shows this hydrogel implant restored axial range of motion in a cadaveric sheep model shortly after being implanted. These results are important, but remind us that this field is still in its infancy. We don't know if the restoration of axial range of motion by this implant would last 30 days, 180 days, 1 year, or indefinitely after the procedure. We also don't know if there would be any clinical benefit to percutaneously injecting such implants into degenerated discs in humans with back pain. I suspect several more studies will be done to address these questions over the next couple of decades.

R. Riesenburger, MD

Incidental durotomy after spinal surgery: a prospective study in an academic institution: Presented at the 2012 Joint Spine Section Meeting

McMahon P, Dididze M, Levi AD (Univ of Miami Miller School of Medicine, FL)

J Neurosurg Spine 17:30-36, 2012

Object.—Incidental durotomies (IDs) are an unfortunate but anticipated potential complication of spinal surgery. The authors surveyed the frequency of IDs for a single spine surgeon and analyzed the major risk factors as well as the impact on long-term patient outcomes.

Methods.—The authors conducted a prospective review of elective spinal surgeries performed over a 15-year period. Any surgery involving peripheral nerve only, intradural procedures, or dural tears due to trauma were excluded from analysis. The incidence of ID was categorized by surgery type including primary surgery, revision surgery, and so forth. Incidence of ID was also examined in the context of years of physician experience and training. Furthermore, the incidence and types of sequelae were examined in patients with an ID.

Results.—Among 3000 elective spinal surgery cases, 3.5% (104) had an ID. The incidence of ID during minimally invasive procedures (3.3%) was similar, but no patients experienced long-term sequelae. The incidence of ID during revision surgery (6.5%) was higher. There was a marked difference in incidence between cervical (1.3%) and thoracolumbar (5.1%)

cases. The incidence was lower for cases involving instrumentation (2.4%). When physician training was examined, residents were responsible for 49% of all IDs, whereas fellows were responsible for 26% and the attending for 25%. Among all of the cases that involved an ID, 7.7% of patients went on to experience a neurological deficit as compared with 1.5% of those without an ID. The overall failure rate of dural repair was 6.9%, and failure was almost 3 times higher (13%) in revision surgery as compared with a primary procedure (5%).

Conclusions.—The authors established a reliable baseline incidence for durotomy after spine surgery: 3.5%. They also identified risk factors that can increase the likelihood of a durotomy, including location of the spinal procedure, type of procedure performed, and the implementation of a new procedure. The years of physician training or resident experience did not appear to be a major risk for ID.

▶ The authors of this study reviewed incidental durotomies (IDs) in Allan Levi's prospective database of elective spine operations done over a 15-year period. This is the largest study that I know of that looks at incidental durotomy incidence in a prospective fashion. This is the major strength of the study. While there have been larger studies reviewing IDs, the retrospective nature of these studies raises the possibility of durotomy underreporting. Since the 3000 patients in this study were collected prospectively and the author is a well-respected spine surgeon, underreporting is not a concern.

ID was defined by the authors as "any disruption of dural integrity with egress of CSF [cerebrospinal fluid] that was recognized during the spinal procedure (102 patients). It also included any patient presenting with symptoms of CSF leakage following a recent spinal procedure (2 cases) without recognition of a durotomy at the time of surgery. Visualization of arachnoid and/or outpouching of arachnoid associated with a loss of dural integrity was not counted as an ID unless CSF was also visualized." ID occurred in 104 patients (3.5%).

The authors broke down ID incidence in several different ways, and all of this information is interesting. The incidence of durotomy was 1.3% in cervical operations, 6.6% in thoracic operations, and 4.9% in lumbar operations. The incidence of IDs was 3.1% in primary operations, 6.5% in revision operations, 2.4% in instrumented operations, and 3.3% in minimally invasive operations. The incidence of a failed repair of an ID was 7 of 102 (6.9%). This is a useful number for patients to know prior to spine surgery. As the authors write, "to put this in perspective, when explaining the risks prior to surgery, only 7 (0.23%) of 3000 patients presented with delayed CSF leakage requiring additional surgical intervention."

Eight of 104 patients (7.7%) developed neurologic deficits following an incidental durotomy. Only 1.5% (45 of 2896) of the patients without an ID developed a postoperative deficit. This difference was statistically significant.

The most common instrument to cause an ID was the Kerrison punch. Second most common was the curette, with the drill being the least common.

R. Riesenburger, MD

Perioperative and delayed complications associated with the surgical treatment of cervical spondylotic myelopathy based on 302 patients from the AOSpine North America Cervical Spondylotic Myelopathy Study: Presented at the 2011 Spine Section Meeting

Fehlings MG, Smith JS, Kopjar B, et al (Univ of Toronto, Ontario, Canada; Univ of Virginia Health System, Charlottesville; Univ of Washington, Seattle; et al)

J Neurosurg Spine 16:425-432, 2012

Object.—Rates of complications associated with the surgical treatment of cervical spondylotic myelopathy (CSM) are not clear. Appreciating these risks is important for patient counseling and quality improvement. The authors sought to assess the rates of and risk factors associated with perioperative and delayed complications associated with the surgical treatment of CSM.

Methods.—Data from the AOSpine North America Cervical Spondylotic Myelopathy Study, a prospective, multicenter study, were analyzed. Outcomes data, including adverse events, were collected in a standardized manner and externally monitored. Rates of perioperative complications (within 30 days of surgery) and delayed complications (31 days to 2 years following surgery) were tabulated and stratified based on clinical factors.

Results.—The study enrolled 302 patients (mean age 57 years, range 29–86) years. Of 332 reported adverse events, 73 were classified as perioperative complications (25 major and 48 minor) in 47 patients (overall perioperative complication rate of 15.6%). The most common perioperative complications included minor cardiopulmonary events (3.0%), dysphagia (3.0%), and superficial wound infection (2.3%). Perioperative worsening of myelopathy was reported in 4 patients (1.3%). Based on 275 patients who completed 2 years of follow-up, there were 14 delayed complications (8 minor, 6 major) in 12 patients, for an overall delayed complication rate of 4.4%. Of patients treated with anterior-only ($n = 176$), posterior-only ($n = 107$), and combined anterior-posterior ($n = 19$) procedures, 11%, 19%, and 37%, respectively, had 1 or more perioperative complications. Compared with anterior-only approaches, posterior-only approaches had a higher rate of wound infection (0.6% vs 4.7%, $p = 0.030$). Dysphagia was more common with combined anterior-posterior procedures (21.1%) compared with anterior-only procedures (2.3%) or posterior-only procedures (0.9%) ($p < 0.001$). The incidence of C-5 radiculopathy was not associated with the surgical approach ($p = 0.8$). The occurrence of perioperative complications was associated with increased age ($p = 0.006$), combined anterior-posterior procedures ($p = 0.016$), increased operative time ($p = 0.009$), and increased operative blood loss ($p = 0.005$), but it was not associated with comorbidity score, body mass index, modified Japanese Orthopaedic Association score, smoking status, anterior-only versus posterior-only approach, or specific procedures. Multivariate analysis of factors associated with minor or major complications identified age (OR 1.029, 95% CI 1.002–1.057, $p = 0.035$) and operative time (OR 1.005, 95% CI 1.002–1.008, $p = 0.001$). Multivariate analysis of factors associated with major complications identified age (OR 1.054, 95% CI 1.015–1.094, $p = 0.006$) and combined anterior-posterior procedures (OR 5.297, 95% CI 1.626–17.256, $p = 0.006$).

Conclusions.—For the surgical treatment of CSM, the vast majority of complications were treatable and without long-term impact. Multivariate factors associated with an increased risk of complications include greater age, increased operative time, and use of combined anterior-posterior procedures.

▶ The authors of this prospective multicenter study operated on 302 adult patients for cervical spondylotic myelopathy (CSM). Of these 302 patients, 275 completed the 2-year follow-up. Perioperative complications (within 30 days of surgery) and delayed complications (between 30 days and 2 years following surgery) were then analyzed. Complications were further subdivided into minor and major complications. Major complications were defined as those that required invasive intervention, resulted in permanent or prolonged morbidity, or resulted in substantial prolongation of hospital stay.

The overall perioperative complication rate was 15.6%. The overall delayed complication rate was 4.4%. Further analysis showed a major perioperative complication rate of 7%, including one perioperative death (0.3%) secondary to cardiopulmonary arrest. The most common major perioperative complication was worsened myelopathy, which occurred in 1.3% of patients. The most common major delayed complication was pseudarthrosis, which occurred in 1.8% of patients.

The rate of postoperative dysphagia was much higher in the combined anterior-posterior surgery (21.1%) when compared to anterior only surgery (2.3%) or posterior only surgery (0.9%). Further analysis showed an increased complication rate for CSM in older patients, those who had longer operations, and anterior-posterior combined operations. Although sometimes necessary based on patient pathology, the increased complication rate of anterior-posterior surgery should be kept in mind before subjecting a patient to this combined approach.

R. Riesenburger, MD

Microscope Sterility During Spine Surgery

Bible JE, O'Neill KR, Crosby CG, et al (Vanderbilt Univ School of Medicine, Nashville, TN)

Spine 37:623-627, 2012

Study Design.—Prospective study.

Objective.—Assess the contamination rates of sterile microscope drapes after spine surgery.

Summary of Background Data.—The use of the operating microscope has become more prevalent in certain spine procedures, providing superior magnification, visualization, and illumination of the operative field. However, it may represent an additional source of bacterial contamination and increase the risk of developing a postoperative infection.

Methods.—This study included 25 surgical spine cases performed by a single spine surgeon that required the use of the operative microscope. Sterile culture swabs were used to obtain samples from 7 defined locations on the microscope drape after its use during the operation. The undraped technician's console was sampled in each case as a positive control, and an additional 25 microscope drapes were swabbed immediately after they were applied to the microscope to obtain negative controls. Swab samples were assessed for bacterial growth on 5% sheep blood Columbia agar plates using a semiquantitative technique.

Results.—No growth was observed on any of the 25 negative control drapes. In contrast, 100% of preoperative and 96% of postoperative positive controls demonstrated obvious contamination. In the postoperative group, all 7 sites of evaluation were found to be contaminated with rates of 12% to 44%. Four of the 7 evaluated locations were found to have significant contamination rates compared with negative controls, including the shafts of the optic eyepieces on the main surgeon side (24%, $P = 0.022$), "forehead" portion on both the main surgeon (24%, $P = 0.022$) and assistant sides (28%, $P = 0.010$), and "overhead" portion of the drape (44%, $P = 0.0002$).

Conclusion.—Bacterial contamination of the operative microscope was found to be significant after spine surgery. Contamination was more common around the optic eyepieces, likely due to inadvertent touching of unsterile portions. Similarly, all regions above the eyepieces also have a propensity for contamination because of unknown contact with unsterile parts of the surgeon. Therefore, we believe that changing gloves after making adjustments to the optic eyepieces and avoid handling any portion of the drape above the eyepieces may decrease the risks of intraoperative contamination and possibly postoperative infection as well.

▶ The authors of this article used sterile culture swabs to perform a microbiological assessment of the microscope drape following 25 spinal operations. Seven areas were swabbed after each operation: the microscope objective lens, both operating handles and controls, the shafts of both optic eyepieces on the main surgeon side and the assistant side, the forehead area on the main surgeon side and the assistant side, and the inferior portion of the microscope arm.

The authors wisely sampled the same areas of 25 microscope drapes immediately after draping to serve as a control group. No growth was observed on the 25 control microscope drapes.

Of the drapes sampled after use during spinal operations, the authors found significantly higher contamination rates compared with the corresponding negative controls. Not surprisingly, these were the shafts of the optic eyepieces for the main surgeon, the forehead area for both the main surgeon and the assistant, and the inferior portion of the microscope arm. Of note, significantly higher rates were not seen on the handles or controls part of the microscope.

Based on these findings, the authors recommend changing gloves after each optic eyepiece adjustment. I think this study provides interesting data, and it probably makes sense to change gloves if several eyepiece adjustments are made in a short time. However, it may not be practical to change gloves after each eyepiece adjustment. In my hands, I may only change the eyepieces once or twice during a lumbar microdiscectomy, but will change it probably in excess of 30 times during tumor removal or a multilevel miniopen lumbar fusion or decompression. When possible, I admittedly try to adjust the eyepieces by moving my head up or down, but this is not always possible.

Although I think it is important to do everything to minimize infection rate, this study does not prove a lower postoperative infection rate with frequent glove changes. It is reassuring that the operating handles and controls did not have significantly higher contamination rates. Although the eyepiece area may be contaminated, it does not necessarily make it to the handles, where it would be most likely to repeatedly contaminate the surgeon's gloves. Also, although anecdotal, in our training program, some cranial neurosurgeons use the operating microscope mouthpiece, which means the drape gets contaminated 100% of the time, while others do not use the mouthpiece. We have never formally studied it, but I have not noticed a higher infection rate in the mouthpiece users. Therefore, it may not be correct to extrapolate the microbiological data in this study to actual rates of postoperative infection. In spine, the route of the operation is likely a more important factor. Minimally invasive cases through a paramedian muscle splitting incision have lower rates of infection compared to open midline operations, likely because of lessened postoperative dead space. This is also likely the reason for the incredibly low infection rate observed after anterior cervical discectomy and fusion. The microscope should continue to be used for these operations, while keeping the field as sterile as possible.

R. Riesenburger, MD

C2 Nerve Root Sectioning in Posterior C1-2 Instrumented Fusions

Kang MM, Anderer EG, Elliott RE, et al (New York Univ Langone Med Ctr)

World Neurosurg 78:170-177, 2012

Objective.—To analyze qualitatively C2 nerve dysfunction after its transection in C1-2 posterolateral instrumented fusions.

Methods.—From 2002–2010, 20 consecutive patients underwent posterolateral instrumented fusions using C1 lateral mass and C2 pars or pedicle screws, mainly for type 2 dens fractures. Screws were placed under lateral fluoroscopic guidance using standard techniques. Bilateral C2 nerve roots were coagulated and transected in all patients. Mean follow-up was 30.7 months and consisted of clinical and radiographic examinations, telephone interviews, and mailed visual analogue scale (VAS) questionnaires assessing C2 nerve dysfunction.

Results.—One patient was lost to follow-up after the initial postoperative visit. Fusion was evident in all patients with 12 months of follow-up and two of three patients with <12 months of follow-up. There were no instances of unintended neurologic deficits, vascular injury, cerebrospinal fluid (CSF) leak, or hardware malfunction or malposition. By the 2-week or 6-week office visit, 4 of 20 patients complained of sensory disturbance,

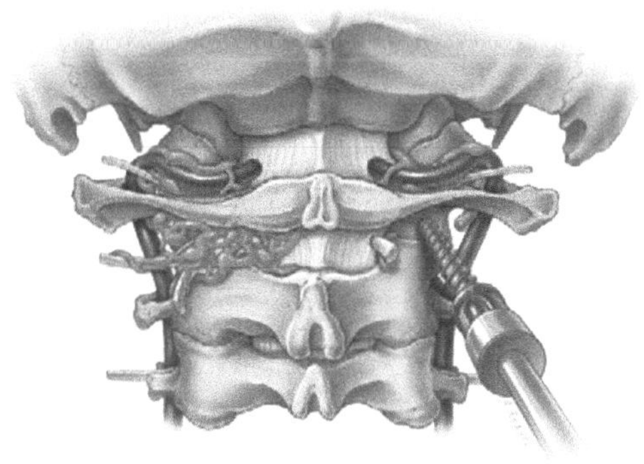

FIGURE 1.—Illustration showing the placement of a C1 lateral mass screw on the right side after sectioning the C2 nerve root on that side and coagulating the large venous plexus that typically resides in this region. (Reprinted from Kang MM, Anderer EG, Elliott RE, et al. C2 nerve root sectioning in posterior C1-2 instrumented fusions. *World Neurosurg*. 2012;78:170-177, with permission from Elsevier.)

and 2 had paresthesias in the C2 distribution. After longer follow-up, one additional patient developed mild sensory symptoms. Quality of life was adversely affected in only one patient. No patient developed neuropathic pain at any time after C2 sectioning.

Conclusions.—This study is the first series to describe C2 nerve function after posterior atlantoaxial instrumented fusion in adults of all ages. Sacrifice of the C2 nerve root increases fusion surface, allows for better preparation and decortication of the atlantoaxial joint, improves visualization for screw placement, and decreases blood loss and operative time without major clinical consequences (Fig 1).

▶ The authors of this study review bilateral C2 nerve root sacrifice in 20 patients. All of these patients underwent C1-2 posterior fusion with C1 lateral mass screws and C2 pars or pedicle screws. C2 nerve root sacrifice was performed bilaterally in all cases. The authors describe the intraoperative advantages of sacrificing the C2 nerve roots: increased exposure of the C1 lateral mass for easier C1 screw placement, no need for traction on the C2 roots during C1 screw placement (which may cause dysesthetic pain), improved ability to detect an anomalous vertebral artery at the C1-2 level, and excellent exposure to the C1-2 joint for C1-2 synovectomy and arthrodesis.

The authors state they transect the C2 root "directly posterior to the midpoint of the atlantoaxial joint and C1 lateral mass to avoid cerebrospinal fluid leak. The technique for nerve root section consists of progressive bipolar electrocauterization and incision with Malis scissors. Deep to the nerve, the ventral portion of the venous plexus is encountered and coagulated, exposing the posterior cortex of the lateral mass of C1 just below the posterior arch." At this time, the authors were ready for placement of the C1 lateral mass screws (Fig 1).

The authors report no cerebrospinal fluid leaks or vascular injuries during these operations. With early follow-up, 20% of patients reported occipital numbness, and 10% had C2 paresthesias. An additional patient complained of delayed occipital numbness. Only one patient in the series reported the "numbness adversely affected his quality of life and affected him on a daily basis." No other patients in the series reported the C2 symptoms negatively affecting their quality of life.

Given the above information, I think I will utilize this technique in my practice. I think a reasonable approach is to initially attempt the C1 lateral mass screws by retracting the C2 nerve root caudally. If it is difficult to obtain good exposure, C2 nerve root sectioning would then be performed to increase the working space for placing a C1 lateral mass screw. Patients should, of course, be counseled about this preoperatively.

R. Riesenburger, MD

16 Surgical Techniques

Intradural anterior petrosectomy for petroclival meningiomas: a new surgical technique and results in 5 patients

Gupta SK, Salunke P (Postgraduate Inst for Med Education and Res, Chandigarh, India)

J Neurosurg 117:1007-1012, 2012

Excision of petroclival meningiomas remains a surgical challenge. Extradural anterior petrosectomy is widely used as a skull base approach for these tumors; however, this approach has significant procedure-related morbidity. The authors describe an alternative technique of tailored intradural petrosectomy for removal of petroclival meningiomas. This technique was used successfully in 5 patients. Gross-total or near-total resection was possible in 2 patients, whereas a subtotal removal was achieved in 3 patients, without significant morbidity. The petrous drilling was tailored depending on the extent of tumor. Transsylvian intradural anterior petrosectomy is a safe approach for petroclival meningiomas. This approach avoids problems related to subtemporal retraction and rationalizes the degree of bone drilling.

▶ The authors describe a technique for intradural anterior petrosectomy during frontotemporal orbitozygomatic transsylvian approaches to petroclival meningiomas (see Fig 2 in the original article). Compared with the extradural anterior petrosectomy techniques (extended middle fossa, Kawase's approach), the intradural technique avoids subtemporal retraction and potential injury to the vein of Labbe, and removal of the anterior petrous bone is dictated by the tumor's pathologic characteristics. After wide splitting of the sylvian fissure, the draining veins from the anterior temporal lobe going into the sphenocavernous sinus are divided to allow mobilization of the temporal lobe posteriorly and laterally to expose the tentorial edge. The tentorium is then divided posterior to the entry of the fourth nerve to further expose tumor that is situated infratentorially. Decompression of the posterior fossa component of tumor is carried out, and the dura over the petrous bone is cauterized and cut out with care to coagulate the superior petrosal sinus. After identifying the gasserian ganglion and trigeminal nerve, drilling of the anterior petrous bone can begin lateral to the ganglion. The extent of bone removal is tailored to the patient based on what is necessary to deliver the tumor from the exposed working corridor. This technique appears to be a helpful adjunct in the surgical resection of petroclival meningiomas. Nevertheless, for extensive petroclival tumors that are situated well below the internal auditory canal, one should be prepared to add a posterior petrosal approach or retrosigmoid approach.

J. K. Liu, MD

Validation of the superior interhemispheric approach for tuberculum sellae meningioma

Curey S, Derrey S, Hannequin P, et al (Rouen Univ Hosp, France; et al)
J Neurosurg 117:1013-1021, 2012

Object.—The objective of this study was to evaluate the ophthalmological outcome, nonvisual morbidity, and surgical complications after tuberculum sellae meningioma (TSM) removal using a superior interhemispheric approach.

Methods.—In the last decade, 20 consecutive patients with TSM underwent operations using the superior interhemispheric approach. Visual acuity, visual field, and ocular fundus examination were assessed both preoperatively and 6-months postoperatively. Nonvisual morbidity was determined at an early postoperative period and at 6 months based on assessment of the Karnofsky Performance Scale score, leakage of CSF, endocrinological status, and olfactory function, which was assessed using a visual analog scale (VAS). The potential brain injury related to the approach was assessed by MRI at 6 months. Magnetic resonance imaging was then performed yearly to detect a recurrence. The mean follow up was 56.3 ± 34 months.

Results.—The primary presenting symptom for diagnosis of TSM in 20 patients (female:male ratio of 6.6:1, mean age 59.1 ± 11.1 years) was visual disturbance in 12 patients (60%), headache in 4 (20%), cognitive alteration in 1 (5%), epilepsy in 2 (10%), and accidental in 1 (5%). In a total of 40 eyes, 17 eyes in 11 patients presented with preoperative deterioration of visual acuity. Postoperatively, the visual acuity improved in 13 eyes in 8 patients (72.8%), remained unchanged in 3 eyes in 2 patients (18.2%) and deteriorated in 1 patient (9%). The nonvisual morbidity included olfactory deterioration in 7 patients (35%), and panhypopituitarism in 1 patient (5%). No patients experienced a CSF leak. The impact of olfactory deterioration on the quality of life, as estimated by a VAS score (range 0–10), was a mean of 5.7 ± 2.2 (95% CI 4.1–7.3). On the follow-up MRI, no additional lesions or recurrences were observed on the medial aspect of the frontal lobe along the surgical corridor.

Conclusions.—The superior interhemispheric approach appears to be effective in resolving the problem of visual deterioration due to a TSM, without inducing surgical injury on the brain surface along the surgical corridor. Olfactory deterioration remained the challenging predominant nonvisual morbidity using this approach.

▶ The authors present their 10-year experience of treating 20 tuberculum sellae meningiomas (all World Health Organization grade I) via the superior interhemispheric approach. The results are excellent (95% achieving Simpson grade I or II complete resection, 72.8% visual improvement, 18.2 visual stability, 0% recurrence) with low rates of complication: 0% cerebrospinal fluid leak rate, visual deterioration in only 1 patient (9%), and panhypopituitarism in 1 patient. Olfaction deterioration was the most common postoperative complication, which occurred in 7 patients (35%) who had large and medium-sized tumors. The impact of this on the quality of life was estimated using a visual analog scale, resulting in a mean score of 5.7 (moderate influence or consequence to patient's life). This approach through interhemispheric fissure appears to increase the risk of the olfactory tracts because these structures are located within the surgical working corridor. In contrast, by coming from a lateral transsylvian or subfrontal approach, such as an orbitozygomatic, orbitopterional, or pterional approach, one tends to spare the olfactory tracts and avoids subsequent injury. Only 3 patients required optic canal unroofing to access tumor involvement in the optic canal. This is an important surgical consideration because these tumors often grow into the optic canal, and leaving tumor behind in an unexplored optic canal can result in postoperative visual worsening and a source of recurrent tumor.

I support early optic nerve decompression in these tumors and usually perform an extradural optic canal unroofing with anterior clinoidectomy when using an orbitozygomatic approach or perform bilateral medial optic canal unroofing when using an endoscopic endonasal transplanum transtuberculum approach. When performing interhemispheric approaches, I have found that positioning the patient in the lateral position allows gravity to facilitate fissure dissection and allows one to do the surgery without fixed brain retractors. Although the advantages of midline orientation are somewhat lost, this can be readily accommodated with more experience.

J. K. Liu, MD

Article Index

Chapter 1: Epilepsy and Other Seizure Disorders

Chapter 2: Headache

Chapter 3: Infectious Diseases of the Nervous System

Chapter 4: Movement Disorders

Chapter 5: Multiple Sclerosis and Other Demyelinating Diseases

Chapter 6: Neoplastic Disease

Chapter 7: Neuromuscular Disease

Chapter 8: Neuro-otology

Chapter 9: Pediatric Neurology

Chapter 10: Sleep Disorders

Chapter 11: Miscellaneous

Chapter 12: Brain Tumors

Chapter 14: Pediatric Neurosurgery

Chapter 15: Spine

Chapter 16: Surgical Techniques

Author Index

FSC
www.fsc.org
MIX
Papier | Fördert gute Waldnutzung
FSC® C083411

Kolibri 360 GmbH
Ferdinand-Jühlke-Straße 7
99095 Erfurt, Deutschland
produktsicherheit@kolibri360.de